ERRATUM

The wording to the first page of the Preface is incorrect. Below please note the corrected text.

PREFACE

What will the legacy of the 20th century be to medicine? For the first time in human history, genetic and molecular mechanisms of pathogenesis as well as demonstrably effective treatments of many diseases have been discovered. Early in this century, X-ray made it possible to look into the human body; now with CT and MRI we can even look at slices of the body without cutting it. These and other exciting developments in medical technology ushered in an explosion of knowledge in the biomedical sciences. With technology came superspecialization and fragmentation in patient care. The primary concern of the superspecialist was often the diseased tissue or organ rather than the patient as a person. The *biopsychosocial model* (as an alternative to the *biomedical model*) was proposed by George Engel in mid-century as an attempt to restore an appreciation of the psychological and social aspects of the patient in the pathogenesis and treatment of disease.

The *biopsychosocial model*, at its best, embodies an *ideal* of medical practice. A skilled biopsychosocial physician would be somewhat like the old-fashioned family doctor, who knows the patient, his/her family, occupation, subculture, as well as the patient's coping style. He/she would ask the patient about ongoing problems, recent stresses, and the impact of the illness on the family and workplace. The physician would, then, take all these factors into consideration in recommending and implementing state of the art treatment. Although this type of comprehensive evaluation and treatment may be more time consuming than a purely problem-oriented focused examination, the reimbursement for a comprehensive evaluation in a fee-for-service environment would partially compensate for the time spent. The satisfaction of providing state-of-the-art service may make up the difference.

Though there are numerous theoretical and practical problems in the *biopsychosocial model* (these problems are discussed in some detail in this book), the major threat to this ideal comes from the *managed care environment,* the epidemic that is fundamentally transforming the practice of medicine. At its worst, managed care, with its preoccupation with efficiency and cost-containment, forces the physician to focus on the single presenting complaint, and to ameliorate it least expensively in the shortest amount of time. Why ask about stresses that will surely take more of the physician's time, and possibly lead to more expensive tests for other stress-related diseases? At its best, however, managed care may encourage biopsychosocially directed prevention and early treatment of disease. As early detection and treatment of depression and anxiety reduce the overall health care cost of the patients, managed care systems should welcome primary physicians who can perform a competent biopsychosocial evaluation of a patient efficiently, and then proceed either to treat the patient directly, or to make judicious referrals.

Biopsychosocial Approaches in Primary Care
Edited by Hoyle Leigh

0-306-45582-X
Plenum Press, New York, 1997

Biopsychosocial Approaches in Primary Care

State of the Art and Challenges for the 21st Century

Biopsychosocial Approaches in Primary Care

State of the Art and Challenges for the 21st Century

Edited by

Hoyle Leigh

University of California, San Francisco
Fresno, California

PLENUM PRESS • NEW YORK AND LONDON

Library of Congress Cataloging-in-Publication Data

Biopsychosocial approaches in primary care : state of the art and
challenges for the 21st century / edited by Hoyle Leigh.
p. cm.
Includes bibliographical references and index.
ISBN 0-306-45582-X
1. Psychiatry--Congresses. 2. Primary care (Medicine)-
-Congresses. 3. Medicine, Psychosomatic--Congresses. I. Leigh,
Hoyle, 1942- .
RC454.4.B57 1997
616.89--dc21 97-3397
CIP

Based on proceedings of the 13th World Congress of the International College of Psychosomatic Medicine, held September 10–15, 1995, in Jerusalem, Israel

ISBN 0-306-45582-X

A Division of Plenum Publishing Corporation
233 Spring Street, New York, N.Y. 10013

http://www.plenum.com

10 9 8 7 6 5 4 3 2 1

Printed in the United States of America

FOR VINNIE AND ALEXANDER

PREFACE

What the legacy of the 20th century be to medicine? For the first time in human history, genetic and molecular mechanisms of pathogenesis as well as demonstrably effective treatments of many diseases have been discovered. Early in this century, X-ray made it possible to look into the human body; now with CT and MRI we can even look at slices of the body without cutting it. These and other exciting developments in medical technology ushered in an explosion of knowledge in the biomedical sciences. With technology came superspecialization and fragmentation in patient care. The primary concern of the superspecialist was often the diseased tissue or organ rather than the patient as a person. The *biopsychosocial model* (as an alternative to the *biomedical model*) was proposed by George Engel in mid-century as an attempt to restore an appreciation of the psychological and social aspects of the patient in the pathogenesis and treatment of disease.

The *biopsychosocial model*, at its best, embodies an *ideal* of medical practice. A skilled biopsychosocial physician would be somewhat like the old-fashioned family doctor, who knows the patient, his/her family, occupation, subculture, as well as the patient's coping style. He/she would ask the patient about ongoing problems, recent stresses, and the impact of the illness on the family and workplace. The physician would, then, take all these factors into consideration in recommending and implementing state of the art treatment. Although this type of comprehensive evaluation and treatment may be more time consuming than a purely problem-oriented focused examination, the reimbursement for a comprehensive evaluation in a fee-for-service environment would partially compensate for the time spent. The satisfaction of providing state-of-the-art service may make up the difference.

Though there are numerous theoretical and practical problems in the *biopsychosocial model* (these problems are discussed in some detail in this book), the major threat to this ideal comes from the *managed care environment,* the epidemic that is fundamentally transforming the practice of medicine. At its worst, managed care, with its preoccupation with efficiency and cost-containment, forces the physician to focus on the single presenting complaint, and to ameliorate it least expensively in the shortest amount of time. Why ask about stresses that will surely take more of the physician's time, and possibly lead to more expensive tests for other stress-related diseases? At its best, however, managed care may encourage biopsychosocially directed prevention and early treatment of disease. As early detection and treatment of depression and anxiety reduce the overall health care cost of the patients, managed care systems should welcome primary physicians who can perform a competent biopsychosocial evaluation of a patient efficiently, and then proceed either to treat the patient directly, or to make judicious referrals.

This book is intended to show the primary care physicians, and psychiatrists who work with primary physicians, that it is possible to provide state-of-the-art biopsychosocial care to patients efficiently, even in a managed care setting. Part I of this book, **State of the Art,** therefore, presents succinct discussions of the psychiatric syndromes often encountered in the primary care setting, and how the primary care physician might evaluate and treat them effectively and efficiently. Another purpose of the book is to take stock of the theoretical aspects of the *biopsychosocial model*, and to stimulate a discussion among our colleagues about how best to preserve our ideal of comprehensive care into the 21st century. Part II, **Challenges for the 21st Century,** presents theoretical and conceptual chapters on some of the many remaining tasks for medicine if it is to maintain what is best of the biopsychosocial model. Symposia presented at the 13th World Congress of the International College of Psychosomatic Medicine, held in Jerusalem, in 1994, provided the nidus for this volume, but this book is far more than just proceedings of the conference. Many contributors to this volume did not attend the conference, and all the presentations have been updated and rewritten. (Please see Introduction for further discussion of the contents of the book).

This book is for primary care physicians, medical students, and mental health workers who work closely with primary care physicians. It is also for psychiatrists and students of philosophy of medicine, and, especially, for administrators of health care organizations (who I hope will gain an insight into the necessity and efficiency of a biopsychosocial approach).

I am grateful to my colleagues and students who have provided me with ideas and feedback to my presentations, lectures, and writings. I am also grateful to Ms. Eileen Bermingham and Mr. Robert Wheeler at Plenum Press for their assistance in preparing and producing this book.

Hoyle Leigh, M.D.
Fresno, California

CONTENTS

Part II. Challenges for the 21st Century

INTRODUCTION

MEDICINE IN A CHANGING UNIVERSE AT THE THRESHOLD OF THE 21ST CENTURY

Hoyle Leigh, M.D.[1]

Professor of Psychiatry
University of California, San Francisco,
and Fresno VA Medical Center

INTRODUCTION

During my lifetime, the universe has changed beyond recognition. The universe into which I was born, in the first half of the 20th century, was still infinite, permanent, orderly, and tranquil --- a universe that worked like a masterfully constructed clock. Matter and energy followed Newton's laws of conservation. Shortly after my birth, Hiroshima proved, with a big bang, that matter was no longer permanent, everything was relative. Einstein had also shown that everything that happened was local, that is, there was an event horizon beyond which no information could reach as nothing can travel faster than light. When I was growing up, the moon was for lovers, and going there was an impossible dream.

Cosmologically, the Big Bang theory that postulates that the universe was born out of an explosion some 10-15 billion years ago from a primordial point won over steady state. It has been expanding ever since, although the ultimate fate of the universe is still unknown - whether it will keep on expanding resulting in a perpetual state of heat death, or will at some point start contracting, resulting in a big crunch of gravitational collapse ending in a single black hole out of space, time, and existence.

Quantum theory has defeated even Einstein's genius and proven that God indeed plays dice. Probability reigns supreme, not only in subatomic particles as had been originally thought, but in macrouniverse as well. According to quantum theory, particles fleetingly come into existence out of nothing, and disappear into nothing. Pairs of particles that are light years away are somehow connected, so that the observation of one's characteristic (for example, the direction of its spin) simultaneously results in the other particle assuming a complementary characteristic, even though there is no way any information could have been

[1]Correspondence: Department of Psychiatry, UCSF-Fresno, 2615 E. Clinton Ave; Fresno, CA 93703

Biopsychosocial Approaches in Primary Care: State of the Art and Challenges for the 21st Century, Edited by H. Leigh, Plenum Press, New York, 1997

transmitted between the particles. This "spooky action at a distance" was what troubled Einstein to no end. But it is there.

Quantum theory has forced physical science to accept, albeit reluctantly, two astounding ideas: (1) the universe is somehow interconnected as a whole, so that what happens in one area is intricately tied to what happens in all the rest of the universe, (2) the observer can no longer be considered outside of what is being observed. Put in another way, by the mere fact of observation, the wave function collapses and matter emerges, literally. The observation need not be human, it could be by a machine or any other recording device.

What does all of this have to do with the practice of medicine? Medical science, that has been so successful in ushering in modern medicine (as Newton's laws have ushered in modern physics), must take into account the notion that consciousness and observation must be considered as a part and parcel of the art and science of medicine. Medicine, through the act of observation of the patient by the physician, and eventually by the patient learning to observe herself or himself, creates medical realities. This insight renders strong support to a comprehensive approach to patients, the essence of *biopsychosocial model.*

Comprehensive approaches to the patient was first articulated by Hippocrates, and, more recently, reemphasized by Menninger and Engel coined the term, biopsychosocial model as an alternative to the *biomedical model*, which he felt was reductionistic. The multiaxial approach of DSM III and IV usefully incorporates the biopsychosocial model. Complexity is inherent in the model, and some wish for a simpler, more elegant, reductionistic model that is equally effective in patient care. Genetic engineering, receptor-oriented pharmacology, and other breakthroughs in medicine and neurosciences may promise to provide effective cure and prevention of disease through unidimensional intervention. Just as Newtonian physics is still useful in putting persons on the moon, and shuttling into space, so may unidimensional, reductionistic approaches in the treatment of specific diseases.

When I was in high school, the smallest units of matter were electrons, neutrons, and protons. Now there is a family of quarks, some up, some down, some others are strange, and some even charmed, that make up existence in the universe. We now live in a universe where virtual particles come and go with no rhyme or reason, and where eleven dimensions are enfolded into an atom. If this sounds a bit chaotic, chaos theory is one of the hottest topics in science. We live in exciting times.

In the health care arena, however, chaos does not have the charm or beauty of the physical science. It is nevertheless the dominant force in the transition of medicine. When I was growing up, the one person I could look up to was the family doctor. She always had the time to come to see me in my bed at home when I was running a fever. When I was curious about my Mom's being pregnant, she explained to me all about how babies are conceived and delivered, using atlases and plaster models that she had in her office. I wonder how much the managed care companies would now pay her for the things she did for me.

The term, *doctor*, has Greek origins derived from the term, *teacher*. Doctors' primary function has always been to enlighten, and to help. Doctors valued autonomy and personal integrity. Profit-making and the "bottom line" have been alien concepts to physicians, but they are exactly the concepts that will be driving the medical profession through "managed care".

We use the term *managed care* loosely, but who manages what? Bureaucrats manage doctors and patients by controlling the delivery of health care - what, where, when, by whom, and how, for how much. The sole reason for managed care is money. People are unwilling to pay what they have been paying for medical care. Why? After all, people will pay huge sums of money for homes, cars, vacations, TV sets. Is medical care any less essential than a house or a car?

The problem with medicine is that no one really "enjoys" medical care. It's no fun to see a doctor, or be in a hospital, or have surgery. Paying medical bills is like paying taxes. Of course, we the medical profession is not blameless in causing this state of affairs. Unnecessary procedures and attempts to prolong life with expensive machines during the end stages of life are examples of why the cost of health care has skyrocketed in the United States. But if the people are willing to pay for a worthwhile cause, then they will, no matter how expensive. Consider going to the moon. It is more the ethos of the times, 1990's, that is just saying "no" both to NASA and to the health care system.

Work force estimations that are needed for the future vary, but all experts seem to agree that there are just too many doctors, both specialists and primary physicians, for the next century. Of course, in the 1960s and 70s, there were dire predictions made of the physician shortage in this country, and federal subsidies for building more medical schools and training programs. But that was then, and now is now. As many as one fifth of the medical schools may have to close during the next decade, and about half of the inpatient beds of all hospitals is considered unnecessary.

So whither the biopsychosocial model in an age of chaos and stringency?
Perhaps, there are two scenarios:

Scenario One: In the 21st century, productivity shall reign supreme, at the expense of time spent with patients. Provide brief and focused care at the expense of comprehensive approach. The physician of the future will be a technician who will be content to work long hours for the managed care company at about half of 20th century physician salary. He/she will be efficient with patients by keeping conversation to a minimum, routinizing the work, processing the patients as in an assembly line, using the absolute minimum of laboratory tests, procedures, and medications. Our hero will associate with administrative people, but not with colleagues, because colleagues may suggest consultations or other expensive things. When asked about "biopsychosocial model", our hero replies, "We don't do such antiquated things. Biopsychosocial model went out the window with home visits and million-dollar work-ups".

Scenario Two: In the brave new world of the 21st century, there will be a resurgence of comprehensive approach to patients, and demand for doctors who will listen, who will teach, and who will understand. The patients, the people who were saying "no" to the expense of medical care, will be fed up by the specter of the monster of managed health care at the turn of the century, and demand that doctors be doctors again. By this time, efficiency is built into the practice of medicine through the use of computers and artificial intelligence, so that doctors can be primarily doctors - listeners, healers, and teachers. Comprehensive or biopsychosocial approach is also operationalized and computerized, so that the doctor of the 21st century is both efficient and comprehensive, both scientist and artist.

It is my hope that this book will, in some small measure, help realize the second scenario.

BIOPSYCHOSOCIAL APPROACHES IN PRIMARY CARE

This volume is based on two symposia I chaired during the 13th World Congress of the International College of Psychosomatic Medicine, held in Jerusalem, Israel, in 1995, and another symposium co-chaired by Professors Benjamin Maoz and Wolfram Schüffel during the same Congress. The symposia were on the topics of "The Biopsychosocial Model : Challenges for the 21st Century", "Teaching of Psychosomatic Medicine", and "*Salutogenesis* : The Creation of Health" and were presented by distinguished leaders in psychosomatic medicine and biopsychosocial education around the world. This book is, however, much more than simple proceedings. A number of distinguished educators and researchers who could not attend the Congress have contributed to this volume. A number of chapters have been added to present a *state of the art* of comprehensive practice of medicine as applied to psychiatric syndromes and special populations such as the geriatric, pediatric, and chronic patients.

Part I of the book, *State of the Art,* presents the most up-to-date application of the biopsychosocial model in the diagnosis and management of patients. Wise presents the basic principles underlying psychiatric diagnosis in the primary care setting, and discusses the *Diagnostic and Statistical Manual of Mental Disorders, 4th Edition, Primary Care (DSM- IV-PC)* that he and his colleagues developed. Leigh presents biopsychosocial analyses of the *anxiety and depressive syndromes,* and presents practical algorithms for primary care physicians in managing these syndromes. Beck and Tong provide a comprehensive and practical discussion of managing *patients with chronic diseases, including terminal disease.* Eisendrath discusses one of the most vexing class of problems in medicine - *factitious disorders.* His discussion includes practical suggestions concerning psychological and pharmacological management of factitious disorders in the managed care setting. Streltzer provides a comprehensive and practical approach to managing another major biopsychosocial syndrome in the primary care setting, *chronic pain.* Human population as a whole is aging around the world. Around 2,030 AD, the elderly population in the United States is expected to reach twenty percent. A significantly larger proportion of the elderly suffer from a variety of psychiatric disorders including dementia, delirium, depression, and anxiety as compared to the younger population. Ahmed and Takeshita discusses these timely subjects that includes elder abuse, and provides practical suggestions for the primary care physician. This chapter is followed by an intriguing research paper by V. Leigh and her colleagues, who have shown that simple changes in the nursing practices of a geriatric unit, that included increasing the amount of sugar provided for their patients, resulted in a significant reversal of a serious quality of life problem of institutionalized geriatric patients, weight loss. Part I ends with a discussion by Fox of the practice of an expanded biopsychosocial model in child psychiatry in the managed care environment.

Part II of the book deals with the challenges that must be faced by medical theoreticians as well as by comprehensive practitioners in the next century. They include the challenge of redefining the concepts and operationalizing the biopsychosocial model. Leigh argues that Engel's biopsychosocial model is confusing because of a lack of clear distinction among *biopsychosocial models of disease, of psychiatric illness, and of the patient* and proposes a new field of integration and research about the patient that he calls *Patientology.* He believes that biopsychosocial approaches are most useful in psychiatric illness and in understanding and managing *patients* (rather than diseases), and proposes an operational and computerized method of biopsychosocial analysis of patients. Howsepian, a psychiatric resident and a Ph.D. candidate in philosophy, discusses the metaphysical implications of the biopsychosocial model, especially *emergentism* implicit in its embrace of the *general systems theory,* and finds that biopsychosocial model has contributed to a revitalization of *reductionism.* Maoz & Shüffel, distinguished psychosomatic researchers and educators in Israel and Germany, respectively, summarizes a symposium during the World Congress that discussed a much neglected aspect of a comprehensive approach in medicine so far - that of *salutogenesis* or creation of health. They show that a *sense of coherence* plays an important role in *salutogenesis,* and discuss models of teaching a comprehensive psychosomatic curriculum. Waldfogel comprehensively discusses another much neglected area, the role of religion (*both positive and negative)* in medicine and health. His suggestion concerning *cultural brokers* may be especially valuable for primary care physicians who must relate with and manage patients of diverse backgrounds and cultures. This volume ends with a discussion of *Managed Care*, perhaps the most significant paradigmatic change in medical practice since the advent of antibiotics.

PART I. STATE OF THE ART

1

PSYCHIATRIC DIAGNOSIS IN PRIMARY CARE: THE BIOPSYCHOSOCIAL PERSPECTIVE

Thomas N. Wise, M.D.[1]

Chairman, Department of Psychiatry
The Fairfax Hospital
Professor and Vice Chair
Department of Psychiatry
Georgetown University School of Medicine

INTRODUCTION

Twenty-eight percent of the adult population within the United States is afflicted with a psychiatric or addictive disorder (Regier, 1993). Only half will seek care for such problems and the majority of those that do will attend primary care settings for treatment. Unfortunately low detection rates for psychiatric disorders mandate the development of newer models to help the primary care provider better understand and diagnose psychiatric disorders that present in this setting (Borus, 1989). In addition, there are many "subthreshold" disorders seen in primary care that do not meet the formal operational criteria for mental disorder in DSM-IV or ICD 9. Subthreshold disorders must be better studied to develop effective treatments for these entities. This chapter will discuss the diagnostic process in primary care and describe the DSM-IV-Primary Care version (DSM-IV-PC), which offers a useful vehicle for the primary care provider to better diagnose such problems.

Correct recognition of emotional disorders in primary care is essential. First, to prevent the suffering and dysfunction that any disease causes is mandate of the physician, i.e., *primum non nocere*. Psychiatric disorders promote disability equivalent to many common medical disorders (Wells, 1989). Second, the actual economic consequences, both direct and indirect, due to psychiatric disorders are significant. The cost of direct psychiatric and mental health services in the United States approaches $67 billion annually but does not measure the other economic consequences such as lost productivity, increased mortality, and

[1]Correspondence: Department of Psychiatry, Fairfax Hospital, 3300 Gallows Road, Falls Church, VA 22046

Biopsychosocial Approaches in Primary Care: State of the Art and Challenges for the 21st Century, Edited by H. Leigh, Plenum Press, New York, 1997

disruption within family and society (Johnson, 1992). Finally, individuals with psychiatric disorders are at increased risk for general medical comorbidity while patients in general medical settings with concurrent psychiatric disorders have longer hospital stays, increased procedures and greater total health care cost. One clear example is the significant comorbidity between vehicular accidents and psychiatric disorders such as substance abuse (Noyes, 1985).

The three elements that lead to under-recognition of psychiatric disorders include patient factors, physician-related issues, and barriers within the health care system itself (Borus, 1989). Patient attitudes can prevent accurate psychiatric diagnosis if patients are sufficiently embarrassed or ashamed not to disclose psychiatric symptoms. This may be due to the stigma attached to a psychiatric disorder or financial concerns that foster fear in admitting to such a disorder (Wise, 1984). The second element that prevents effective diagnosis and treatment is the insufficient skills of many physicians in ascertaining accurate psychiatric diagnoses or lack of knowledge about psychiatry (Thompson, 1982). Such knowledge and technical deficits, combined with negative attitudes about psychiatry, abet under-recognition. Physicians, much like their patients, are often uncomfortable in discussing emotional issues for fear of stigmatizing their patients. This compromises the ability to obtain a full psychosocial history. For example, the utilization of direct or closed-end questions hinders the patient from explaining distressing affective states or fully explaining the use of addictive medications. Unfortunately, few primary care training programs require significant periods of time for ambulatory psychiatric services. Inadequate knowledge about proper psychopharmacologic management hinders treatment even when the disorder such as depression is recognized (Katon, 1992). Finally, the present health care system inherently presents a barrier to effective recognition. The time pressures in ambulatory primary care are inadequate for proper psychosocial or substance abuse evaluation. The reimbursement system offers little incentive for the treatment of psychiatric disorders; and in rural areas, there is a limited availability of psychiatric physicians. Future health policy must address such barriers if effective recognition in the treatment of emotional disorders is to improve significantly.

THE DIAGNOSTIC PROCESS

Inherent within the diagnostic process is the dyadic relationship between doctor and patient. Balint has elegantly described this process by demonstrating that patients present in a disorganized phase of an illness (Balint, 1973). Thus, patients will come to their physician with a variety of symptoms and ideas about the cause of their distress. In primary care settings, family members will also accompany the patient and provide corroborating or contradicting information. It is the task of the physician via questions, physical examinations, and laboratory tests to better "organize" the illness into a discrete category and determine whether a diagnosable disorder, whether medical and/or psychiatric, or both, is present.

The strategies for accurate categorical designation are not as precise as one might wish. A diagnosis represents a coherent cluster of signs and symptoms, i.e., a syndrome which the physician has learned via his or her medical education or has accrued from clinical experience. Thus, symptoms of fatigue, shortness of breath, and observable signs such as pedal edema, tachycardia, and pulmonary rales can be recognized syndromically as suggestive heart failure. The specific subcellular abnormality is not always apparent. As with medical diseases, psychological disorders can also be organized by clustering of signs and symptoms. The individual who presents with a sad face and complains of fatigability, difficulty sleeping, and decreased appetitive symptoms in the realms of appetite, sleep, and sexuality may be suffering from an affective disorder but also may have a chronic infectious process such as Lyme disease. Koran has demonstrated the limited reliability of subjective interpretations of observable signs in medical illnesses (Koran, 1968). He concludes that physicians show greater disagreement among diagnostic categories considered to be less severe, as well as disagreeing about judgements which are dimensional as opposed to categorical. This has important implications for psychological difficulties. The clinician might relegate emotional difficulties to a less serious position than physical illnesses. Furthermore, psychological distress is measured along a continuum, such as greater or lesser anxiety instead of a categorical state such as Generalized Anxiety Disorder. The mind-body dualism is embodied in the dialectic of understanding versus explanation (McHugh, 1982). It is often easy to "understand" why a patient might appear sad and depressed if they have serious difficulties in their life circumstances, such as an unhappy marriage or relevant losses. It does not explain, however, the lowered energy level, suicidal ramifications, and weight loss that all could be etiologically related to the individual's affective disorder. Such empathic understanding often minimizes the role of accurate treatment in categorical psychiatric illnesses as major mood disorders or generalized anxiety disorders.

George Engel has urged physicians to utilize a biopsychosocial model that would include psychological issues as well as social phenomena in addition to the biologic data that allows them to better understand the problems with which patients present (Engel, 1977). Thus, patients must be viewed as more than purely biological substrates. McHugh and Slavney have extended such an approach by demonstrating that psychiatry must be viewed from multiple perspectives, each of which has its own specific logic and internal grammar (McHugh, 1983). They challenge the biopsychosocial model by suggesting that whether the various perspectives, biological, psychological and social, are not fluid systems but are dysjunctive. Thus, there is no clear transduction between the social realm and the biological spheres in many patient problems. Nevertheless, the clinician must understand each perspective and its inherent strengths and weaknesses in order to best assess and manage the complex clinical problems routinely encountered. The four perspectives that are outlined include the disease model; the life history method; the intersubject differences; and motivated behaviors.

The *disease model* is that most familiar to physicians. This approach is based upon the medical model and utilizes syndromic categorization to organize the presenting symptoms and observable signs which allow categories to be developed. Such categorization allows reliability that can eventually lead to syndromic validation via family studies, response to specific treatments, and eventual pathophysiologic correlation (Robins, 1970). When such pathophysiologic causes are discovered, the disorder can be explained and a rational treatment can often be developed. Syndromes are studied via the five phases of diagnostic validation that include careful clinical description utilizing demographic and clinical factors, laboratory studies, genetic studies, follow-up studies to ascertain the course of the disorder and response to various treatments. The disease approach is readily exemplified by the patient who presents with fatigue, weight loss and problems concentrating. If the full evaluation reveals abnormal thyroid function, the diagnosis of hyperthyroidism is made and rational treatment can be initiated. In another individual, however, similar symptoms with normal thyroid tests may lead the clinician to conclude the individual has a mood disorder with a very different treatment approach. It is the disease approach that is best exemplified by the DSM-IV and the primary care version (Pincus, 1995).

LIFE HISTORY APPROACH

The next perspective is that of the life history method, which is commonly found in a variety of psychotherapeutic endeavors (Slavney, 1985). In this approach, each individual is treated as a unique subject rather than a biologic object (McHugh, 1982). The physician tries to understand how the patient reacts to various life events and developmental vicissitudes. Basically, this approach is one of idiographic investigation wherein a subject is looked at as a single case in depth rather than in a nomothetic manner which denotes norms and averages of a large population. Via empathetic listening, the physician tries to link the meaningful events in a patient's life that illuminate their history and correlate with present feeling states and behaviors. Such connections, however, do not explain in a formal causal sense as do the natural sciences. The life history approach allows us to understand why a patient may seek treatment at this point in time and how they subjectively experience a variety of stressors including biologic events such as disease states. Many psychiatric phenomena that are seen in primary care may be operationally defined and utilized in the life history perspective (Fava, 1995). Thus, abnormal illness behaviors that lead to health anxieties, denial of illness, or phobic fears of various diseases should be elicited. Anniversary reactions often trouble patients when memories, both conscious and unconscious, of the losses of important family members or people in their lives occur. That such events from the past may be currently operant in the individual's life are essential to recognize. The clinician must also understand the various tasks within the patient's life cycle (Glick, 1980). Thus is the individual in the beginning of a childbearing age. Is the decision to have children creating a marital difficulty or the failure to procreate causing distresses and sorrows of infertility. Is the individual coping with marital problems due to the absence of children who are grown or coping with retirement and aging. It is thus important for the clinician to map out the various phases of adult development as outlined by Glick and Kessler (Glick, 1980). The clinician utilizing the life history methodology begins to understand the patient's autobiography and may utilize the life-cycle tasks as chapters in each patient's life story. This will help make meaningful connections between the data presented and behaviors and feelings observed. By understanding such information, the physician may help explain to the patient why they are feeling or behaving as they do now or better offer support to an individual with a psychiatric disorder. The limits of the life history methodology are that what may be true for one individual is not always true for another. Although early childhood abuse may often create problems for the individual when they reach adulthood, it does not explain why other individuals are not so affected. Nevertheless, broad maxims such as early life traumas may create problems later in one's life are truisms that must be incorporated into daily clinical work via a careful psychiatric history.

The next perspective found in psychiatry is that of intersubject differences. Many phenomena found in medicine and psychiatry are dimensional, i.e., they exist along a continuum rather than a discrete category. Height, weight, blood pressure, and intelligence all demonstrate such a nomothetic perspective wherein the variable can be compared quantitatively along a measurable dimension. Thus, electrolytes are measured as greater or lesser, and a certain level is considered abnormal. Likewise, personality traits can be measured in this manner (Wise, 1995). An individual may be more or less outgoing, social, and energetic or more or less prone to anxiety, hostility, depression, and dysphoria. A variety of traits characterize an individual's personality, a descriptive term that tries to document their propensity for behavior when provoked by a variety of tasks. Thus, a very conscientious and organized person will react to a school examination with systematic study, where someone less organized will wait until the last minute. Someone prone to anxiety will worry about such an examination for weeks prior to the actual test, whereas those low on this trait will not worry but may study in a calm and reflective manner. Alexithymia exemplifies a personality trait that is often important in primary care settings (Wise, 1992). This style denotes a tendency to somatize, utilize external concrete details and to have a diminished ability to abstract and fantasize. Such individuals are often prone to anxiety and worry and may repeatedly seek medical care without connecting other life circumstances. It is important for the primary care physician to understand intersubject differences as they relate to personality. If they can utilize coherent personality approaches such as the five-factor model, which emphasizes neuroticism, extroversion, agreeableness, conscientiousness, and openness to new ideas, it becomes relatively easy for such clinicians to develop a "personality fingerprint" for their respective patients (McCrae, 1990). Such personality traits need not be pathologic but descriptive. The clinician can understand the strengths and vulnerabilities of each individual.

The final perspective is that of *motivated behaviors*, which are goal-directed activities that lead to reduction in tension (McHugh, 1982). Such behaviors include eating, sleeping, and sexual drives which are natural physiologic elements. This perspective can also be invoked to better understand a variety of behaviors such as obesity, sexual deviations, or repeated self harm, such as the persistent wrist cutting in patients with borderline personalities. The perspective of motivated behaviors is helpful in considering in addictive problems. Individuals prone to alcoholism may have intense cravings for intoxicating substances which reduce tension states, whereas those without such vulnerabilities will not experience such tension. Although the construct of motivated behaviors is complex, it is helpful in understanding a variety of addictive behaviors that are frequently under-recognized in primary care settings.

DSM-IV-PC

The introduction of reliable syndromes via DSM-III, IIIR, and IV have greatly changed the approach to psychiatric classification during the past two decades. This diagnostic taxonomy reifies the medical basis of psychiatry. Unfortunately, the DSM iterations, including the present DSM-IV, are difficult to use for primary care physicians. The detailed information in the DSM system, as well as the many disorders included that are rarely observed in general medical settings, can become cumbersome for primary care providers. Furthermore, the DSM is organized along major subclasses of disorders which assumes that the user knows which section to initially refer. This presents a difficulty for physicians who are not familiar with symptom patterns to appropriately classify these patients. Finally, the DSM-IV may not contain information sufficiently valuable to the primary care physician, such as details on typical presentations of psychiatric disorders in primary care and how to best differentiate among disorders with similar symptom presentations. For these reasons, it was felt that a guide based on presenting symptoms that emphasizes recognition and differential diagnosis would be more useful to the primary care physician. Representatives from various primary care organizations developed the DSM-IV-PC. Representatives from internal medicine (Society of General Internal Medicine, the American College of Physicians); family practice (American Academy of Family Practice, Association of Departments of Family Medicine, American Board of Family Practice, Society of Teachers of Family Medicine); obstetrics (American College of Obstetrics and Gynecology); pediatrics (American Academy of Pediatrics); psychiatry (American Psychiatric Association) and the American Medical Association organized a committee to develop such a manual.

At the outset, the group established a list of principles to guide the manual's development. These included the following: a) the manual must be organized in such a way that is compatible with how a physician manages the primary care visit, for example, by presenting symptoms. the manual must be user-friendly--it must be succinct, given restricted consultation time, and must be designed for easy use; b) it should provide a rubric for differential diagnosis and provide "clinical pointers"; c) it should provide an appropriate cross-reference to research criteria sets in the DSM-IV Appendix B for subthreshold presentations seen commonly in the primary care setting, for example, minor depressive disorder; d) it should be compatible with the DSM-IV and also the ICD-9-CM to ensure correct medical record-keeping and to facilitate communication.

DEVELOPMENT PROCESS

From the main committee, sub work groups were formed to focus on major diagnostic classes. These included 1) a mood/anxiety sub work group; 2) a somatoform sub work group (somatoform disorders and disorders of sleep, sex, eating, and pain); 3) a psychosocial/environmental sub work group (focusing on psychosocial problems that, while not formally mental disorders, are common in primary care); 4) a substance use disorders sub work group; and 5) a childhood disorders sub work group. Disorders that are described in less detail (e.g., disorders of impulse control, dissociative disorders, personality disorders, and other disorders less frequently diagnosed in the primary are setting) were reviewed by all sub work groups.

Each sub work group sorted the DSM-IV disorders into three groups: 1) those that are rarely diagnosed in primary care (e.g., paraphilias) and thus could easily be summarized; 2) those that are adequately described in DSM-IV already (e.g., sleep disorders); and 3) those for which an expanded description would be helpful (e.g., mood disorders, psychosocial problems). This determination was based on the overall prevalence of the disorder, prevalence of the disorder in primary care settings, salience of the condition (e.g., importance of its identification by primary care physicians), evidence of frequently misdiagnosed disorders in primary care, and educational significance. DSM-IV diagnostic definitions were then reworded for utility in the primary care setting. In some cases, this involved simplifying subtypes, providing clear examples of criteria, or defining technical terms. In other cases, information beyond the criteria set (e.g., differential diagnosis pointers) was added. The work groups then grouped the conditions under various symptom clusters, and those symptom clusters common in primary care were used to organize the conditions algorithmically.

Although brief descriptions of DSM-IV disorders diagnosed in childhood and adolescence will be included, a more detailed guide that is structured upon developmental variation will be written. *The Classification of Child and Adolescent Mental Conditions in Primary Care: DSM-PC Child and Adolescent Version* will be coordinated by the American Academy of Pediatrics in conjunction with the American Psychiatric Association and other child health care organizations.

The manual is partitioned into four sections. Section 1 describes those disorders and conditions most frequently encountered in primary care and comprises the majority of the manual. These disorders are presented in nine algorithms. The second section includes psychosocial problems that are a focus of clinical attention but that are not considered a mental disorder (e.g., relational [family] problems, psychological factors affecting general medical conditions). Section 3 describes disorders that are rarely first identified in primary care (e.g., dissociative disorders). These disorders are not presented algorithmically, but they are clustered by common symptomatology. The final section describes, similarly by cluster, disorders usually first diagnosed in infancy, childhood, or adolescence.

A list of presenting symptoms guides the clinician to one or more of the nine major algorithms (e.g., loss of energy leads the clinician to the depressed mood algorithm, difficulty concentrating leads the physician to the impaired memory algorithm). Using presenting symptoms as the organizational basis of the manual is consistent with other diagnostic systems designed for primary care clinicians. Within each algorithm, a series of steps, or "rule out" or "consider" statements, guides the clinician. Each algorithm is organized according to what is most relevant for that group of disorders. The order of the algorithm may be based on prevalence (e.g., disorders encountered more frequently are listed first); salience (e.g., those disorders that are considered more important to clinical care or most important to recognize are listed first); or severity (e.g., the most impairing disorders are listed first). Although the organizational principles differ somewhat across algorithms, consistency across algorithms was maintained in part by having the first step of each algorithm (to first consider if the presenting symptoms may be better accounted for by a general medical condition, substance use, or other mental disorders not included in the grouping) be essentially identical.

Within each step, the code and definition of the condition is highlighted and distinguished (by being boxed) from information that is available for the clinician who wants additional detail. The additional clinical information is indented (to indicate its secondary importance) and may include the following: specifier/subtype information, differential diagnostic pointers, and additional clinical information (e.g., definitions of terms used in the criteria sets, specific examples of the criteria, onset and course information). Disorders are often accompanied by an additional paragraph of text providing coding pointers, if relevant.

An introductory text section also accompanies each algorithm. The text is divided into four sections: 1) epidemiology (e.g., prevalence of the disorders among the general population and/or the primary care population, sex ratio); 2) primary care presentation (e.g., common symptom patterns of patients who might present to the primary care physician); 3) differential diagnosis and common associated conditions; and 4) organization of the algorithm (i.e., explanation of the principles by which the algorithm is organized, such as by prevalence).

In addition to the four sections previously mentioned, sections describing the "Use of the Manual" and "Steps Common to All Algorithms" explain the organization and use of the manual. Included in the front of the manual is a brief distillation of the manual consisting of pictorial summaries of the nine algorithms and a quick coding guide. An Appendix includes aspects of the DSM-IV multiaxial system, that is, the psychosocial/environmental checklist (Axis IV) to remind clinicians to also consider the potential effect of the person's environment on his or her care, and the Global Assessment of Functioning Scale (Axis IV) provides a measure of overall social and occupational functioning. A symptoms index is also included in the Appendix.

Two conceptual issues central to the development of the manual were compatibility and inclusiveness. While ensuring that the manual be as relevant to the primary care practice as possible was a very important goal, compatibility with DSM-IV (and ICD-9-CM) was also necessary. Compatibility does not mean that the systems needed to be identical. For example, a complex set of DSM-IV criteria was often summarized and simplified in DSM-IV-PC but was still consistent in terms of the categorization of cases. Further, in DSM-IV-PC it was at times appropriate to add a sentence or two explaining the disorder's label and how the disorder typically manifests in patients. Because a common complaint about the DSM-III-R was that it was overwhelming, one of the primary goals of the project was to provide a succinct manual. On the other hand, it was important to provide enough information to help the physician recognize a disorder. This issue was resolved by providing a different level of detail for presentation of different sets of conditions; disorders more commonly seen in primary care are more extensively discussed. For example, the inclusion of subtypes differs among disorders in DSM-IV-PC: 1) they were eliminated if they provided limited utility in primary care; 2) they were simplified and mentioned briefly in the additional clinical information section (i.e., purely for informational purposes); or 3) they were retained with definitions and criteria if they had particular relevance to primary care (e.g., specifier related to the postpartum period). One concern expressed by primary care clinicians was the extent to which individuals manifest psychiatric symptoms that fall below the threshold for a specific DSM-IV disorder. Because these presentations may involve impairment in functioning, and because they may represent an increased risk for the development of a disorder that does meet the threshold for a mental disorder, primary care physicians were especially concerned that such presentations be discussed in DSM-IV-PC. For these situations, an NOS category was used that provides a brief description of common subthreshold syndromes (e.g., minor depressive disorder). For those interested in research criteria, a cross-reference citation to the Appendix of DSM-IV is provided.

The DSM-IV process required an extensive empirical review, and changes were made only when they were supported by significant empirical evidence; therefore, DSM-IV-PC was built on that evidence. But because there is much less research on diagnosis and assessment of mental and addictive disorders in primary care, DSM-IV-PC relied more on extrapolation of specialty-setting data and clinical consensus. The process has additionally resulted in the elucidation of a research agenda for primary care.

DISCUSSION

Engel's initial call for a "new medical model" helped to formalize the recognition that diagnosis and evaluation are more than a simple taxonomic ritual to label a pathophysiologic process (Engel, 1977). The biopsychosocial approach reminds the clinician to include psychological and social factors when considering the individual patient. The introduction of various perspectives found in psychiatry is the next logical step, as it provides a logical and coherent approach to better understanding the patient via the four perspectives described above (McHugh, 1982). The DSM-IV-PC best exemplifies the disease model and can be understood by primary care physicians and other health personnel (Pincus, 1995). It reifies the medical tradition and underscores why psychiatry is a medical specialty. It is also essential to understand who the patient is as well as what disorder the patient has. This perspective is best considered as the Life History Methodology. The primary care physician can beneficially utilize the DSM-IV-PC to maximize accuracy in the disease approach. Consideration of other common phenomena, however, found in medical practice demands understanding the intersubject differences embodied in a five-factor model of personality (neuroticism, extroversion, agreeableness, conscientiousness, and openness) (McCrae, 1990). It also demands of the primary care physician to truly understand the individual's life history. Such an understanding should accrue from the longitudinal relationship that embodies the definition of primary care medicine.

REFERENCES

Balint M: *The Doctor, His Patient and the Illness,* Pitman, London, 1973.

Borus JF, Howes MJ, Devins NP et al.: Primary Health Care Providers'Recognition and Diagnosis of Mental Disorders in Their Patients. General Hospital Psychiatry 10:317-321, 1989.

Engel GL: The Need for a New Medical Model: A Challenge for Biomedicine. Science 196:129-136, 1977

Fava GA, Freyberger HJ, Bech P et al.: Diagnostic Criteria for Use in Psychosomatic Research. Psychotherapy Psychosom 61:1-8, 1995

Glick ID, Kessler, DR: *Marital and Family Therapy, second edition*, pp. 30-82. Grune and Stratton: New York 1980.

Johnson J, Weissman MM, Klerman GL: Service Utilization and Social Morbidity Associated with Depressive Symptoms. JAMA 267:1478-1483, 1992.

Katon W, VonKorff M, Lin E, et al . Adequacy and Duration of Antidepressant Treatment in Primary Care. Med Care 30:67-76, 1992.

Koran L: The Reliability of Clinical Methods, Data, and Judgements (Part 2) New England Journal of Medicine 293:462-467, 695-701, 1968.

McCrae RT, Costa PR: *Personality in Adulthood: Emerging Lives, Enduring Dispositions.* Guilford: New York, 1990.

McHugh PR and Slavney PR: Methods of Reasoning in Psychopathology: Conflict and Resolution. Comprehensive Psychiatry 23:197-215, 1982.

McHugh PR and Slavney PR: *The Perspectives of Psychiatry.* Johns Hopkins: Baltimore, 1983. 159 pages.

Noyes R: Motor Vehicle Accidents Related to Psychiatric Impairment. Psychosomatics 26:569-580, 1985.

Pincus HA, Vettorello NE, McQueen LE, et al.: Bridging the Gap Between Psychiatry and Primary Care: The DSM-IV-PC. Psychosomatics 36:328-335, 1995.

Regier DA, Narrow WE, Rae DS et al.: The DeFacto U.S. Mental and Addictive Disorders Service System. Arch General Psychiatry 50:85-94, 1993.

Robins E, Guzes B: Establishment of Diagnostic Validity in Psychiatric Illness. American Journal of Psychiatry 126:107-111, 1970.

Slavney PR, McHugh PR: The Life Story Method in Psychotherapy and Psychiatric Education. American Journal of Psychotherapy 39:57-67, 1985.

Thompson TL: The Psychiatric Education of Primary Care Physicians in Thompson TL, Byyny RL (Editors). *The Education of the General Internist.* University of Colorado, Denver, 89-107, 1982.

Wells KB, Stewart A, Hays RD, et al.: The Functioning and Well-Being of Depressed Patients. JAMA 262:914-919, 1989.

Wise TN, Mann LS, Berlin RM, et al.: Mental Health Referral Patterns by Family Medicine Educators. Comprehensive Psychiatry 25:465-469, 1984.

Wise TN, Mann LS, Shay L: Alexithymia and the Five-Factor Model of Personality. Comprehensive Psychiatry 33:147-151, 1992.

Wise TN: Categories and Dimensions in Primary Care Psychiatry. Psychosomatics 36:326-327, 1995.

2

BIOPSYCHOSOCIAL APPROACHES TO ANXIETY IN PRIMARY CARE

Hoyle Leigh, M.D.[1]

Professor of Psychiatry
University of California, San Francisco and
Fresno VA Medical Center

INTRODUCTION

Anxiety is the most common emotional condition encountered in primary care settings. In fact, a majority of antianxiety drug prescriptions are written by primary care physicians in the United States. Unfortunately, however, the treatment of anxiety rendered by primary care physicians without specialized training tends to be ineffective for two reasons - 1) lack of an understanding of the biopsychosocial approach, and 2) lack of a systematic, phased treatment plan.

In evaluating and managing the complex syndrome of anxiety, a biopsychosocial approach is not an ideology but an indispensable practical approach. No evaluation of a patient with an anxiety can be understood without an assessment of the patient's biological state, genetic influences, developmental factors, and social stresses. No management of such a patient is effective unless the therapy is geared to his/her brain, body, and his/her relationship with the environment (Leigh, Feinstein & Reiser, 1980; Leigh and Reiser, 1992).

THE CONCEPT OF FINAL COMMON PATHWAY

Almost all psychiatric syndromes, including anxiety, depression, delirium/dementia, and psychosis are final common pathway syndromes (Leigh & Reiser, 1992, Leigh, 1983). A final

[1]Correspondence: Department of Psychiatry, University of California, San Francisco-Fresno, and Fresno VA Medical Center, 2615 E. Clinton Ave, Fresno, CA 93703

Biopsychosocial Approaches in Primary Care: State of the Art and Challenges for the 21st Century, Edited by H. Leigh, Plenum Press, New York, 1997

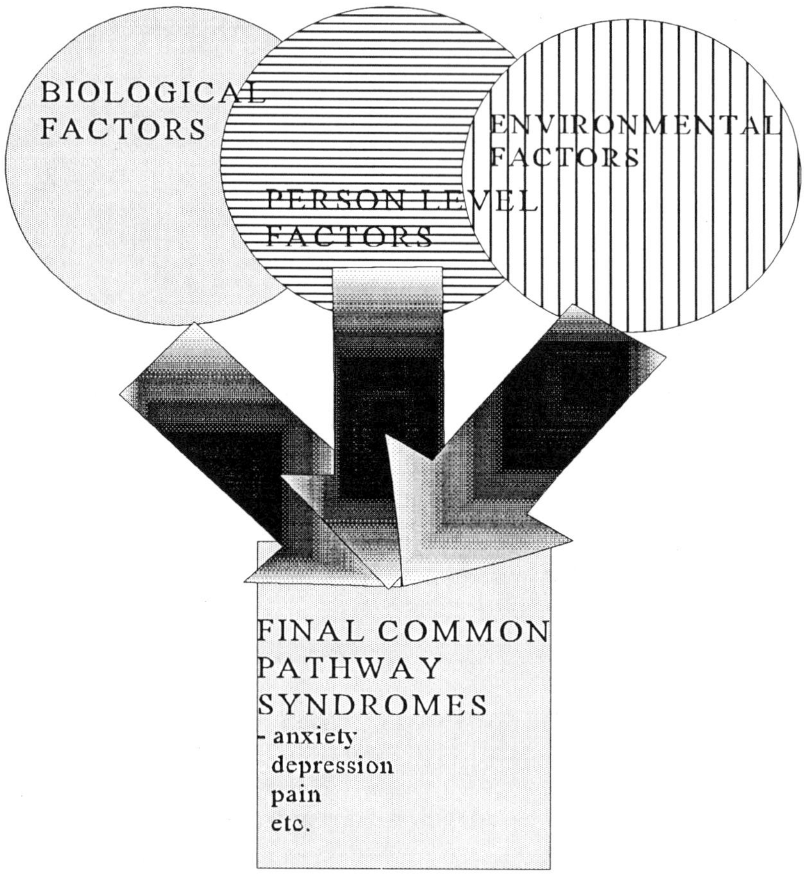
BIOLOGICAL FACTORS
PERSON LEVEL FACTORS
ENVIRONMENTAL FACTORS
FINAL COMMON PATHWAY SYNDROMES
- anxiety
depression
pain
etc.

common pathway syndrome signifies an altered state of the organism that may have many different causes or contributing factors. An example in physiology is fever. Fever may be *caused* by a virus, a bacteria, a toxin, a brain lesion, a metabolic anomaly (e.g. etiocholanolone fever), a neoplasm, etc. Multiple factors may contribute to a patient's fever, e.g., a mild infection in a dehydrated patient. The paths to the final common pathway of anxiety involves environmental stresses, intrapsychic conflicts, personality and disposition of the person, and genetic and other biochemical influences on the limbic system and hypothalamus. Effective management of a final common pathway syndrome (e.g. fever) may be symptomatic (e.g., Aspirin), etiologic (e.g., antibiotics), or both.

The most efficacious way of evaluating the causes or contributing factors of a final common pathway syndrome is to examine the three dimensions of the patient systematically as we will in this chapter.

THE NATURE AND RECOGNITION OF ANXIETY

Characterized by the subjective feelings of dread and/or fear, accompanied by symptoms and signs of physiologic activation (usually sympathetic, with some cholinergic activation such as sweating), anxiety is often a signal that a danger situation exists either in the environment, in the patient's personality system, or in the patient's body. Thus an environmental stressor (e.g., an impending exam), intrapsychic conflicts (e.g., an activation of a repressed and unacceptable wish), or medical disease or symptom (e.g., hyperthyroidism, or the discovery of the presence of a lump in the breast) may all contribute to the danger signal. The final common pathway activation in anxiety seems to be the activation of reticular activating system in the brain, the hypothalamus (*fight-flight reaction*), and the noradrenergic neurons of the locus ceruleus in the pons.

Anxiety, like pain, has a protective function, and is normal within limits. It is to be expected that patients presenting to a doctor's office with a physical symptom would feel a certain amount of anxiety. The physician's gentle, reassuring manner, and a comfortable atmosphere of the office can greatly allay this normal anxiety. Uncertainty generates and exacerbates anxiety. Therefore, the physician can reduce anxiety attendant in the consulting room through *information*, about the nature of his/her findings, plans for further workup, and options concerning treatment. Providing opportunities for the patient to ask questions is another anxiolytic maneuver that physicians often overlook.

An important point for the primary care physician concerning anxiety is that it is often a *catalyst* for help-seeking behavior. Persons who are anxious are more likely to seek help for symptoms that they may have ignored for months or even years. Often they are unaware of the increased anxiety level or attribute the anxiety to the physical symptom, when, in fact, the danger situation may be elsewhere. When a patient comes to the physician complaining of a long-standing or mild symptom, it behooves him/her to ask, "Why now?" and "Is the patient's anxiety level increased, and if so, why?"

While a certain amount of anxiety is normal and even necessary for motivation as in preparation for a major performance, in excessive amounts, anxiety can interfere with and even paralyze normal daily activities. Such *dysregulation* of anxiety may occur by one or more of the following factors:

A. Biological Dimension:

1. Genetic predisposition
2. A biologic condition or disease, such as:
   - any endocrinopathy (e.g., hyperthyroidism, Cushing's syndrome, etc)
   - any metabolic disorder (e.g. diabetes mellitus, hypoglycemia, hypoxia)
   - infections (e.g., HIV)

neoplasms (e.g., carcinoid syndrome, pheochromocytoma)
seizure disorders

3. Substance-related conditions, such as:
CNS stimulant use/abuse (e.g., cocaine, amphetamines, caffeinism)

withdrawal from a CNS depressant (e.g., opiate withdrawal, alcohol withdrawal)
side effect of a prescribed drug

B. Psychological Dimension

1. Specific Anxiety Disorders[2]

Specific anxiety disorders are anxiety syndromes with characteristic symptoms that, in turn, are determined by biopsychosocial factors. The one year prevalence rate of anxiety disorders is about 12.6 %. Social Phobia is most common, with a lifetime rates of 10-11 %.

Panic disorder *(Panic Disorder without Agoraphobia: DSM IV Code: 300.01)*
recurrent panic attacks, often associated with fear of
open spaces (agoraphobia) *(Panic Disorder with Agoraphobia: DSM IV Code: 300.21)*
A panic attack is a discrete period of intense fear or discomfort, often with cardiopulmonary (e.g., shortness of breath, palpitations), autonomic (e.g., sweating), gastrointestinal (e.g., choking sensation, nausea), neurologic (e.g., trembling, dizziness, paresthesia), and psychiatric symptoms (e.g., derealization, fear of dying).

Social Phobia *(DSM IV Code: 300.23)*
avoidance of social situations with fear of embarrassment

Specific Phobia *(DSM IV Code: 300.29)*
avoidance of specific object or situation, e.g, high places, cats

Separation Anxiety Disorder *(DSM IV Code: 309.21)*
anxiety concerning separation from major attachment figure

Obsessive Compulsive Disorder *(DSM IV Code: 300.3)*
recurrent and persistent bothersome thoughts (obsessions) and/or
ritualistic behaviors or recurrent mental acts (compulsions)

Posttraumatic Stress Disorder (PTSD) *(DSM IV Code: 309.81)* and Acute Stress Disorder *(DSM IV Code: 308.3)*
re-experiencing highly traumatic events
if symptoms persist for at least 4 weeks, PTSD

Generalized Anxiety Disorder *(DSM IV Code: 300.02)*
pervasive symptoms of anxiety and worry associated with a variety of
events or situations, persisting for at least 6 months

---

[2]After American Psychiatric Association (1995): DSM IV-PC, pp 47-49

2. Anxiety as a symptom of other major psychiatric disorders

Anxiety is a common symptom of most major psychiatric disorders including mood disorders (depression, mania), psychoses including schizophrenia, somatoform disorders, and substance use disorders. In these cases, there are characteristic history, symptoms, and signs of the other major psychiatric disorder in addition to anxiety.

C. Social/Environmental Dimension

1. Social/Environmental Stresses

bereavement, separation, job change, change in residence, etc.

2. Anticipated Stresses

The terms, *Adjustment Disorder with Anxiety (DSM IV Code: 309.24)* or *Adjustment Disorder with Mixed Anxiety and Depressed Mood (DSM IV Code: 309.28),* may be used when the stressed-related anxiety is excessive.

MANAGEMENT OF ANXIETY

Rational management of anxiety is based on an understanding of the nature of the anxiety to be managed. Reasonable degree of anxiety associated with an external stressor usually requires little intervention, other than identifying the stressor and recognizing the anxiety as a signal, and making appropriate plans for dealing with the stress. On the other hand, excessive or even paralyzing anxiety, even as a result of an everyday stress, may require vigorous management. It is important to note that the management of anxiety is not necessarily isodimensional to the cause of anxiety. For example, anxiety associated with a physical condition (biological dimension) might be managed effectively with a relaxation technique (psychological intervention), while panic associated with an external stressor (environmental dimension) might be treated most efficaciously with a medication (biological dimension). Effective treatment modalities exist in all three dimensions of the patient.

SPECIFIC TREATMENT MODALITIES

Biological Dimension

Antianxiety drugs

Benzodiazepines: diazepam, lorazepam, clonazepam, alprazolam, etc.

These are effective antianxiety agents that bind to the benzodiazepine receptors, functionally linked to the GABA receptors to form the GABA-benzodiazepine-chloride ionophore complex (Paul et al, 1981). They are also sedating (may be used as a hypnotic), and are muscle relaxants and respiratory depressants, especially if combined with alcohol. They are also habit forming, and if used in large doses for a prolonged period, abrupt cessation may result in potentially dangerous physiologic withdrawal symptoms. A typical dose for diazepam is 5 mg p.o., h.s. or b.i.d. or t.i.d. (p.r.n.) It is important to caution patients about the sedative properties of benzodiazepines, interaction with alcohol, especially in relationship to driving, and possible dependence. If the patient has been receiving benzodiazepines for more than approximately 3 months regularly, it should be tapered gradually (by about 10% a week).

Buspirone: A partial serotonin presynaptic autoreceptor (5-HT_{1A}) agonist, buspirone seems to reduce serotonin neurotransmission (Lucki, 1996). Buspirone's effect occurs in approximately 2 weeks of continuous therapy (typical dose: 20 mg p.o., b.i.d.), but is neither sedating nor habit-forming.

Beta-Adrenergic Blocking Agents (e.g., propranolol): Beta blockers are effective in reducing the peripheral manifestations of anxiety due to sympathetic activation, such as palpitations, tremor, and sweating. They are particularly useful in certain social phobias, and in performance anxiety (e.g., giving a speech). A typical dose of propranolol for performance anxiety is 10 mg 30 min-1 hr before the performance.

Specific Anti-Obsessive-Compulsive Drugs : Certain tricyclic antidepressants such as clomipramine and specific serotonin reuptake blockers (SSRI) such as fluoxetine may be especially effective in treating the anxiety disorder, Obsessive-Compulsive Disorder (OCD). OCD is a serious psychiatric disorder, and its pharmacotherapy (as well as psychotherapy) should be performed under the supervision of a trained psychiatrist.

Antipanic Drugs: The benzodiazepine alprazolam and antidepressant drugs, especially specific serotonin reuptake blockers such as fluoxetine, sertraline, and paroxetine may be particularly effective in the treatment of panic disorders. Treatment of panic disorders should be performed under the supervision of a trained psychiatrist.

Sedatives: Barbiturates, antihistaminics, and other sedatives have been used to treat anxiety or as a hypnotic, mainly utilizing their nonspecific sedative qualities. They are less effective than specific antianxiety drugs in the treatment of moderate to severe anxiety.

Psychosurgery: Cingulotomy may be effective in intractable Obsessive-Compulsive Disorder in approximately 25-30% of cases (Baer, Rauch, Ballantine et al, 1995).

Personal (Psychological) Dimension

Relaxation Techniques (e.g., Relaxation Response, Self-Hypnosis, Meditation, Autogenic Training, etc.) : These are techniques that the patient learns to use to relieve anxiety. The techniques are relatively simple, and may be self-taught or be taught by a trained therapist. It may be useful for a primary physician to train a nurse or a paraprofessional to teach patients one of the relaxation techniques.

Biofeedback: Requiring EEG, EMG, skin conductance, and/or skin temperature feedback equipment and a trained professional, biofeedback may be useful for specific end-organ symptoms associated with anxiety (e.g. tension headache, migraine). The primary physician should be aware of community resources that perform biofeedback.

Psychotherapies:

General Psychotherapy

Simply seeing a physician is often psychotherapeutic for the patient who is anxious that he/she may have a serious disease, provided the physician reassures that patient that no serious disease has been found. Simple laying of hands by the physician as well as complete physical examination followed by an explanation of a line of approach and treatment for a symptom can be more effective in relieving anxiety and providing a sense of mastery for the patient than any antianxiety drug. Thus, realistic **sympathetic listening, physical examination, reassurance** and **explanation** about diagnostic and therapeutic approaches are psychotherapeutic maneuvers that any primary care physician should be able to provide.

Specific Psychotherapies

Psychotherapy by a trained mental health professional is indicated for specific anxiety disorders described above. Psychotherapy for anxiety may be cognitively or behaviorally oriented or psychodynamically oriented depending on the nature of the anxiety syndrome. For most phobias, behaviorally oriented therapy is most effective (e.g., desensitization). Obsessive-Compulsive Disorder(OCD) also responds to behaviorally oriented psychotherapy utilizing the principles of exposure and response-prevention (Baer & Minichiello, 1990) as well as to medications (see above). It is of note that positron emission tomography (PET) studies demonstrate that local cerebral metabolic rates for glucose in the head of the right caudate nucleus in OCD patients decreased significantly in responders of *both drug and behavior therapy* (Baxter, Schwartz, Bergman, et al, 1992; Schwartz, Stoessel, Baxter, et al, 1996). This is a clear indication that the prolonged biologic abnormalities in the brain associated with OCD change with behavioral as well as pharmacologic treatment. For anxiety associated with deep-seated psychological conflicts (e.g., a pattern of excessive anxiety in the presence of authority figures), psychodynamically oriented psychotherapy may be in order.

Environmental (Social) Dimension

Hospitalization: This is seldom indicated in anxiety disorders with the exception of severe agoraphobia with or without panic attacks, severe panic disorder, and severe (paralyzing) Obsessive-Compulsive Disorder.

Group Therapy: Group therapy may be effective either alone, in conjunction with individual psychotherapy, and/or medications.

Environmental Change: Anxiety associated with stress may respond well to vacation, change in occupation or residence. Any major and permanent change in the environment is best discussed in advance in a psychotherapeutic session.

ALGORITHM FOR MANAGING ANXIETY

1. Determine if the anxiety is associated with a *general medical condition* (e.g., thyrotoxicosis, hypoglycemia).
   If yes, treat the medical disease. If anxiety is overwhelming during the course of the treatment of the underlying disease, treat the anxiety with *antianxiety agents* (see above) until the underlying disease has been treated successfully. If anxiety persists after successful treatment of the underlying disease, provide *behavioral treatment* (see above) and/or antianxiety agents with at least 6 month follow-ups.

2. Determine if the anxiety is associated with a *transient stressor* (e.g., impending exam).
   If yes, determine if the anxiety is severe enough to interfere with optimal function.
   If it is severe enough, then provide *behavioral treatment* and/or *antianxiety agents* until the stressor and its effects have passed (e.g., the exam is over and the patient passed it; the patient has recovered from acute grief).

3. Determine if the anxiety is part of the symptoms of Acute Stress Disorder or Posttraumatic Stress Disorder following an extraordinary stressor.
   If yes, the patient should be evaluated by a mental health professional and psychotherapy (individual and group) and pharmacotherapy should be coordinated by a psychiatrist.

4. Determine if excessive physiologic activation associated with mild/moderate anxiety of everyday living (e.g., irritable bowel syndrome, hyperventilation syndrome, stress-related hyperacidity) is the main problem.
   If yes, provide specific end-organ directed treatment if available (e.g., antidiarrheal drugs, paper-bag rebreathing technique for hyperventilation, H2 blockers for hyperacidity).

   If the specific end-organ directed treatment is not fully effective, provide *behavioral treatment* and/or *antianxiety agents* in sufficient doses and for an indefinite period as long as there is a recurrence of the excessive physiologic activation when the medication is reduced or stopped.

5. Determine if a specific Anxiety Disorder (see Psychological Dimension, above) is present.
   If yes, a psychiatric referral should be made for specific treatment of the anxiety disorder. The psychiatrist, after evaluation, may collaborate with the primary care physician in treating the patient.

Acknowledgment

The author thanks Trevor Glenn, M.D., Clinical Professor of Psychiatry, University of California, San Francisco, for his valuable feedback and suggestions for this chapter.

REFERENCES

American Psychiatric Association: *Diagnostic and Statistical Manual of Mental Disorders, 4th Edition, Primary Care Version (DSM IV-PC)*, American Psychiatric Association Press, Washington, DC, 1995

Baer L, Rauch SL, Ballantine HT, Martuza R, Cosgrove R, Cassem E, Giriunas I, Manzo PA, Dimino C, Jenike MA: Cingulotomy for intractable obsessive-compulsive disorder.
Arch Gen Psychiatry 52:384-392, 1995

Baer L, Minichiello WE: Behavior therapy for obsessive-compulsive disorder. in Jenike MA, Baer L, Minichiello WE, (eds): *Obsessive-Compulsive Disorders: Theory and Management*, 2nd ed.
St Louis, Mo. Mosby-Year Book, 1990, pp 1117-1126

Baxter, Jr LR, Schwartz JF, Bergman KS, Szuba MP, Guze BH, Mazziotta JC, Alazraki A, Selin CE, Ferng HK, Munford P, Phelps ME: Caudate glucose metabolic rate changes with both drug and behavior therapy for obsessive-compulsive disorder.
Arch Gen Psychiatry 49:681-689, 1992

Leigh H, Feinstein AR, and Reiser MF: The Patient Evaluation Grid: A Systematic Approach to Comprehensive Care.
General Hospital Psychiatry. 2:3-9, 1980.

Leigh H: The Clinical Applications of the Biopsychosocial Model, in Krakowski, AJ and Kimball CP (editors): *Psychosomatic Medicine*
Plenum Publishing Co, New York, 1983, pp. 541-549

Leigh H & Reiser, MF: *The Patient. Biological, Psychological, and Social Dimensions of Medical Practice, 3rd Edition,* Plenum, New York, 1992

Lucki I: Serotonin receptor specificity in anxiety disorders.
J Clin Psychiatry 57 (suppl 6): 5-10, 1996

Paul SM, Marangos PJ, Skolnick P: The benzodiazepine-GABA-chloride ionophore receptor complex: Common site of minor tranquilizer action. Biol Psychiatry 16:213-229, 1981

Schwartz JM, Stoessel PW, Baxter Jr LR, Martin KM, Phelps ME: Systematic changes in cerebral glucose metabolic rate after successful behavior modification treatment of obsessive-compulsive disorder. Arch Gen Psychiatry 53:109-113, 1996

3

BIOPSYCHOSOCIAL APPROACHES TO DEPRESSION

Hoyle Leigh, M.D.[1]

Professor of Psychiatry
University of California, San Francisco, and
Fresno VA Medical Center

INTRODUCTION

Depression is the most common psychiatric syndrome in primary care medicine. With a one year prevalence rate of approximately 5% for major depression, and 5.4% for dysthymic disorder, depressive symptomatology is seen in about 10% (8-18%) of the general population in a one year period (DSM IV-PC, 1995; Gotlib, 1993). The life time risk for major depression is approximately 10-25% in women and 5-12% in men.

The diagnosis of depression is often missed in primary care settings because the patients' presenting symptoms are often somatic (especially pain) and not emotional. In many cultures, depression is experienced as somatic symptoms. In fact, it should be remembered that depression is as much a somatic illness as it is an affective illness.

NATURE OF DEPRESSION

Depression is a psychiatric condition that is at one end of the affective spectrum that includes sadness, being blue, euthymia, feeling happy, euphoria, and ecstasy. The psychiatric condition occupying the other end of the spectrum is mania. As anxiety is a signal of a danger situation, this spectrum of emotions serves as a signal that a loss has taken place or a joyful event has occurred. Sadness and joy are necessary ingredients in personality development and emotional health. Depressive Syndrome (as is the Manic Syndrome), on the other hand, is an abnormal condition caused by a dysregulation of the mood modulation mechanism of the brain that requires medical attention and treatment.

The *catecholamine hypothesis* was one of the earliest theories concerning the brain mechanisms of mood disorders based on the observation that drugs that deplete catecholamines in the brain such as reserpine often cause depression, while drugs that

---

[1]Correspondence: Department of Psychiatry, University of California, San Francisco Fresno Division and Fresno VA Medical Center, 2615 E Clinton Ave, Fresno, CA 93703

Biopsychosocial Approaches in Primary Care: State of the Art and Challenges for the 21st Century, Edited by H. Leigh, Plenum Press, New York, 1997

increase the their functional levels are effective in reversing depression. Later studies found, however, that the brain mechanisms of mood regulation are not that simple. Nevertheless, the final common pathway in the brain for mood dysregulation appears to be affected by the neurotransmitter pathways involving the monoamines (serotonin, norepinephrine, dopamine). Long-term treatment with most antidepressants decrease β-adrenergic receptor density and function, enhances the α_1-adrenergic receptor responsiveness, and decrease the function of presynaptic α_2-adrenergic autoreceptors (McManus, Greenshaw, 1991; Sapena R, Morin D, Zini R et al., 1992; Delgado, Price, Heninger et al., 1992; Miller, Delgado, Salomon et al., 1996). Antidepressant therapy appears to have complex effects on dopamine receptors; mesolimbic dopamine function seems to be enhanced by antidepressant therapy. Enhancement of the serotonergic systems seem to occur with antidepressant therapy, but there is evidence that there may be an abnormality in a neuronal system that remains to be yet discovered, that is highly regulated by the monoamine systems. Corticotropin-releasing hormone and neuropeptide Y are regulated by the monoamines and may be involved in the mechanism of depression. It is hypothesized that corticotropin-releasing hormone and neuropeptide Y may exert a reciprocal regulation of emotional responsiveness, via an interaction of these systems in the amygdala (Miller, Delgado, Salomon et al., 1996; Helig, Kook, Edman et al., 1994).

PATHS TO DEPRESSION

What factors may, then, in combination or sequence, lead to the final common pathway of depression?

Biological Dimension

Genetic factors certainly play an important role (Gershon, 1990). There is a high concordance rate for monozygotic twins than in dizygotic twins, especially for bipolar disorder. The risk of major affective disorder of an offspring of a bipolar parent is about 30%; the risk rises to 74% when both parents have affective illness, with one of them bipolar.

Various medical diseases may cause depression. All endocrinopathies (e.g., hypo- and hyper-thyroidism), metabolic disorders (e.g., diabetes mellitus), many neoplasms (especially visceral cancers), infections (e.g., infectious mononucleosis, HIV), and head trauma may cause various features of the depressive syndrome. Especially of note is the cancer of the tail of the pancreas, in which depression may be the presenting symptom.

Both endogenous and exogenous substances may cause depression either by their presence (e.g., alcohol), excess (e.g., uremia, hypercalcemia), deficiency (e.g., hypoglycemia, pellagra), or withdrawal (e.g., cocaine). It is important to note that the substance causing depression may be a prescribed medication (e.g., reserpine, propranolol, cimetidine, corticosteroids, etc.)

Psychological and Environmental Dimensions

Many patients who develop depression may have a cognitive set of negative views of self, environment, and the future, which is called *Beck's Cognitive Triad* (1979). These patients view themselves as being defective and worthless, the environment as being hostile and unsupportive, and the future as hopeless, offering nothing but failure and frustration. Early adverse experiences may establish these negative concepts (*schemas*) that may be reactivated by life events. Depression, then, would be a result of this faulty thinking (cognition).

Animal studies show that early separation from mothers may result not only in despair in infancy, but long-standing difficulties in adulthood, especially in socialization and sexual activity. Without substitute mothering, such early experiences may predispose an individual to maladaptation in adulthood predisposing to adverse events and depression. Dogs exposed to unavoidable electric shock eventually developed an unwillingness even to attempt to avoid the shock (Seligman, 1967). This *learned helplessness* might also characterize a psychological pathway to depression in humans.

Intrapsychic conflicts over achievement, success, and independence may also predispose some individuals to depression, as well as conflicts over dependency and hostility. A sense of loss is characteristic of depression. The loss may be the real loss of a loved one or possession, or it may be symbolic, anticipatory, or purely intrapsychic (disappointment in a person leading to a loss of love).

Environmental (Social) Dimension

The phenomenology of acute grief following separation and bereavement is very similar to that of depression. Parkes (1972) described *three phases of bereavement*: the phase of numbness, followed by pining, followed in turn by depression. Although the course of normal grief is usually considered to be four to eight weeks, a substantial proportion of the bereaved continue to feel distress up to one or two years after the death of a spouse. Grief is, in fact, a potent stimulus for the development of depressive syndrome. Clayton and her associates showed that 35% of a bereaved population were definitely or probably depressed at one month after bereavement, and 17% at 13 months (Leigh & Reiser, 1992).

Other stressful life events, particularly interpersonal rejection and disappointments or failures often precipitate a depressive episode.

Toxins, excessive noise, and other noxious factors in the physical environment may also contribute to the pathogenesis of depression.

RECOGNITION OF DEPRESSION

How does the primary care physician recognize the presence of depression? If the patient presents with emotional symptoms, such as sadness or feelings of helplessness, the physician would immediately suspect depression. Patients with depression, however, often do not recognize that they are depressed, and do not present with emotional complaints. Instead, they often present to the health care system with somatic symptoms. The somatic symptoms include pain, especially vague and ill-defined pain, discomfort, fatigue, constipation, indigestion, insomnia, weight loss, anorexia, loss of libido, etc. Sometimes, the patient may complain of hypersomnia and/or weight gain. When a patient presents with vague complaints, fatigue, or any of the above symptoms in the absence of apparent physical disease to explain them, the index of suspicion should be raised for depressive syndrome.

Once depressive syndrome is suspected, a careful evaluation should be performed to document whether the patient has a depressive syndrome that warrants pharmacotherapy or partial depressive mood (e.g., sadness) that may respond better to the support of family and friend without medication.

Diagnosing depressive syndrome is somewhat like building a house - it requires a foundation, four (at least two or three) walls, and a roof:

A. The *foundation* is the family history and past history of the patient. Depression is a familial disorder and a recurrent disorder. Positive family and/or past history for depression greatly increases the probability that the patient currently has a depressive syndrome.

B. *Walls*

1. Behavior and Appearance: Sad or apathetic appearance, loss of interest in work, hobbies, and other activities that used to be enjoyable, evidence of self-neglect, agitation or psychomotor retardation, suicidal behavior, giving away possessions (in patients who decided on suicide)

2. Affect and Mood: Does the patient feel sad, blue, down-in-the-dumps? Does he/she feel like crying?

3. Cognition (Thought): Does the patient feel that the future is bleak? Low self-esteem? Thoughts of death or suicide? Difficulty in concentrating? Difficulty in remembering things? Small tasks appear monumental, impossible to achieve? Difficulty in making decisions?

4. Physiologic function (Neurovegetative signs): Symptoms and signs of hypothalamic dysfunction including fatigue, anhedonia (lack of pleasure in activities that used to provide pleasure), loss of appetite (sometimes increase in appetite), weight loss (sometimes gain), insomnia (sometimes hypersomnia), lack of libido, constipation, dry skin, dry mouth

C. *Roof*: Mental Status Examination

The mental status examination systematically documents the current status of the patient's mental state. In depressed patients, it may document unkempt appearance (self neglect), presence of psychomotor retardation, speech may be slow and labored, blunted affect with depressed mood, and content of thought may be characterized by pessimistic and nihilistic thoughts and *suicidal ideation*, the patient may admit delusions that are congruent with the mood (e.g., "My brain is rotting"), and even hallucinations (e.g., "I smell foul odor"). The patient may show a low degree of motivation to do simple tasks (e.g., serial 7's), poor attention and concentration (e.g., digit span, simple calculations), presenting a dementiform picture (*pseudodementia of depression)*.

RECOGNITION AND EVALUATION OF SUICIDALITY

Any patient suspected of having depression should be queried about suicidal ideation specifically and directly. The fear that some interviewers have that they might be suggesting suicide if they ask patients about such thoughts is groundless. The questions might be: Have you had times when you thought you might be better off dead? Any thoughts of harming yourself such as taking an overdose? Any other such thoughts? If you had such thoughts, do you have any plans now? If so, how? Have you ever made plans of suicide in the past? Have you ever attempted suicide in the past? If so, how? Have you ever had thoughts of harming someone else? If so, how?

Approximately 15% of depressed patients ultimately commit suicide. About 45% of persons who committed suicide have a depressive disorder (Leigh & Reiser, 1992). Many people who ultimately commit suicide have recently sought help from a doctor. Seventy percent of depressed persons committing suicide were in touch with a physician within thirty days of their death, and nearly half during the preceding week.

The **risk factors** for suicide include:

1) Psychological Condition: presence of depressive syndrome, suicidal ideation, especially suicidal plans, presence of severe anxiety, agitation, and/or panic, exhaustion

2) Demographic risk factors: male sex; single, divorced, or widowed; living alone; protestant

3) Recent Changes:

A) Behavioral warnings of suicide - seeking help, talking about suicide, giving away possessions, putting personal affairs in order, hoarding drugs, buying weapons, etc.

B) Apparent lifting of depression without cause - this may be a sign that the person has decided on suicide as a solution

C) Losses and failures: job, loved one, etc.

4) Medical Condition: presence of a painful condition or other chronic medical disease

5) Alcohol or other drug use

6) History: previous suicide attempt, history of depression, family history of suicide and/or depression

7) Environment: ready availability of the means of suicide, for example, large quantities of prescribed medication or a rifle hanging in the den

Note: If the patient has definite suicidal plans, or if the patient has definite suicidal ideations and has a high risk (approximately more than three of the above categories positive for high risk), consider hospitalization (see Management below).

DIAGNOSIS OF DEPRESSION

Once the primary physician has recognized a depressive syndrome (even a partial one, but at least with two walls to stand on), the following procedures may be followed for further diagnosis:

1. Is there a medical condition that may cause depression?

All Endocrinopathies
All Metabolic disorders
Infection (esp. viral, or CNS)
Neoplasms (esp. visceral, e.g., pancreas)
Head trauma

If yes, diagnose *Mood Disorder Due to a General Medical Condition (DSM IV Code:293.83 and indicate the medical disease)*
If no, go to 2.

2. Is there a substance that may cause depression?

Substances of abuse (both intoxication and withdrawal)
Prescribed drugs

If yes, diagnose *Substance-Induced Mood Disorder (for DSM IV, look up code for specific substance)*
If no, go to 3.

3. Is the depression a partial depressive syndrome (Not all 4 walls are complete)

If not (complete depressive syndrome), go to 4.
If so (partial depressive syndrome):

(A) Was there the death of a loved one? If so, is the duration of the depression less than 2 months and the depressive syndrome partial?

If so, diagnose *Bereavement* (Not a psychiatric disorder) *(DSM IV:V62.82).*
If not, go to (B).

(B). Is there an identifiable stressor that may have precipitated the depression?

If so, diagnose *Adjustment Disorder with Depressed Mood (DSM IV:309.0)*
If not, has the patient had depressed mood for at least 2 years or longer?
If yes, diagnose *Dysthymic Disorder (Chronic Depression) (DSM IV:300.4)*
If not, diagnose *Depressive Disorder Not Otherwise Specified (DSM IV:311)*

4. Is the depressive syndrome at least of 2 week's duration?

If so, diagnose *Major Depressive Episode*
In addition, does the patient have periods of mania or hypomania (elevated mood, energy, speeded-up thoughts, no need to sleep, etc)?

If so, diagnose *Major Depressive Episode, in Bipolar Disorder (DSM IV: 296.50 if there was mania at any time, i.e.,Bipolar I; 296.89 if only history of hypomania in past, i.e., Bipolar II)*
If not, diagnose *Major Depressive Episode, in Major Depressive (Unipolar) Disorder (DSM IV: 296.30 if recurrent; 296.20 if single episode)*
If not, diagnose *Depressive Disorder Not Otherwise Specified (DSM IV: 311)*

PRINCIPLES OF MANAGEMENT OF DEPRESSION

Once the diagnosis of depression has been made, the physician must decide on a plan of management:

The first decision that has to be made is in the environmental dimension - ***to hospitalize or not.***
Hospitalization may be imperative if the patient is acutely suicidal. Even if the patient may not be acutely suicidal, patients with serious suicidal ideations or plans with high risk factors for suicide should be seriously considered for hospitalization (See below, Environmental Dimension, for further discussion of hospitalization).

If the decision is not to hospitalize the patient, then:

Simple depressive mood or mild partial depressive syndrome associated with an environmental stress (*Adjustment Disorder with Depressed Mood)* may be managed successfully by mobilizing the support of family and friends. This may be done through a discussion with the patient, and/or with the patient's family.

Bereavement is usually time-limited, and social and family support will usually suffice. It has to be kept in mind, however, that a significant proportion of the bereaved develop major depression requiring definitive treatment.

Mood Disorder due to a General Medical Condition should be treated by treating the underlying medical disease, such as hypothyroidism or hyperparathyroidism. If the depressive syndrome persists even after successful treatment of the underlying disease, or if the depression is so severe as to be paralyzing or life-threatening (e.g., suicidal behavior), pharmacotherapy for the depression per se may be indicated as in major depression.

Substance-Induced Mood Disorder is best managed by treating the underlying substance abuse or, in case the substance is a prescribed drug, by switching to a different medication. If the mood disorder persists in spite of successful treatment, a course of pharmacotherapy may be indicated. The primary care physician should be familiar with community resources for the treatment of substance abuse problems and make appropriate referrals.

Dysthymic Disorder is a chronic condition, almost a personality style, that is usually resistant to definitive treatment. If the patient is motivated for treatment, referral to a psychiatrist is indicated. The psychiatrist may choose to treat the patient with chronic administration of an antidepressant. Such maintenance therapy with periodic exam may be undertaken by the primary physician. The primary physician should be aware that many dysthymic patients also develop periods of acute exacerbation, resulting in major depressive episodes. Such episodes respond to specific treatment for major depression, allowing the patient to return to his/her baseline dysthymic state. The primary care physician should also be aware that many dysthymic patients tend to present themselves to the health care system with *chronic multiple somatic symptoms*. Avoiding unnecessary, repeated, and often painful lab tests is an important consideration for such patients.

Major Depression, in Bipolar Disorder, is a highly genetically-determined, highly recurrent disorder with a high incidence of suicide, that often requires hospitalization, and is best treated by a psychiatrist. During the maintenance stage, the primary care physician may be the primary provider with the psychiatrist as a consultant. The biological treatment of Bipolar disorders includes mood stabilizers such as lithium carbonate, valproic acid, and carbamazepine, as well as antidepressant drugs and electroconvulsive therapy (see below). Antidepressant treatment of depression in bipolar disorder may precipitate a manic attack. Therefore the management of both depression and mania in bipolar disorder require very close monitoring and rapid and flexible treatment.

Major Depression, in Major Depressive (Unipolar) Disorder

The primary care physician, often the first physician that a patient with major depressive disorder consults, is in a position to treat such a patient effectively, especially if a psychiatrist is available for consultation when necessary.

As previously discussed, major depression is a final common pathway syndrome whose management requires considerations in all three dimensions of the patient. No medication is effective unless it is taken by the patient. A depressed patient is someone who sees no hope, who feels everything is futile, feels he/she has no energy, and often wishes to die. Such a patient is unlikely to take any drug, especially antidepressant drug because the latter often has uncomfortable side effects, and the antidepressant effect usually does not even appear for at least 2-4 weeks. Careful explanation of the rationale and what to expect from the medication as well as personal encouragement by the prescribing physician is essential even to achieve compliance in an antidepressant drug therapy of the depressed patient.

Involvement of the family is often crucial in the treatment of major depression. In addition to providing encouragement and support, the family may be able to remind the patient when to take the medication, and ensure that he/she does take it. The family may also observe the patient for suicidal behavior, remove potential suicide tools from the environment (e.g., guns), and monitor the progress of therapy.

We shall now discuss specific treatment modalities for the depressive syndrome (major depression) in each dimension.

SPECIFIC TREATMENT MODALITIES FOR THE DEPRESSIVE SYNDROME

A) Biological Dimension

Antidepressant Drugs

Categories of Drugs

Tricyclic Antidepressants (TCA): amitriptyline, nortriptyline, desipramine, etc.
Monoamine Oxidase Inhibitors (MAOI): phenelzine, tranylcypromine, etc.
Serotonin Specific Reuptake Inhibitors (SSRI): fluoxetine, sertraline, paroxetine, etc.
Other newer antidepressants: venlafaxine, nefazadone, etc.

Choice of Drug

The decision as to which antidepressant to use depends to a large extent on the patient's symptoms, the side effect profile of the drug, and the physician's familiarity with the drugs. For example, for a patient with severe insomnia, the sedating side effect of amitriptyline may obviate the need of an additional hypnotic drug. On the other hand, for patients with narrow-angle glaucoma, amitriptyline may be contraindicated because of its anticholinergic side effect.

Because of the relatively benign side-effect profile, serotonin specific reuptake inhibitors (SSRI) are widely used in the primary care setting, followed by tricyclic antidepressants. It should be remembered, however, that SSRI's tend to inhibit the drug-metabolizing liver isoenzyme cytochrome P450IID6 (debrisoquin hydroxylase) and thus elevate the blood levels of other drugs that are metabolized by this isoenzyme. Especially of concern are such drugs that have a narrow therapeutic index, such as flecainide (and other type 1C antiarrhythmics), vinblastine, carbamazepine, and tricyclic antidepressants. Other drugs that may be significantly affected include antipsychotics such as fluphenazine, risperidone, clozapine and quinidine. Co-administration of monoamine oxidase inhibitors with SSRI's is contraindicated. If a patient has been receiving a monoamine oxidase inhibitor, there should be at least two weeks' washout period before commencing an SSRI. At least six weeks should elapse after the last dose of fluoxetine before an MAOI is instituted. Because of multiple interactions with other drugs (especially sympathomimetics) and tyramine-containing foods, monoamine oxidase inhibitors should be used with extreme caution under the supervision of a psychiatrist.

Initiation and Maintenance of Drug

Antidepressant drug therapy in the primary care setting is often ineffective because of 1) inadequate instructions to the patient, 2) insufficient dosing, and/or 3) insufficient length of therapeutic trial. Patients must be instructed to take the antidepressant drug *regularly* (not only when he/she feels depressed), even though the patient will not feel any appreciable change in mood for at least four weeks or longer. The dosing must be built up adequately, especially in using a tricyclic antidepressant. SSRI's tend to be effective at the starting dose level provided the duration of treatment is adequate. The antidepressant effect of antidepressant drugs, as opposed to the side effects such as sedation, is usually not fully manifest until six to eight weeks of therapy. Premature termination in the drug regimen, either by the patient or by the physician for apparent lack of efficacy is therefore a major cause of treatment failure.

[An Algorithm for Antidepressant Therapy for the Primary Care Physician]

1. Is the patient seriously considering suicide, or showing signs of severe psychomotor agitation or retardation? AND/OR

2. Is the patient unable to function in his/her occupation or home because of depression?

    If so, refer the patient to a psychiatrist for possible hospitalization and/or joint management with antidepressant drugs and/or electroconvulsive therapy (ECT).

    If the patient does not meet the above two criteria, the primary care physician might attempt to treat the patient as follows:

3. Which symptoms of Major Depression are most pronounced in the patient?
    If insomnia is not pronounced, then go to A.
    If insomnia is pronounced, then go to B.

A. Serotonin Specific Reuptake Inhibitor (SSRI) Treatment

If anxiety is pronounced, choose sertraline or paroxetine as fluoxetine may exacerbate anxiety and cause insomnia. Treat with sertraline 50 mg or paroxetine 20 mg in AM or HS (depending on whether the patient tends to feel sedated or more alert after taking the drug).

If anxiety is not pronounced, and the patient may have psychomotor retardation, or there is hypersomnia and/or weight gain, choose fluoxetine as it tends to be alerting, reduces drowsiness, and cause weight loss. Treat with fluoxetine 20 mg in AM per day.

Regardless of the specific SSRI chosen:
The patient should be followed at least weekly and instructed to call the physician if significant side effects develop, such as nausea, vomiting, diarrhea, rash, sexual dysfunction, etc. In the absence of significant side effects,
At 4 weeks, if there is some improvement, continue for another 4 weeks.
At 4 weeks, if there is no improvement, double the dose and continue for another 4 weeks.
At end of 8 weeks, if there is still no or little improvement, **go to B, OR**
Change to another SSRI and treat for another 4 weeks.
If at the end of this 4 week period, there is little or no improvement, double the dose and continue for another 4 weeks.
After 4 weeks, if there is little or no improvement, refer to a psychiatrist.
At end of 8 weeks, if there is improvement, go to C.

The following apply to all SSRI's concerning side effects:

If significant side effect occurs, switch to the another SSRI (ie,- from sertraline to paroxetine or from paroxetine to fluoxetine, etc) after one to 3 day's washout (longer washout for switching from fluoxetine to another SSRI). Continue regimen for 4 weeks. Double the dose if insufficient response
and continue for another four weeks. At end of 8 weeks, if there still no or little improvement, go to B.

If significant side effect occurs again with the second SSRI, go to B.

B. Tricyclic Antidepressant Treatment

Amitriptyline: For patients who are over the age of 45, or who have histories or symptoms referable to the cardiovascular system, obtain an EKG before starting therapy. Patients who have narrow-angle glaucoma, urinary retention, known arrhythmias, or hypersensitivity to another tricyclic should not receive amitriptyline. For such patients, consider SSRI, as above, or referral to a psychiatrist with joint management may be indicated.
In the absence of above, or EKG evidence of arrhythmias:

Table 1. Some Commonly Used Antidepressants

Category	Name	Usual Dose/d	Common Side Effects	Approx Half-life
SSRI	Fluoxetine	10-40 mg Typical: 20 mg in AM	anxiety, restlessness headache, insomnia drowsiness, nausea, vomiting, diarrhea, anorexia, sexual dysfunction (delayed ejaculation, anorgasmia)	2-3 days(active metabolite 7-9 d) *strongly inhibits cytochrome P450IID6
SSRI	Sertraline	50-100 mg Typical: 50 mg in AM or HS	nausea, diarrhea, dyspepsia, tremor, dizziness, insomnia, somnolence, male delayed ejaculation	26 hrs *less inhibition of cytochrome P450IID6 than fluoxetine or paroxetine
SSRI	Paroxetine	20-40 mg Typical: 20 mg in AM or HS	asthenia, sweating, nausea, anorexia, somnolence, dizziness, insomnia, tremor, nervousness, delayed ejaculation	21 hrs *moderately inhibits cytochrome P450IID6
TCA	Amitriptyline	75-150 mg	sedation, anticholinergic action, esp blurred vision, constipation, dry mouth, dysuria, paresthesias, orthostatic hypotension quinidine-like cardiac action, weight gain, seizures	24 hrs *metabolized by cytochrome P450IID6

After Physician's Desk Reference and Kaplan, Sadock, & Grebb, 1994

Note: As with SSRI's, patients who are on a regimen of TCA should be seen at least once a week, with instructions to report any significant side effects. Inquire into alcohol use. The sedative effect of amitriptyline is strongly potentiated with alcohol. Warn the patient about driving and/or operating machinery while on amitriptyline. The patient should never drink and drive while on amitriptyline. Further, the patients should be told that certain mild to moderate side effects are to be expected, such as dryness of mouth and blurry vision. They should be cautioned against getting up suddenly from a supine or sitting position as dizziness may occur. It is important for the physician ***not to prescribe a lethal amount*** *of tricyclic antidepressants (usually the patient should not have more than a week's supply) to potentially suicidal patients.*

Start with 25 mg of amitriptyline, HS, and in the absence of rash, severe orthostatic hypotension, dizziness, palpitation, increase by 25 mg HS per day until the patient receives 75 mg HS. If the patient oversleeps with this regimen or too sedated in the morning, administer the medication in divided doses (e.g., 25 mg t.i.d.)

Re-evaluate progress in 4 weeks.
If there seems to be no or little response,
- increase the medication by 25 mg per week until the patient is receiving 150 mg per day. Maintain this dose for another four weeks.

Re-evaluate in 8 weeks of treatment.
- If the patient still shows minimal or no response, refer to a psychiatrist.
- If there is good response, go to C.

C. Antidepressant Drug Maintenance Therapy

The patient should be maintained on the drug regimen that has been effective for at least a symptom-free 6-12 month period. At the end of this period, the antidepressant drug may be tapered gradually (by 5-10 mg of fluoxetine or paroxetine a day per week, or 25 mg of amitriptyline per day per week). Rapid discontinuation of antidepressant drugs may result in withdrawal symptoms such as anxiety, gastrointestinal disturbance, insomnia, and recurrence of depression. If there is a recurrence of depression or withdrawal symptoms, the drug should be increased to the maintenance dose and a more gradual tapering may be attempted after stabilization. For recurrent depression, maintenance for longer periods are indicated (Prien & Kupfer, 1986; Frank et al. 1990).

Electroconvulsive Therapy (ECT)

The primary care physician should be aware that ECT is an important and effective treatment modality for depression, even though the procedure itself should be performed by a psychiatrist with the assistance of an anesthesiologist. Modern ECT is performed while the patient is intravenously anesthetized, with the skeletal muscles relaxed with succinylcholine. Therefore, the patient suffers minimal or no discomfort from the procedure. ECT is usually performed about three times a week, and, on the average, approximately nine ECT's are sufficient for optimal effect. Therefore, a patient may be successfully treated within three weeks of treatment, comparing favorably to the 6-8 weeks necessary for antidepressant drug therapy. The only significant side effect of ECT is transient recent memory loss. The only relative contraindication for ECT is increased intracranial pressure. Before the advent of antidepressants with minimal side effects such as SSRI's, ECT was the treatment of choice for patients with serious medical diseases. ECT still remains a safe and effective treatment modality for seriously ill depressed patients and those patients who have failed a trial of drug therapy.

B) Personal (Psychological) Dimension

As indicated before, nonspecific doctor-patient relationship and caring and concerned examination by the primary care physician, including the mental status examination, and regular follow-up appointments have important psychotherapeutic value. In addition, specific psychotherapeutic modalities are available for depressed patients. For patients who do not require hospitalization, psychotherapy alone or in combination with antidepressant medication may be indicated. Treatment outcomes for depressed patients with high levels of cognitive dysfunction are better treated with medication and cognitive-behavioral therapies than medication alone (Clarkin et al. 1996). Psychotherapy may be an alternative to medication for patients when drug treatment is not suitable or feasible, e.g., during pregnancy, while breast-feeding, before or during major surgery, etc. A combination of pharmacotherapy and maintenance interpersonal therapy (IPT) has been shown to be effective in preventing recurrence in persons with a history of recurrent depression (Frank et al, 1991).

Specific psychotherapies should, in general, be performed by trained mental health professionals. Interested primary care physician may familiarize himself/herself with a manual-assisted psychotherapy such as the interpersonal psychotherapy (IPT). Referral for psychotherapy may be made by the primary care physician if he/she is familiar with the qualifications of the mental health professional (psychiatrist, psychologist, licensed psychiatric social worker, psychiatric nurse practitioner). Otherwise, the referral should be to a psychiatrist, who may, in turn, refer the patient for psychotherapy to an allied mental health professional. A brief discussion of some of the specific therapies follows:

Counseling is effective for mild depressive mood associated with life events and stresses and in normal grief reactions. This modality is geared to providing interpersonal support for the patient, and help him/her cope with the stress or grief.

Cognitive Therapy, developed by Aaron Beck, is brief, usually lasting twelve to sixteen sessions. It postulates that the affective response in depression is a result of the way the patient perceives experience as a result of an emergence of maladaptive cognitive themes. Depressed patients have negative concepts about themselves and their future. The therapy, then, is to identify these false beliefs, and to correct them through rational analysis and home work.

Behavioral Therapy for depression is usually conducted in about twelve sessions. Behavior therapy is based on the notion that a low rate of positive reinforcement may elicit certain aspects of the depressive syndrome. It may be predictable by how the individual behaves in the face of lack of available positive reinforcement as well as negative reinforcing events in the environment. The treatment, then, would be to change the behavior so that there would be an increase in positive reinforcements in the environment. Social skills therapy, assertiveness training, pleasant events therapy (focusing on pleasant and rewarding experiences), and self-control therapy are examples of therapies based on behavioral principles.

Interpersonal Therapy, developed in its current form by Klerman, Weissman, and their colleagues (1984), lasts usually about nine to twelve sessions. It has two fetuses: to reduce depressive symptoms and to deal with the social and interpersonal problems associated with the onset of the symptoms. Using the medical model, the depression is given a name, the patient is given the "sick role", and the need for medication is assessed. Then depression is related to appropriate losses or interpersonal problems, and resolution is attempted through clarification, reassurance, inventory, and other here-and-now directed methods.

Long-Term Psychodynamic Psychotherapy may be useful in patients who have a pattern of putting themselves in situations that result in grief, loss, or stress. It is, in general, not appropriate for acute severe depression.

C) Environmental (Social) Dimension

A major environmental dimension treatment for the depressed patient is ***hospitalization.*** Hospitalization is indicated if a) the patient is a danger to self or others and/or b) the patient is unable to care for self. Definite suicidal plans, or profound psychomotor retardation or agitation are examples of depressive symptoms necessitating hospitalization. *Involuntary hospitalization* may be needed in some seriously depressed patients. State laws differ concerning involuntary hospitalization of psychiatric patients. Primary care physicians should familiarize themselves with state laws about involuntary hospitalization as such psychiatric emergencies do occasionally arise in the primary care setting. Recruiting the support of the family is often essential in patients requiring emergency psychiatric care such as hospitalization.

Hospitalization for depression serves several functions: a) it protects the dangerous patient (from both suicidality and homocidality), b) it ensures appropriate biological dimension treatment (e.g., drugs or ECT), c) it begins to provide the patient with psychotherapy/therapeutic milieu, and d) it begins the process of resocialization of the patient. In this era of managed care, however, hospitalization tends to serve primarily the first two functions of protection and crisis intervention. Outpatient follow-up is therefore crucial for optimal treatment of the hospitalized patient.

Environmental change other than hospitalization may be salutary in several respects. Patients with mild depression associated with environmental stressors may find vacation to be an effective treatment. Change of occupation, residence, or school may be indicated in some patients - usually such major changes are best contemplated with the help of a psychotherapist or counselor. Environmental change to reduce the social isolation of depressed patients, such as support groups or group-living situations might be considered.

Acknowledgment: The author thanks Trevor Glenn, M.D., Clinical Professor of Psychiatry at University of California, San Francisco, for his valuable input and feedback for this chapter.

REFERENCES

Beck AT, Rush AJ, Shaw BF, Emery G: *Cognitive Therapy of Depression*
Guilford, New York, 1979

Clarkin JF, Pilkonis PA, Magruder KM: Psychotherapy of depression: Implications for reform of the health care system
Arch Gen Psychiatry 53:717-723, 1996

Delgado PL, Price LH, Heninger GR, Charney DS: Neurochemistry of affective disorders, in Paykel ES, (Ed) *Handbook of Affective Disorders*, Churchill Livingstone, New York, 1992, pp219-253

Frank E, Kupfer DJ, Perel JM, et al. Three-year outcomes for maintenance therapies in recurrent depression
Arch Gen Psychiatry 47:1093-1099, 1990

Frank E, Kupfer DJ, Wagner EF, McEachran AB, Cornes C: Efficacy of interpersonal psychotherapy as a maintenance treatment of recurrent depression.
Arch Gen Psychiatry 48:1053-1059, 1991

Gershon ES: Genetics, in Goodwin FK, Jamison KR (Editors): *Manic Depressive Illness*
Oxford University Press, New York, 1990, pp373-401

Gotlib IH: Depressive disorders, in Bellack AS, Hensen M, (Editors): *Psychopathology in Adulthood.* Allyn & Bacon, Inc, Boston, 1993, pp 179-194

Helig M, Kook GF, Edoman R, Britton KT: Corticotropin-releasing factor and neuropeptide's role in emotional integration.
Trends Neurol Sci 17:80-85, 1994

Kaplan HI, Sadock BJ, Grebb JA: *Kaplan And Sadock's Synopsis of Psychiatry, Behavioral Sciences, Clinical Psychiatry, 7th Edition*
Williams & Wilkins, Baltimore, 1994

Klerman GL, Weissman MM, Rounsaville BJ, Chevron ES: *Interpersonal Psychotherapy of Depression*
Basic Books, New York, 1984

Leigh H, Reiser MF: *The Patient: Biological, Psychological, and Social Dimensions of Medical Practice, 3rd Edition.*
Plenum Press, New York, 1992 pp 101-144

Miller HL, Delgado PL, Salomon RM, Berman R, Krystal JH, Heninger GR, Charney DS: Clinical and biochemical effects of catecholamine depletion on antidepressant-induced remission of depression.
Arch Gen Psychiatry 53:117-128, 1996

McManus DJ, Greenshaw AJ: Differrential effects of chronic antidepressants in behavioral tests of β-adrenergic and GABA3 receptor function.
Psychopharmacology 103:204-208, 1991

Parkes CM: *Bereavement: Studies of Grief in Adult Life*
International Universities Press, New York, 1972

Prien RF, Kupfer DJ: Continuation drug therapy for major depression episodes: how long should it be maintained? Am J Psychiatry 143:18-23, 1986

Sapena R, Morin D, Zini R, Tillement JP: Evaluation of central adrenergic receptor signal transmission after an antidepressant administration to the rat.
Biochem Pharmacol 44:1067-1072, 1992

4

PSYCHIATRY IN THE PRIMARY CARE SETTING: MANAGING CHRONIC ILLNESS: PSYCHIATRIC ISSUES [1]

Stuart Beck, M.D.

Clinical Instructor in Psychiatry
University of California, San Francisco
Psychiatry Service, San Francisco Veterans Affairs Medical Center

Lowell Tong, M.D.

Assistant Clinical Professor of Psychiatry
Department of Psychiatry, University of California, San Francisco

INTRODUCTION

What makes managing patients with chronic medical illnesses different? The difference is that patients with chronic medical illness are expected to take on an active role in their own health care over an extended period of time, and therefore they have an essentially different relationship with their illness and with their health care clinicians. A patient with an acute illness is expected to be largely passive, talking only to answer the physician's focused questions, and following through compliantly with examinations, procedures, and treatments. More often than not, little concern is given to the impact of the acute medical problem on the rest of the patient's overall life.

In contrast, the chronic illness patient learns about the chronic illness over the course of many years either by instruction or through self motivation. In addition to learning more factual information about the illness, the patient usually has years to learn experientially about the impact of the illness and its treatment on the patient's body and life.

The chronic illness patient is expected to take active responsibility for the ongoing management of the illness: glucose checks, self exams, peritoneal dialysis exchanges, etc. With experience, patients can become more expert than the physician on what works and

Correspondence: Lowell Tong, M.D., Department of Psychiatry, School of Medicine
University of California, San Francisco, 401 Parnassus Road, San Francisco, CA 94143-0984

what doesn't, and may be able to notice changes in their medical status before there are any overt or objective findings. Armed with these abilities, the chronic illness patient can take a more active and beneficial role in their own health care. In order for this to happen, however, primary care clinicians must develop a full repertoire of roles which they can bring to the delivery of care. These roles can include consultant, colleague, adviser, coach, and friend.

The psychiatric consultant may be called by the primary clinician at any time during the course of a chronic illness. From the period before the patient is notified of an illness to the final stages of disease, the psychiatric consultant is in a unique position to help both the patient and the care givers with their situation. The following discussion covers the following: 1) general concepts of chronic illness, 2) specific chronic illnesses, and 3) conclusions. The goal of this chapter is to provide a framework for dealing with chronic illness in the primary care setting.

CONCEPTS

The Doctor-Patient Relationship

The term doctor-patient relationship is meant to include the relationship between the patient, patient's family, and any health care clinicians central to the patient's ongoing care. Two key elements to a good doctor-patient relationship are 1) understanding that there are *stages of a chronic illness* from the patient's perspective and 2) good *communication* between all parties concerned.

Stages of Chronic Illness

There are a number of stages that chronic illness patients may experience, each with its own cognitive and psychological impact.

Pre-diagnosis: Even before a chronic illness develops, patients can be aware of risk through knowledge of genetics or health related behavior like smoking or unprotected sexual activities. In addition to this sort of general awareness of risk level, there are many options for today's patient to assess specific risk of having or developing a chronic illness. HIV antibody testing and genetic testing for neurological disorders or BRCA1 are examples of medical diagnostic advances that can bring profound and swift confirmation or news.

Diagnosis: The diagnosis may present the patient with clarity, crisis, or premonition of course of illness and prognosis. This may be the initial point at which a medical diagnosis or treatment regimen becomes incorporated into a person's sense of identity, in addition to gender, age, occupation, or religion. Person with AIDS or Dialysis Patient: This may be the start of an additional conversion in which a "person" becomes a "patient."

Symptoms: There may be three types of symptom stages, each with its own meaning for the patient. The asymptomatic stage is after diagnosis, when the patient feels little different physically. At some point there are manifestations of first symptoms. Then come progressive symptoms.

Disability: At some point during most chronic illness, the patient becomes disabled. Functional disabilities precede occupational disability. At some point, most patients inevitably must leave work and the physician may additionally become the gatekeeper to long term work disability insurance benefits. A unique situation occurs if neurocognitive symptoms develop, as in a dementing process, since the patient's ability to understand the illness becomes itself impaired.

Treatment: The patient may have little more than periodic contact with clinicians until treatment actually begins. Once treatment starts, however, whether directed towards prophylaxis, attempted cure or against progression, patients become acutely aware of the centrality of illness in their lives.

Terminal: At some point in the progression of chronic illness, the vaguely defined "terminal" phase begins. For some it can be a premonition, for others it is an obvious precipitous change in condition. During this stage, preparation for dying often becomes the central theme.

Communication

Doctors generally overestimate the amount of time that they think they spend with their patients, overestimate how comfortable their patients are asking questions, underestimate the amount of information that patients want, and very frequently interrupt while their patients are talking. In an era of managed care and other forces which push for "efficiency" and high volume patient turnover, it is important to utilize styles of communication which facilitate true efficiency: understanding patients' symptoms and needs, providing enough information for patients to make comfortable decisions and making patients feel understood. Good communication need not mean longer expenditure of time in the long run, since good communication can lead to better patient cooperation and compliance, and improved doctor and patient satisfaction.

Most effective communication styles with patients include:

Open ended questioning: Whenever possible, ask questions which require a qualitative answer, instead of merely a yes-no answer. This facilitates much fuller input from the patient. For instance, the clinician can ask "what kind of pain do you have now?" instead of "do you have any pain now?" A specific form of open-ended questioning method is *reflection*. In the reflection method of inquiry, the patient is asked to reflect on what the clinician has just talked about. Instead of limiting communication to technical data gathering, the clinician should frequently ask for the patient's opinions and understanding about what is unfolding. This is applicable to all phases of the typical patient visit: data gathering, ongoing education and specific treatment instruction phases. As described above, the chronic illness patients have a very long time to become acquainted with their illness, their symptoms, their bodies and effects of treatment. The patients have invaluable information which may go unheard if speaking is not encouraged.

Clear instructions: The more straightforward and streamlined the instructions, the more cooperative and compliant a patient can be. Instead of relying on massive pre-written patient educational and instructional materials, substituting or adding a straightforward, neatly written summary of instructions can be extremely helpful to patients and to those who help them at home.

Reality-based treatment plans: Expect that patients, no matter how well motivated, are still human. Assume that no patient can be perfect, and that there will be at least some level of non-compliance, for reasons ranging from oversight to outright denial. Adjust treatment plans accordingly.

The following example illustrates how switching to a reality based plan led to improved compliance:

A 40 year old male with insulin-requiring diabetes mellitus was unable to abstain from occasional splurges of alcohol, with resultant poor glucose control. Both patient and doctor wanted tight control of the diabetes, since the patient wanted to avoid the serious disabling consequences of his father's poorly controlled diabetes. The treatment plan, suggested by doctor and accepted by patient, included strict caloric intake, steady exercise and abstention from alcohol. The patient had successfully modified his food intake and had started a steady physical exercise regimen. It turned out that the patient and his entire family were serious wine enthusiasts. He would be successful with abstention for many weeks at a time, and then would periodically consume a bottle of wine. After consultation for ideas of how to achieve abstention from alcohol in such a highly motivated patient, it was instead decided to reconfigure insulin doses to allow for, and actually require, a regular regimen of one glass of wine every day. The patient was at first reluctant to try this because his father had been a heavy drinker, but ultimately accepted this plan with the encouragement of his doctor, and glucose control became much more successful, and there were no further "binges" of wine.

Psychological Coping

Chronic illness taxes the most energetic of care givers and committed of patients. The longevity of illness and severity of disease stretch the limits of coping strategies. In chronic illness, coping shifts from immediate problem-solving to dealing with existential issues and problems without solutions. Both the care givers and the patient are equally challenged and require careful evaluation and management by the psychiatric consultant.

Chronic illness brings up the classic existential issues of death, freedom, isolation and meaninglessness. It also raises concerns around disability, self-esteem, dependence, and rejection. In the face of such tremendous problems, psychological defense mechanisms may start to deteriorate or fail altogether. Less mature defenses may begin to appear, and it may become more difficult for the patient to develop new coping options as their illness continues. Whatever the case, the psychiatric consultant is tasked with moving the patient and care givers from pessimism, rigidity, reluctance, and passivity towards optimism, flexibility, resourcefulness, and practicality. Any intervention must improve coping with potential problems beyond the limits of illness itself.

As the care giver enters into a relationship with a patient suffering from a chronic illness, the best provision of care must start with the provider. Care givers need to understand their own assumptions and attitudes about their work, and possess a good understanding of why they do what they do. A self-inventory of capabilities, motivations, strengths and weaknesses is the beginning of an appropriate working alliance and a successful treatment course. It is has been established that doctor's integrity and informed compassion are the most important factors in patient's experiences of care giving and ability to cope with their illness. This requires open-ended communication and self-awareness (Martin, 1995).

Many patients are blamed for not being able to cope well with their illness. It is important to keep in mind that if a patient can not cope, they are not inadequate. They just need help. Mounting frustration is common when cure is not possible, as much for the patient as for their care givers. Attempting to align care behavior with the coping style of the patient can provide the necessary support for the development of more useful and effective coping strategies. It must be remembered, however, that sickness can be a solution for those who have difficulty coping with life in the first place. Change of coping style for these individuals may provoke an increase in psychiatric symptoms and a decreased sense of well-being.

With a clear sense of self, the care giver is then in a position to work effectively with the patient. Before looking at the patient's pathology, begin by paying attention to the patient's positive attributes. These strengths may be the key to successful adaptation and coping strategies. Courage, confidence, loyalty, intelligence, hope, dedication, and generosity are only a few qualities that patients can use to their advantage. Although these desirable qualities may fluctuate over the course of illness and with the stresses of life, any efforts made at recognizing and fostering them are rewarded with improved coping at many different levels.

Coping responses are often spontaneous, as people do what comes naturally to them and what has worked in the past. These efforts will not be enough at times, and there is little correlation between specific illness stressors and success of the strategy employed (Newman, 1993). This means that patients must look carefully at their individual coping mechanisms and their usefulness in coping with the specific aspects of their illness. Easier said than done, this type of examination requires good communication within an open doctor-patient relationship, as previously mentioned.

Just as care givers must cope by redefining the meaning of their relationship with their patients, the patients must redefine their relationship to their illnesses to cope better. The first area to examine with them is social. Clinicians can start by asking patients about their family and significant relationships, their job and financial situation, community, and religion. Casting this broad net may capture areas of vulnerability that will require resources beyond the psychiatric consultant. Social work consultation, family meetings, collaboration with clergy or community organizations may be helpful. Social support and adaptive coping strategies predict fewer depressive episodes (Holahan, 1995).

The next area to examine is medical. When there is uncertainty related to diagnosis, etiology, disease activity, treatment, and prognosis, patients will have greater difficulty coping with their illness. Education, support, and reassurance can go a long way in helping patients deal with chronic illness. Most of the time, patients will ask for this themselves, but if speaking and questioning is not supported, this most straightforward of assistance may be ignored. Clarification and resolution of uncertainty in this area will both assist the patient in figuring out what they need, but also in setting the stage for more active involvement in their care.

The final area to examine is personal. A patient's self-image is severely assaulted by chronic illness. Exploring how they view themselves and their relationship to their illness is critical in understanding how they cope. Although severity of "illness" changes over time, there is worse subjective "disease" with loss of control and less acceptance. Individuals accepting their illness display less guilt, tension, and more endurance. Patients who feel empowered to maintain control and to enhance the quality of life are able to create extensive repertoires of coping skills. Make sure that security, future orientation, and loneliness are evaluated as well. Those who feel able to persevere and want to live an active life show a more positive belief in the future and less indolence (Bredtsen, 1994).

Specific issues to consider during this process of evaluation include healthy denial, power, control, and restoration. Keep in mind that the goal of coping is to provide relief and ultimately a new equilibrium. Patients have to live with chronic illness for a long time, so a solution is not only specific change, but a solution may be learning how to become involved with and effect an ongoing process of change. Endurance is central to the successful management of illness and disease. Do not take away healthy denial without being prepared to create something stronger in its place. Finally, the promotion of empowerment and a sense of well-being in the patient is the most important goal in coping with chronic illness.

Family Systems

Just as physicians generally expect the acute illness patient to be passive and compliant, so do family members expect the patient with the new diagnosis to be "sick". This might include playing the standard sick roles of lying in bed, being catered to, following directions, relieved of routine domestic and occupational routines. At some point in the course of living with a chronic illness patient, however, family members can switch from benevolent care givers to resenters of the patient and the special sick role. This may emerge during a period when the patient has stable symptoms and the family members envy the patient's role which allows for suspension of contributions to normal family life. This also may be the result of family members simply becoming tired of treating the patient as special, assisting with care, and the patient being the focus of attention.

Financial hardship can occur when the patient's income has been a major source of total family income, as well as when care for the patient becomes a drain on family time and financial savings. Careful inquiry into and screening of patient's resources are essential, and a social work referral or consult can be invaluable. Patients and families can also gain much help from support groups, often built around a particular diagnosis. These groups can give not only emotional support, but can be helpful information clearinghouses about resources and practical advice.

Communication between the patient, health care workers and family members cannot always be assumed to be straightforward. Inadvertent carelessness of who has told what to whom, poor previous family communication style, and different "agendas" can all contribute to misinformation or incomplete information. This can lead to suboptimal patient care because of withholding consent, decisions based on irrational fears, or confusion over the treatment plan. Health care professionals need to coordinate their approach to the patient's care, choosing one clinician to be the primary communicator with the patient. Bringing the patient's closest support, whether spouse, partner, family member or friend into the information loop will also optimize good communication.

It is important to remember that the family of the chronic illness patient may not be "traditional" in composition. The extended family is one example, especially in families that have recently immigrated to this country. There may be numerous siblings, children, cousins, parents, aunts, uncles and in-laws involved in family meetings or paying lengthy visits whenever the patient is hospitalized or has a special procedure administered. In these cases, it may be wise to ask the patient and family to choose one or two spokespersons for the larger family, and the health care clinicians can focus their communication with this more manageable number. Other examples of non-traditional families in the medical setting would be common-law spouses, step-children/parents, domestic partners (of any gender combination), significant others, grandparents playing the primary parental role. While legally sanctioned relationships may have a hierarchically important role, for example in the incompetent patient without an advance directive, in general it is prudent to be aware of whom the patient considers to be important or close "family" and not to force only traditional notions of what comprises an authentic family onto to the patient. It is, after all, generally those whom the *patient* defines as family who are the most helpful providers of at-home care and patient support.

Compliance

Compliance is the barometer of the multidimensional structure required for the management of chronic illness. How well a patient can adhere to and cooperate with their treatment plan reveals a great deal about self-efficacy and self-management. Many conflicts can be acted out through noncompliance and overcompliance, and these can include problems with medical judgment, communication, coping, family dynamics, and acceptance.

Better compliance is related to accurate knowledge of the treatment plan, agreement with the prescribed treatment, easy access to care givers, less fear of illness, ability to read and understand information about the illness and treatment, understanding what the care giver has said, and living within a family network (Lorenc, 1993). There are conflicting reports of age as a factor affecting compliance, and this appears to be confounded by which issues related to age are examined. Adequate social support is clearly helpful with compliance, and this may come in the form of extended family, community groups, support groups, educational classes, or friends. Social support has been related to measures of depression and perception of illness, which have a direct bearing on the ability of a patient to be compliant. Compliance patterns are stable over months in patients (Kimmel, 1995).

Noncompliance behavior may be separated into two groups: active and passive. This grouping blurs when patients are passive-aggressive about their treatment. This last category includes a variety of active and passive behaviors intended to rid the patient of the anger and frustration which they cannot easily tolerate. Unlike more straightforward compliance problems, passive-aggressive behaviors require that the care givers do not identify with the projected material, and that the patients assume responsibility for their own feelings. Suffice it to say, this area provides a great challenge for the psychiatric consultant within the matrix of care givers and patient.

Active compliance behaviors include sincere engagement in the management of illness, which is to be supported, and overt choices that the patient makes which undermine the management plans. The patient may be only partially aware of the reasons for their behavior, and it is the task of the psychiatric consultant to help the patient clarify why they are doing what they are doing. It is important to note that patient autonomy must be respected, despite disagreement from other involved parties, as long as the patient is competent to make decisions. Skipping appointments and shortening treatment courses are common and active compliance problems. Because they can be detrimental to the patient's medical status, they must be addressed whenever they come up. Changes in the treatment plan or reconfiguration of treatment goals may need to be considered.

Passive compliance behaviors include benign acceptance of treatment or ignoring treatment recommendations. These as well as active behaviors may not be fully in the patients conscious awareness, and may reflect poor attitudes about the patient, care givers, and the illness. Even when the patient is agreeable to receiving the prescribed care, passive acceptance may reflect a system of denial or minimization which could surface later to the detriment of the patient. Another danger is that passive compliance behaviors may reflect underlying depression, factitious behavior or malingering. Secondary gain may come in the form of resistance to health and medical noncompliance. People may be quite invested in maintaining a level of disease so as to preserve the sick role for themselves. Depression needs to be evaluated and treated if it is contributing to poor compliance with needed care.

Working with compliance problems requires an assessment of objective behaviors and correlation of these behaviors with the issues they reflect. This correlation may be both highly individual and representative of group or family dynamics. Resetting treatment goals from cure to survival and setting personal limits are important. Treating coexisting psychiatric illness will enhance treatment outcome and compliance (Fullwood, 1995). Specific interventions might include behavioral rewards, careful monitoring, and contingency contracting (Koch, 1993).

Sexuality and Body Image

Sexuality is an essential component throughout most normal people's lives, and an important facet to their interpersonal relations. Sexual activity is one important part of sexuality. Chronic illness can directly affect sexuality through dysfunction, pain, alteration or removal of actual sex organs. In addition to these obvious effects, sexuality can be affected indirectly.

Misinformation: Some patients possess the idea that during the course of certain treatments, or even for the duration of a particular illness, sexual activity must be suspended. These patients or their sexual partners may be too embarrassed to mention or ask about this.

Body image: A patient's self image and sense of desirability can be affected greatly merely by being given a serious or chronic illness diagnosis. Actual alterations in skin complexion, weight or hair appearance can contribute further to patients' senses of undesirability through shame, depression, not feeling whole, and assumptions about how others regard them. Amputation or alteration of body parts beyond sex organs, for example amputation of an extremity or even a digit, can have similar effects.

Sexuality issues can affect levels of compliance with medical treatment. Most patients are willing to put up without sexual activity for short periods of time, as in an acute illness, injury or hospitalization. Fatigue and pain almost always affect sexuality through impaired libido and sexual activity. Over time, however, it would be natural for chronically ill patients and their partners to be interested in pursuing an active sexual life again. Ongoing treatments which interfere with sexual functioning are targets for lower compliance rates. These may be medication side effects, such as anorgasmia, dry mucous membranes or erectile dysfunction.

In the following example, important surgery was delayed because of misunderstanding of the patient's sexual needs:

A 55 year old recently divorced male was deemed a good candidate for curative resection of colorectal cancer. He was reluctant to proceed, and in fact missed several routine pre-operative appointments. During his admission for the surgery, he had much ambivalence about the surgery, and delayed signing consent for the procedure. The surgeons and staff assumed that anxiety and perhaps even some cognitive deficits were causes of the ambivalence and delay. A psychiatry consultation revealed that the patient was extremely worried about the anatomical consequences of the surgery. He had once mustered up the courage to inquire about the after effects of the surgery on his sex life. Evidently the surgeon had kindly reassured him that impotence was an unlikely side effect, and the patient had not felt comfortable inquiring further. He had been informed about the likelihood of a colostomy, and had been too embarrassed to ask about whether he would ever again be able to engage in anal intercourse (as recipient), his preferred form of sexual activity with a long time partner. With this additional information, the psychiatrist and the surgeon were then able to engage the patient in a frank discussion about his sexual concerns, and what post-operative reconstructions were possible. The patient consented to surgery without further delay.

Here are some suggestions for a clinician to facilitate a useful discussion about sexuality with patients.

Normalize sexuality and sexual activity as a topic to be discussed candidly like other important topics. For instance, the clinician can lead with the statement that many patients engaged in a particular treatment often experience dry mucous membranes, which can cause thirst, difficulty with contact lenses and uncomfortable sex. Instead of asking "are you having any sexual dysfunction?" the clinician might say, "so many of my diabetes patients have difficulty with erections and feeling sensations in their skin, you must be having at least some of these kinds of problems too?"

Instead of making assumptions about a patient's sexual life, the clinician should ask open ended questions. For instance, instead of limiting questions to male-female vaginal intercourse, the clinician should inquire about what sorts of sexual concerns the patient has, framing the question as though to expect sexual activity beyond male-female vaginal intercourse. While labels of sexual orientation can have some usefulness, the clinician should remember that for many, sexuality is more fluid than marital status and defined sexual orientation may imply.

Even when there are limited remedies to sexual dysfunction from chronic illness and their treatments, inquiry into and conversation about the sexual dimension in the lives on chronic illness patients can make them feel better understood, with more satisfactory doctor-patient relations and improved cooperation with treatment.

Depression and Anxiety

The degree to which the patient loses either physical or psychological function, and through such losses is impaired by illness, depressive symptoms and anxiety of some kind will undoubtedly arise. Chronic illness spreads loss out over many years, making depression a factor to contend with almost for the rest of ones life. Anxiety is a ubiquitous symptoms with many causes, but is another theme that surfaces every time a change occurs in the level of function or medical status of the patient.

There has been much written about depression and anxiety in the medically ill, but chronic illness brings a new dimension to the problem because the illness usually does not go away. To help the patient with depression and anxiety, it is important to develop an understanding of the patient's subjective experience. Diagnostic and Statistical Manual of Mental Disorders (DSM) criteria for depression and anxiety only scratch the surface of the issues, and can lead the psychiatric consultant away from effective interventions. Diagnostic criteria are hard to interpret because of the nature of chronic illness. As stated previously, neurovegetative symptoms are normal in chronic illness and do not necessarily herald major depression. Anxiety states are also part of the normal human response to stress, and chronic illness poses ongoing stresses for a long time. To help with the diagnostic task, the DSM for Primary Clinicians offers wording, definitions and explanations specifically designed for use primary care clinicians.

If a patient does seem to meet criteria for depression or anxiety, then going forward with treatment is indicated. It must be remembered that depressive symptoms do not mean necessarily that a patient has major depression. As the psychiatric consultant considers medications, it is helpful to think about pharmacological agents that address both depression and anxiety. Tricyclic antidepressants also help with anxiety, as do the newer serotonin reuptake inhibitors. Make sure that additional medications in no way complicate the patient's status. Coach care givers in ways to minimize patient anxiety through what they say and how they provide care. Also, discuss ways for depressive symptoms to be acknowledged, monitored, and folded back into the ongoing treatment plan.

If anxiety and depression distort the patient's ability to accept or to cooperate with their treatment plan, then aggressive psychiatric treatment is imperative. If resolution of symptoms does not occur in time for critical medical interventions, then be sure to enlist the support of all involved parties. Beyond this, an ethics consult might prove helpful in sorting out the most appropriate course of action.

Finally, what can the psychiatric consultant do to understand the patient's experience beyond sorting out objective diagnostic criteria? First, look directly at the overlapping areas of depression and anxiety. They are often caused by the threat of death, the most grievous loss one can imagine. Ask directly about the fear of dying. Attempt to ascertain what kind of denial mode they predominantly use to deal with their mortality. Death anxiety can take many forms, and some of the most common concerns are abandonment, uncontrollable pain, and disability.

As the patient starts to talk, listen to how the patient is presenting information. Listen for points in the patient's descriptions where an unobtrusive question might lead to empathic contact. This will open new areas for discussion, but more importantly will give the patient the sense that you are hearing what they have to say about their life, and thereby respect them for who they are. This in itself can help alleviate anxiety and depressive symptoms. Trying to figure out what to say when a patient is feeling depressed or anxious is much less effective than focusing on listening as carefully as possible to what the patient is saying. Genuine compassion and concern are communicated not by speaking, but by hearing.

Cognitive Changes and Competency

Chronic illnesses like diabetes, renal disease, HIV, hypertension, and malignancies can contribute to neurocognitive decline. This can happen both directly and indirectly, for example through neurotoxic mechanisms or through increased risk for stroke and therefore multi-infarct dementia. Memory problems, dementing syndromes and other cognitive dysfunction sequelae pose unique complications for the patient with chronic illness, since the patient's *understanding* of the illness, its treatment and course are affected. Problems with consent, cooperation and compliance can follow.

It is important fairly early on in the course of the chronic illness to educate the patient not only about the basics of the illness and its treatment, but also about any cognitive impairment that is likely to develop. Patients at risk for becoming cognitively impaired need to be advised that they can have some control over how they will be treated at the point of incompetence, through declaring their wishes while still cognitively intact, assigning future decision making powers to someone else, or both.

Patients may complete a "Living Will" or similar document like a Durable Power of Attorney (for health care issues). These documents allow for discussion and document of patient instructions for health care options, and to assign decision making capacity to another person, to take effect when the patient is no longer capable of making reasoned decisions.

Competency is a legal decision, usually following guidelines in State Probate-type codes. The clinical version of competency is the clinical assessment of the patient's ability to make reasoned decisions. In the chronic illness patient population, the question of whether a patient should be "allowed" to die may surface. Often, the question of "incompetence" is related to whether or not the patient is depressed.

The following example illustrates some of the principles to consider in these types of situations:

The patient had multiple chronic medical problems and had been on dialysis for many years. He wanted to stop dialysis in order to die peacefully at home with his family. He sometimes cried when he spoke about this to the dialysis staff, who did not really think that he was depressed, but a consultation was requested as a second opinion. The patient revealed that one major goal of dialysis had been for him to stay alive to see his granddaughter graduate from college, the first member of the family to do so. He had paid a significant portion of her tuition. She had successfully graduated, and he decided that it was now time to end his suffering from debilitating illnesses. He was not in any significant amount of physical pain, but was tired of being "an invalid." His wife and family reported that for several years he had spoken of stopping dialysis after the granddaughter's graduation, and they were saddened by but respectful of his wishes. His outlook on life was realistic; he was able to describe certain pleasurable and satisfying qualities of his life, including the pride of his granddaughter's achievements. He was saddened by the prospect of saying a final good-bye to his family, but knew that they were well taken care of. He had no significant recent change in appetite, sleep, energy or interpersonal engagement. Several factors led to the conclusion that while he certainly had some depressive symptoms (some sadness with tearfulness), he did not have a depressive disorder: he did not have a predominantly depressed mood, his decision was not an impulsive or even recent one, he was not preoccupied with morbid thoughts, he did not feel helpless or hopeless, he had a good sense of self worth and accomplishment over his lifetime, there was no sense of coercion by others including his family members. His was a fully informed decision. It was decided that this patient had the capacity for reasoned decision making, and his family was in agreement with his decision. He spent the next month making preparations for his death, and then stopped dialysis and died at home.

Terminal Phase, Death, and Dying

Health professionals in all settings are there to help those who need care. Although helping a patient through death may seem antithetical to the primary goal of preserving life, caring for a patient during the process of dying can be one of the most profound and important aspects of chronic illness.

People die as they have lived, and health care professionals handle death as they have been trained. Since most physicians have considerable experience with dying patients, a psychiatric consult request most likely reflects a significant problem. A full psychiatric consultation can be invaluable. This must include the usual evaluation, with particular attention paid to reviewing medications, evaluating for depression and delirium, screening cognition, and allowing time for the patient to express themselves. An early assessment of the patients coping style and concepts of death, as well as the attitudes and abilities of the care-givers will help to provide a road map for navigating this last and crucial phase of illness.

If there is concern that the patient is suffering from depression, it is imperative to remember that neurovegetative symptoms are hard to interpret in the face of severe illness. Terminal illness frequently decreases appetite, quality of sleep, libido, energy and interest in pleasurable activities. A normal response to dying may very well include periods of sadness, tearfulness, guilt, rumination, and remorse. The psychiatric consultant, therefore, must be attuned to sustained depressed mood, helplessness, hopelessness, worthlessness, and a sense of being a burden. If there seems to be evidence for major depression, initiating pharmacologic treatment needs to be tempered with quality of life issues. In most cases, major depression should be treated, but not at the cost of a clear sensorium or a stable medical status. Medications should be used if they can provide comfort and help, and definitely not solely because care-givers are having difficulty handling the death of their patient.

Before the terminal phases of illness are reached, an early, frank discussion with the patient and the family is of utmost importance. This discussion should include advance directives, code status, wills, and comfort measures. The patient and the family will also need to know the likely course of the dying process, including information about depression, pain, delirium, confusion, and coma. Having a plan in place will allow care-givers and care-receivers a measure of security and stability during a painful period of pain and loss.

Patients suffering from chronic illness may be forced to confront the reality of their death at any point. It is helpful to bring to mind the classic stages of loss espoused by Elisabeth Kübler-Ross: shock/denial, anger, bargaining, depression and acceptance (Kübler-Ross, 1969). The phases of uncomplicated grief are described in the below (Brown,1983). These stages are not absolute or linear, and may overlap, change order, or mix over the course of a long illness. The psychiatric consultant needs to be careful to distinguish normal grief processes around death from complicated responses. Complicated responses include those where manifestations of grief are absent, are of extreme intensity, are prolonged, develop into major depression, or become distorted. In these situations, the patient and care giving team will need help.

Help may come in the form of the "C's of Cassem": competence, concern, comfort, communication, children, cohesion, cheerfulness, consistency (Cassem). Setting limits with dying patients may be difficult for staff, but they can provide structure and organize an out-of-control situation. The dying patient does not want to be left alone and is generally comfortable talking about death. The importance of religious faith should not be underestimated.

PHASES OF UNCOMPLICATED GRIEF

Phase I	**SHOCK**	denial sense of unreality crying numbness
Phase II	**PREOCCUPATION**	anger sadness insomnia anorexia weakness fatigue dreams anhedonia introversion
Phase III	**RESOLUTION**	recall the past with pleasure regained interest new relationships

[adapted from Brown]

STEPS TO HELPING SURVIVORS

1. Give advance notice
2. Provide privacy
3. Inform as a group
4. Offer chaplaincy
5. Sit with the family
6. Offer appropriate touch
7. Allow for questions
8. Provide for viewing the deceased
9. Consider an anatomical gift
10. Offer an autopsy
11. Know hospital procedures
12. Make appropriate subsequent contact

A 'good' death can mean a great deal to those that remain and sets the model for themselves and can alter their ideas about what life is all about. Effective responses to death can provide increased quality of life for the remaining time a patient might have, decrease the stress on care givers, and reduce the suffering of survivors. With chronic illness, death often brings a sense of relief. This may be difficult for survivors to handle, but it needs to be anticipated and discussed. It is important to remember to offer assistance to family members and care-givers as they may need brief support or access to psychiatric care in the future.

A final issue to consider is euthanasia and assisted suicide. The debate over these areas continues to be polemic and vigorous. For the general psychiatric consultant, making as accurate assessment of the effect that psychiatric disorders has on the patient who wants to die is crucial for further ethical decisions to be made. Euthanasia essentially entails the act of purposely terminating the life of a patient to prevent further suffering. Assisted suicide refers to providing such patients with the means to end their lives with the awareness of the patients intentions to kill themselves (Leigh, 1994). There are no laws currently which protect the physician in participating in these actions. The most crucial distinction for the psychiatrist to make is the degree to which a psychiatric problem such as depression is affecting the patient's decision to end their lives. If depression is prominent, for example, and seems to be affecting decision-making, then treatment of depression would most likely be indicated before allowing the patient to proceed further with willful death.

SPECIFIC CHRONIC ILLNESSES

HIV and AIDS

HIV disease has become an epidemic since the early 1980's. As an epidemic, HIV infection has assumed the mantle of fear, prejudice and concern that great epidemics of the past have created. With new antiviral medications, the life expectancy of HIV infected people has lengthened. This has indeed made HIV disease a chronic illness, but one colored by stigma.

More than one million people in America are infected with HIV, and 1/3 of these people will have neuropsychiatric complications. Vulnerable populations include those who have engaged in homosexual activity, intravenous drug abusers, and those dependent upon blood products. The first two populations have received particularly negative responses from society, and these experiences make the chronic illness of HIV disease more complicated. With the removal of homosexuality from the DSM, there has been a shift in how psychiatrists view their role in the care of homosexual people. There also has been change in how people with substance abuse problems are treated. A historical and sociological accounting must be brought as much to the evaluation of HIV disease as to the interventions that are applied.

The gay male population in particular is an extremely organized cohort of patients. The cohesion of the gay male activism, breadth of support networks and wide-spread education is unprecedented in the arena of chronic illness. This poses two unique issues. The first is that a patient with HIV disease may come to their clinician extremely well-versed in treatment methodology and understanding of disease. They may also bring frustration, anger and resentment related to social issues to the clinical relationship. Many times, they will know about new advances and alternative treatment options before the general clinician does. The second issue is that the patient may not be part of this at all. They may not have availed themselves of the support offered by the gay community for many different reasons. Also, they may not have enough information about HIV disease to cooperate successfully with treatment, monitoring and safe sex practices. Both of the issues need to be anticipated and explored with the HIV patient.

A psychiatric evaluation must include gathering a social and developmental history. Toss out old assumptions of sexual orientation and behavior, drug use and related behaviors, and instead seek to understand each patient within their individual context. Defining the exact nature of support systems and significant others is crucial. Particular attention needs to be given to "coming out" and core sense of self-esteem and self-image, as these issues will resurface with each critical point of disease. HIV disease is a continuum with critical points, each of which may require psychiatric intervention. The critical points include the HIV positive test result, transition from one stage of illness to another, multiple personal and social losses, and disturbances in the support system.

In terms of offering psychiatric assistance to the patient with HIV, it is helpful to consider three basic phases: early, middle and late disease. In early HIV disease, adjustment disorders, depression, anxiety and sleep disturbances can be found. Appropriate interventions might include clarification and interpretation, supporting healthy defenses, offering support groups, and attempting to balance reasonable concern with being overwhelmed and overly preoccupied. If possible, it is prudent to try to avoid psychotropic medications.

Middle HIV disease induces difficulty with adjustment, taking medications, and loss of image as an infected but healthy person. The patient is less able to mobilize denial, handle possible loss of ability to work and be active. Their appearance may change and they may develop major depression. The goals of psychiatric intervention are to facilitate adjustment, to help the patient maintain a positive attitude, and to reframe advancing disease as something other than a personal failure. Antidepressants may be indicated.

Late HIV disease poses more complicated issues. The patient is challenged with coping with severe symptoms, loss of ability to work, loss of ability to care for self, profound decrease in level of functioning, and death. Getting affairs in order, and leave-taking are some of the tasks that need to be addressed. The patient may also suffer from dementia, delirium, and behavioral disturbances. The psychiatric consultant must strive to balance hope with reality of disease, to discuss death and dying, to explore spirituality, and to probe denial very gently. Lower doses of psychotropic medications are generally in order. Benzodiazepines may disinhibit the patient, and the patient may be extra sensitive to antipsychotics. For those patients who do not respond adequately to more traditional antidepressants, psychostimulants may be helpful.

Organic mental disorders include HIV-dementia, secondary affective disturbances or psychosis, and delirium. Symptoms can include memory deficits, concentration impairment, psychomotor changes, motor deficits, apathy, withdrawal, depression, and mania. These entities can be related to primary effects of the virus, neurotoxic products of local CNS responses, indirect consequences of systemic disease, intracranial tumors or infections, and medical treatments. AIDS Dementia Complex (ADC) can produce cognitive, behavioral and motor changes. Cognitive changes can include impaired memory, loss of concentration, and confusion. Behavioral changes can include apathy, social withdrawal, personality change, and organic psychosis. Motor changes can include ataxia, leg weakness, tremor, and loss of fine motor coordination. Patients with HIV may have decreased acuity, slowed mentation, and psychomotor retardation that can resemble depression (Faulstich, 1987).

The psychological problems of anxiety, depression, and suicidal ideation are common. Patients may express anger toward ineffective medical care and perceived public discrimination. They may have guilt about sexual practices or drug abuse. Generally, all HIV patients have reactions to the social isolation and uncertainty of an AIDS diagnosis. Opening up these issues at any phase of the disease can point towards key psychotherapeutic issues, if not effective solutions. Patient activism, community-based support groups and care organizations can provide a great deal relief, satisfaction, and help.

Brief psychotherapy is a viable concept, even while the patient is in the hospital. It requires an active and optimistic stance, rapid assessment of problems, emphasis on "here and now", an interpersonal focus, prompt intervention, and addressing termination. Done well, a brief psychotherapy relationship can help immensely with the common problems of modifying life goals, adjusting to the progression of illness, and bereavement.

A final issue to be aware of is the reaction of the care giving staff. Although it is assumed that medical staff have been trained in the factual information of HIV disease, they may harbor irrational fears, prejudice, or inappropriate assumptions about it. Informal discussions and monitoring the quality of care delivered may provide clues to these issues. If these issues are affecting patient care, then a frank discussion of roles and boundaries can give health providers a chance to get their feelings under better control.

Cancer

Cancer is considered by many to be the most horrific illness that one can suffer. Oncologists regularly encounter difficult emotional situations, and handle them usually without problems. Issues can arise, however, that require the assistance of a psychiatric consultant.

The first issue that may arise is telling that patient their diagnosis. By and large, all patients with cancer should be told the truth. Difficult as this may be, straight talk and simple information is the best route to go. Rehearse what needs to be stated. Be brief, and speak no more than three sentences at a time. Use words like "cancer" instead of "tumor" or "malignancy." Encourage the patient to talk, and reassure continued attention and care. More information and detailed planning for treatment can be reserved for later. Do not forget the beneficial effects of appropriate touch and silence for this first encounter of the patient with their cancer.

Once a patient is told about having cancer, they may display symptoms from any of the phases of grief previously described. One of the differences, however, is that cancer has been felt in the past to be the result of emotional distress or personality attributes. At the same time, it is a disease that cannot be controlled by the patient. Unlike heart disease, COPD, diabetes, etc., patients have no control over their disease. They really can do very little to alter the course of their disease, and they are more dependent upon the physician for survival. This puts added stress on the care givers, and leaves the patient more vulnerable than with other chronic illnesses. The opposing issues of responsibility and helplessness can leave the patient with ambivalent feelings about themselves and their treatment options.

One-quarter to one-half of patients with cancer develop psychiatric syndromes. Depression is the most common, and anxiety is also seen. CNS effects of the tumor or its treatment can bring about mental disorders. The cancer diagnosis and related psychosocial stresses also can contribute to emotional problems. Metastases to the head can occur with primary cancer of the lung, breast, gastrointestinal system, kidneys and prostate. Delirium can be caused by chemotherapeutic agents and any other organic process related to the cancer or treatment.

The dynamic and symbolic concepts of cancer, however, can be equally powerful in developing interventions for cancer patients in crisis. One of these concepts is that of the body turning on itself. This can bring up issues of guilt and self-punishment, as well as feelings that the cancer is deserved retribution for past sins. As such, helping the patient turn the tables can be helpful. Learning to view cancer as the physiological development of cells gone astray can both relieve internal conflict about the reasons for getting cancer and allow for new images of healing to develop. There have been interesting reports about using guided imagery and mental constructs to enhance the efficacy of cancer treatments. It has become accepted that positive thinking and optimism can make a great deal of difference to the long-term success of oncological interventions.

Along with altered internal body image, changes in external appearance also have an effect on the patient battling cancer. When hair and weight loss become evident, a patient may have a harder time maintaining a system of denial. Other people as well will begin to see the patient as "sick". Although this may work to the patient's advantage in allowing them to assume the sick role, it is a time when the patient may need supportive care to realign their coping strategies and to bolster their self-esteem.

Pain is a very common experience for cancer patients. In chronic courses of cancer, inadequate pain control can be a source of great anxiety and fear, as well as a very real detriment to quality of life. It must be emphasized that fears of addiction have no place in the treatment of cancer patients. Only a small percentage of patients will develop addiction problems with the use of narcotic agents, and even if a cancer patient were to develop an addiction, in general this can be handled with less discomfort than if less analgesics were used in the first place. Non-medication strategies to enhance the management of pain should be considered for the chronic patient as well.

Renal Failure and Dialysis

The progressive renal failure patient may have many months or years to ponder the day when dialysis becomes essential to continue life. Anxiety, depression and philosophical questions are common, sometimes related to the especially obviously "artificial" and technologically complex regimen that dialysis will bring.

An example, although somewhat extreme, will illustrate:

A 44 year old male with idiopathic progressive glomerulonephropathy over the course of several years reached the point where dialysis became indicated and recommended. The patient became increasingly dysphoric and anxious, and was extremely ambivalent about starting dialysis. His psychiatric symptoms increased to the point where he expressed suicidal thoughts to his nephrologist of many years, and a psychiatric consultation was requested. He had been a championship body-builder well into his renal failure years, and saw dialysis as admitting to having a weakness of which he was mightily ashamed. He also reported that dialysis was not part of his ethnically based "culture." He was fully informed about dialysis and its indications, benefits, disadvantages, outcomes and alternatives, but did have some distorted ideas about life with dialysis. For instance, he thought that dialysis treatment meant that he could never leave his hometown on travel. He knew that he was being offered a "trial" of dialysis, and that he could always decide to stop dialysis treatment at any time. His response was "why bother to start if you may stop down the road?" The diagnosis of an anxiety-based syndrome was made, and the patient was willing to continue psychotherapeutic interactions but did not want to try medications. Eventually, a reframing from dialysis as a weakness to dialysis as a challenge that required strength of character and discipline helped convince the patient that he should start a dialysis trial. His decision was also facilitated by strong persuasions from family members.

Once *on* dialysis, the patient has unique stressors to contend with for the duration of life: very frequent dialysis treatments or exchanges with the constant reminder of dependency on extremely invasive technology. The dialysis patient must actively engage in a highly artificial procedure multiple times weekly or even daily, depending on the type of dialysis. Additionally, the dialysis patient must take a multitude of daily medications, including some, like antacids which are taken in large quantities, that cause uncomfortable side effects such as constipation, and give no immediate benefit apparent to the patient.

The dialysis patient spends an enormous amount of time over years in close contact with health care clinicians, especially dialysis unit nurses. The psychological "health" of the treatment team is particularly important, since the dialysis patient is often attuned to even the subtlest nuances in behaviors, moods and relations amongst staff.

Rheumatology and Arthritis

Not all chronic illnesses follow the progressive cancer or HIV model with the expected "terminal" phase. Rheumatoid arthritis patients experience different and unique problems as a result of the extremely chronic and rarely directly mortal nature of their disease (Ross, 1990). They have a considerable duration of illness, much longer than other chronic diseases with a distinct "terminal" phase. As a result they often have decades to become particularly experienced and knowledgeable about their disease process and treatment.

They also generally have continued joint degeneration with concomitant pain and disability even with the best care and compliance with treatment. Therefore, the most useful coping style for patient and clinician is to change desires from cure to very long term management of symptoms. Because of poor outcome in most cases, these patients end up putting a higher value on the interpersonal and psychosocial aspects of their care.

Pain and Substance Abuse

In handling chronic pain, the psychiatric consultant needs to rule out hysteria, depression, anxiety, malingering, and psychosis. Once these issues are clarified, appropriate psychiatric treatment can be instituted if firm diagnoses can be made. Most of the time, however, the chronic pain patient has only some of these symptoms, and continues to pose a challenge for their care givers. The management of chronic pain has a rich literature, but the problem of pain and substance abuse is confounding in practice.

For the health provider, giving patients the least amount of narcotic agents is a good rule of thumb. This practice helps to minimize delirium and over-dependence, while encouraging the patient to learn new ways to handle pain. As mentioned previously, however, only a certain percentage of the population are "addicts" and they typically identify themselves early on. Iatrogenic dependence, however, does not an "addict" make. Although the early identification of the abusive dependence of an "addict" is usually fairly easy, health providers are ever vigilant and tend to minimize analgesic use in the majority of their patients. There is evidence that staff tend to withhold powerful analgesics from patients who regard themselves as ill. In other words, patients who complain more tend to get less pain medication. Health providers also tend to give more analgesics to women, and less to the elderly. There is a marked difference in the perception of pain between care giver and patient.

Needless to say, the accurate assessment of pain is difficult and the appropriate treatment of pain is even more so. For the chronic patient, however, the ability to decrease and to control pain are related to better adjustment (Geisser,1994). If the goal of managing pain in chronic illness is to increase well-being, then it makes no sense to make everyone suffer to prevent addiction in a few. It makes better sense to work very closely with the patients, allowing them as much control and choice as possible, so that a pain regimen makes sense to all parties. Giving enough medication to decrease subjective pain in the patients suffering from a chronic illness may provide much needed relief and improve their endurance in the long run. Remember to consider using tricyclics and serotonin reuptake inhibitors as adjunctive agents, particularly if depression or anxiety are prominent features.

CONCLUSION

Psychiatric aspects of chronic illness depend on the unique combination of the patient's life situation, personality, relationships, and coping style. They are affected by the fluctuating course of the specific illness, the treatments, compliance, and level of function. The psychiatric consultant is in a unique position to help both the patient and the care givers with chronic illness. We have attempted to discuss some general concepts of chronic illness and various areas of interest. Our goal has not been to be exhaustive, but instead to highlight particular issues that can be important in dealing with chronic illness.

Chronic illness creates a rich matrix of people and problems into which the consultant is thrown. Almost all of the sections of this chapter are related to the others, reflecting the nature of chronic illness . Examining as many issues as possible around a given individual with a chronic illness will provide the care givers and consultant with an almost endless array of possible options for creating change and maintaining quality of life. This viewpoint is of great value to a situation where chronicity and frustration can many times leave care givers and patient alike seriously beleaguered. The primary care setting is the ideal environment for the development of a new equilibrium for those involved with chronic illness.

REFERENCES

Bendtsen, P., and Hornquist, J.O., 1994, Rheumatoid Arthritis, Coping, and Well-Being, Scandinavian Journal of Social Medicine, 22 (2):97-106.

Brown, T., and Stoudemire, G.A., 1983, Normal and Pathological Grief, Journal of the American Medical Association, 250:378-382.

Cassem, N.H., 1991, *Handbook of General Hospital Psychiatry*, Third Edition, Mosby Year Book.

Cassem, N.H., and Stewart, R.S., 1975, Management and Care of the Dying Patient, International Journal of Psychiatry in Medicine, 6 (½):293-304.

American Psychiatric Association, 1995, *Diagnostic and Statistical Manual of Mental Disorders, Fourth Edition, Primary Care Version,*
American Psychiatric Association, Washington, D.C.

Faulstich, M.E., 1987, Psychiatric Aspects of AIDS,
American Journal of Psychiatry, 144:551-556.

Fullwood, A., Drossman, D.A., 1995, The Relationship of Psychiatric Illness with Gastrointestinal Disease, Annual Review of Medicine, 46:483-96.

Geisser, M.E., et al. 1994, The Coping Strategies Questionnaire and Chronic Pain Adjustment: A Conceptual and Empirical Reanalysis,
Clinical Journal of Pain, 10(2):98-106.

Holahan, C.J., et al. 1995, Social Support, Coping, and Depressive Symptoms in a Late-Middle-Aged Sample of Patients Reporting Cardiac Illness,
Health Psychology, 14(2):152-63.

Kimmel, P.L., et al. 1995, Behavioral Compliance with Dialysis Prescription in Hemodialysis Patients,
Journal of the American Society of Nephrology, 5(10):1826-34.

Kűbler-Ross, E., 1969, *On Death and Dying*, New York: The Macmillan Company.

Koch, D.A., et al. 1993, Behavioral Contracting to Improve Adherence in Patients with Thalassemia, Journal of Pediatric Nursing, 8(2):106-11.

Leigh, H., 1994, *Consultation-Liaison Psychiatry*, New York, Plenum Press.

Lorenc, L., and Branthwaite, A., 1993, Are Older Adults Less Compliant with Prescribed Medication than Younger Adults?, British Journal of Clinical Psychology, 32:485-92.

Martin, S.D., 1995, *Coping with Chronic Illness*, Home Healthcare Nurse, 13(4):50-4.

Mooradian, A.D., Geriatric Sexuality and Chronic Diseases,
Clinics in Geriatric Medicine, 7(1):113-131.

Newman, S.P., and Revenson, T.A., 1993, Coping with Rheumatoid Arthritis, Baillieres Clinical Rheumatology, 7(2):259-80.

Obrien, M.K., et al. 1992, Adherence to Medication Regimens: Updating a Complex Medical Issue, Medical Care Review, 49(4):435-454.

Ross, C.K., et al. 1990, The Role of Expectations and Preferences in Health Care Satisfaction of Patients with Arthritis, Arthritis Care and Research, 3(2):92-98.

Sharps, M., et al. 1994, Why do doctors find some patients difficult to help?,
Quarterly Journal of Medicine, 87(3):187-193.

Yalom, I.D., 1980, *Existential Psychotherapy*, Basic Books.

5

FACTITIOUS PHYSICAL DISORDERS IN THE MANAGED CARE SETTING

Stuart J. Eisendrath, M.D.[1]

Director, Psychiatric Consultation-Liaison Program
Professor of Clinical Psychiatry
University of California, San Francisco

1. INTRODUCTION

Factitious physical disorders are one of the greatest challenges for both primary care physicians and psychiatric consultants (Nordmeyer, 1994). Although factitious disorders may occur with either physical or psychological presentations, the latter is most common in psychiatric settings. This discussion will focus on the conditions most commonly seen in the general medical setting, factitious physical disorders. Patients with these disorders willfully create signs and symptoms of disease. The current DSM-IV criteria are described in Table 1 (American Psychiatric Association, 1994). In some instances, the feigned illness may be a mild one, in others a full-blown medical crisis may be produced.

The financial and social costs associated with these conditions may be enormous. It is critical for managed health care systems to become better at identifying and treating these patients in order to diminish unnecessary drains on limited health care resources. Powell and Boast (1993) have described the "One million dollar man" in a patient with factitious physical disorder (FPD) in England. Feldman (1994) has similarly described the enormous costs that FPD may be associated with. At the University of California, San Francisco one patient with FPD approached one million dollars with her self-induced aplastic anemia (Bright and Eisendrath, unpublished manuscript). Cohen et al. (1985) have discussed the high cost of not identifying and treating psychiatric disorders when they occur in the medical setting. It is clear that FPD warrants full attention in any system where resources are finite and under scrutiny.

---

[1]Correspondence: Department of Psychiatry, School of Medicine, University of California, San Francisco,401 Parnassus Road, San Francisco, CA 94143-0984

Biopsychosocial Approaches in Primary Care: State of the Art and Challenges for the 21st Century, Edited by H. Leigh, Plenum Press, New York, 1997

Table 1

DSM-IV FACTITIOUS DISORDERS CRITERIA[2]

A. Intentional production or feigning of physical or psychological signs or symptoms.

B. The motivation for the behavior is to assume the sick role.

C. External incentives for the behavior (such as economic gain, avoiding legal responsibility, or improving physical well-being, as in Malingering) are absent.

Code based on type:

300.16 With Predominantly Psychological Signs and Symptoms:
If psychological signs and symptoms predominate in the clinical presentation.

300.19 With Predominantly Physical Signs and Symptoms:
If physical signs and symptoms predominate in the clinical presentation.

300.19 With Combined Psychological and Physical Signs and Symptoms:
If both psychological and physical signs and symptoms are present but neither predominates in the clinical presentation.

300.19 Factitious Disorder Not Otherwise Specified

2. HISTORY

Asher drew attention to FPD with his classic paper, "Munchasusen's Syndrome" in the Lancet (1951). This paper and works by others immediately after, described patients who wandered widely, often telling tall tales of medical illness and complications that seemed highly improbable. Asher's use of the term Munchausen was related to the Baron von Munchausen's tales, which are somewhat analogous to the folk stories of American Paul Bunyan (Nickl 1992). These patients often caught their physicians' attention, but with experience, clinicians became aware that the vast majority of factitious patients did not have the Munchausen characteristics of constant wandering, unceasing hospitalizations, sociopathy and impostorship. Reich and Gottfried (1983) estimated that only 10% of FPD patients have the Munchausen features; the majority of patients come from much more stable social systems. These patients often have established family systems, intermittent factitious episodes, and do not wander in their medical travails. Indeed, they often have worked in the health care field, sometimes holding responsible positions such as being the head nurse in a general hospital.

3. EPIDEMIOLOGY

How large is the problem with FPD? The true answer is unknown. In many instances physicians may fail to identify a FPD for a variety of reasons. In some cases, the physician may fail to officially pronounce a patient as having a FPD. For example, identifying a case as factitious may result in a failure of health care insurance coverage for the medical problems associated with the disorder. In other instances, the physician may fail to identify a case as factitious due to fears of litigation or ethical considerations. In summary, the actual numbers of FPD cases is quite difficult to ascertain.

Nonetheless, some epidemiological studies of specific diseases do shed light on the occurrence of FPD. In one study of fever of unknown origin at the National Institutes of Health (Herzberg and Wolff, 1972), 6.5% of cases were factitious. In another study of the same condition, Aduan et al. (1979) found that 9.3% of cases were factitious. In a more recent study, Knockaert et al. (1992) discovered that 3.5% of cases with fever of unknown origin were factitious; this rate was higher than the percentage associated with drug-related fevers and suggested that FPD is a significant clinical problem to be considered. In another area of medicine, Gault et al (1988) reviewed a large number of urinary calculi. That study revealed that 3.5% of the 10,000 stones analyzed were factitious in origin--consisting of nonhuman origin minerals such as quartz and feldspar. Thus this study also suggests that FPD is a real and substantial problem in clinical medicine.

Studies have suggested certain demographic characteristics of FPD patients. Most authors agree that Munchausen patients tend to be predominantly male in a 2:1 ratio. The majority of non-Munchausen FPD cases, however, tend to have females outnumbering males in a 3:1 ratio. The FPD usually develops during the patient's twenties or thirties, but there are often precursors present earlier. For example, some of these patients will have a history of somatic symptoms arising in childhood without clear-cut organic findings. Others will have histories of telling lies during adolescence that were recognized by other family members.

FPD patients generally are not overtly psychotic. In many instances they may not appear to have any apparent psychiatric disorder. With some investigation, however, most patients will have some features of personality disorder evident. Nadelson (1979) has suggested that Borderline Personality Disorder may be particularly common in this population. Partly as a consequence of the personality disorders, these patients often generate significant staff splitting on medical surgical floors. Some staff exhibit tremendous support and nurturance of the FPD patient while others angrily reject them. In some instances, FPD has been considered to have depressive features. Geracioti et al. (1987) have noted that episodes of factitious disorder onset may be associated with a loss. A number of authors have described the beneficial use of antidepressants in FPD (Earle and Folks 1986; Schwartz et al 1993). Still other authors (Spivak et al. 1993) have suggested that FPD may represent an individual who is suffering from an underlying psychosis that threatens the survival of a cohesive psyche. The FPD may then serve as an important organizing structure to prevent personality disorganization.

4. CLINICAL FEATURES

Factitious disorders can be produced at three levels: 1) fictitious; 2) simulation; 3) actual creation. In the first instance, a patient gives a deceitful medical history to a physician that is aimed at producing a false diagnosis. In the second instance, the patient may do things like squeeze a drop of blood into a urine specimen to feign having hematuria. In the third category, patients actually create a pathophysiological disease state by doing things such as injecting themselves with foreign substances or taking medications knowingly in an incorrect manner.

Factitious disorders often do not become diagnosed for several years after they first emerge. Often this is related to the physician's lack of considering the factitious etiology as a possibility. This is understandable since most physicians are biased towards believing their patients. Reich and Gottfried (1983) , in reviewing cases of factitious cellulitis, described an average of six years before the factitious diagnosis was made. In addition to not suspecting a factitious disorder, some physicians may miss the diagnosis because they are not familiar with certain clues to the identification of FPD.

One of the most important clues is that the signs or symptoms fail to respond to the appropriate, and often extensive, medical treatment. For example, an abscess or wound with bacteria that are easily cultured in the laboratory, fails to respond to the sensitivity-proven antibiotics repeatedly. Another hint to the diagnosis of a FPD is that there are a remarkable number of diagnostic tests that are often highly invasive, yet the etiology of the condition remains elusive. It is also noteworthy that the FPD patient is unusually willing to undergo the invasive diagnostic and therapeutic interventions.

A common finding in FPD is that the patient is often able to predict exacerbations of the illness. For example, one patient was able to forecast where her next abdominal abscess would occur before there were any findings on physical examination or gallium scan. In FPD, exacerbations are common immediately prior to hospital discharge. Perhaps the most frequent clue is that the patient has either worked in the health care field or is associated with someone who has (such as a family member). An occupational background as a nurse, ward clerk, medical technician, or medical office assistant may be an important factor that the clinician should consider in formulating a clinically puzzling case (Cramer et al. 1971, Aduan 1979).

The clinical laboratory is often an important diagnostic aid to the clinician. Wallach (1994) has reviewed the many types of abnormality that have been produced factitiously. Individuals are often extremely creative. One patient produced elevated urinary amylase by spitting saliva into his urine. Others have produced chronic diarrhea with hyperosmotic agents (Topazian et al, 1994) and pancytopenia with alkylating agents (Ford et al. 1984). Perhaps the most renowned recent case of FPD was a patient with Goodpasture's syndrome reported twice in the New England Journal of Medicine as the "Red Baron" (Ifudu et al. 1992; Duffy 1992). The laboratory may be the key to making a correct diagnosis of FPD and should be utilized to its fullest extent. For example, C-peptide studies may identify exogenous insulin administration in a patient being evaluated for an insulinoma.

The Munchausen syndrome subset of FPD are often easier to identify than other FPD patients because the histories are more striking. They typically have an unceasing record of moving from one hospital to another. They essentially have no life outside that of being a medically ill patient. They are sociopathic, often lying readily or posing as some grandiose figure. This type of grandiosity led Cramer et al. (1971) to describe these patients as having pseudologia fantastica. In some instances the pseudologia may represent an attempt at wish fulfillment or support for a poor self concept (Ford et al. 1988). In other cases the pseudologia is part of the deception the patient utilizes in at attempt to outwit and "defeat" the physician.

5. DIFFERENTIAL DIAGNOSIS

Perhaps the most critical differential diagnosis to consider in evaluating these patients is a genuine but rare medical disease. In most instances this can be accomplished within a short period of time and often by careful review of past medical records. For example, immune deficiency states can readily be excluded as producing a wound that doesn't heal.

Once a genuine disease has been ruled out, the clinician must consider other forms of abnormal illness-affirming behaviors in the differential diagnosis (Pilowsky 1978). These behaviors include malingering, somatization disorder, conversion disorder, hypochondriasis, and pain associated with psychological features (formerly somatoform pain disorder) (Eisendrath, 1996). These conceptual differences are illustrated in Table Two.

Malingering and FPD differ from the other conditions because the signs and symptoms of disease in these states are believed to be consciously produced. This conscious, or voluntary, production is assumed due to the presence of one or more of several factors described by Overholser (1990) - 1) direct patient admission of fabrication; 2) observation of fabrication; 3) signs or symptoms that contradict laboratory testing; 4) nonphysiological response to treatment; or 5) physical evidence such as finding empty syringes at the bedside. Teasell and Shapiro (1994) suggested that a voluntary component is present when the patient must make decisions regarding timing and concealment that require deliberate thought. For example, a patient feigning paraplegia is observed being able to walk when she believes she is not being watched. FPD differs from malingering in terms of the motivation for the voluntary behavior. In FPD there is no motivation apparent to an outside observer except that the individual wishes to obtain the patient role. In FPD, the motivation is generally regarded as unconscious so that the patient herself is not fully aware of what is driving the behavior. An observer would have to speculate about the presence of some psychological motivation, that is generally considered a *primary gain.* With malingering an outside observer who is aware of the individual's circumstances would be able to decide what motivation is present. Typical motivations include relief from a noxious situation (e.g. imprisonment), monetary rewards (e.g. in litigation), or narcotics. In some cases there may be blurring of the boundary between what is a conscious and unconscious motivation.

6. ETIOLOGY

In many respects factitious behavior can be conceptualized across a spectrum from normalcy to severe dysfunction. At one end lies the normal child or adult who may amplify

Table 2
ABNORMAL ILLNESS-AFFIRMING BEHAVIORS[3]

	SIGNS AND SYMPTOMS	
	PRODUCTION	MOTIVATION
MALINGERING	CONSCIOUS	CONSCIOUS
FACTITIOUS DISORDERS	CONSCIOUS	UNCONSCIOUS
CONVERSION DISORDER SOMATIZATION DISORDER HYPOCHONDRIASIS PAIN ASSOCIATED WITH PSYCHOLOGICAL FACTORS	UNCONSCIOUS	UNCONSCIOUS

[3]After Eisendrath, 1984 and Eisendrath, 1996.

somatic complaints to get a need met on a temporary basis.. This individual achieves some psychological goal but then drops the factitious symptom and resumes a healthy life. A child who occasionally amplifies physical symptoms to get parental attention is a common example.

At the other end of the spectrum lies the Munchausen variant. This individual pursues an unbroken life of patienthood that leaves little time for any other development. There are a number of factors that may lead to the development of FPD. There are predominantly two etiologic theories: the first behavioral and the second psychodynamic. In the behavioral conceptualization, FPD appears to result from learned responses. For example a child who gains his or her parents' attention only when he or she is physically ill, may learn that illness is an essential way to get needs met. This type of reinforcement of the sick role may occur with adults as well.

The other conceptualization of FPD etiology rests upon psychodynamic hypotheses about the motivations of these patients. Perhaps the most frequent motivation that appears to underlie FPD behaviors is the patient attempting to achieve some sense of control. For example, an individual who was traumatized by a medical illness as a child may utilize factitious behavior as an adult in an attempt at restoring a semblance of control.

This feature helps explain how a critically ill FPD patient may appear calm and less worried than the doctors caring for him. He feels more in control of the situation than they do.

Masochism is another important motivation in many FPD patients. They often feel a sense of guilt over various feelings such as anger over past sexual abuse and emotional deprivation. The factitious behavior may then serve to provide a sense of atonement to reduce guilt. This view coincides with many clinicians' suggestions that the factitious behavior may be considered parasuicidal (Menninger 1934, Schoenfel et al., 1987). The factitious behavior may serve as a comparatively minor sacrifice compared to actually killing oneself.

The FPD may symbolically replicate early abuse with physicians and nurses assuming parental roles. Physicians, while attempting to provide good care, may step into providing the patient a sense of abuse being reenacted with invasive diagnostic or therapeutic procedures. The FPD may then provide the patient with the opportunity to express rage over the symbolic abuse as well as the earlier real childhood traumas. The rage is evident in the patient feeling a sense of victory over the duped physician. This is manifest in the patient leaving clues to factitious etiology. For example, one patient with an unusual lymphedema of one leg eventually was diagnosed with FPD when a tourniquet was found at her bedside. This type of discovery was necessary for the patient to demonstrate her triumph. Obviously, such a victory is a pyrrhic one.

In some instances the FPD serves other psychodynamic themes. Geracioti et al (1987) noted that factitious disorder episodes may be activated by a loss. In this conceptualization, the FPD may serve as a way to avoid the sense of loss. The perpetuation of a relationship with a medical caregiver may help the patient avoid confronting a devastating loss directly.

Some authors (Spivak et al., 1994) have suggested FPD behavior may play another role in preserving the self. Although it is rare to see a FPD patient with overt psychosis, some clinicians have found during intensive psychotherapy that the FPD performs a central organizing role. Without the structure of the FPD, the patient feels overwhelmed with chaotic interpersonal relationships (Freyberger et al., 1994). The FPD thus allows the patient to synthesize a stable world.

7. MANAGEMENT

Although physicians have been aware of FPD for centuries (Gavin,1843), Asher's description of the Munchausen syndrome in 1951 really initiated coordinated efforts at treatment. Shortly after Asher's article, Birch (1951) suggested the formation of blacklists to identify Munchausen patients in an attempt to prevent iatrogenic injuries and follow patients. Other physicians (Ifudu, 1992) have also suggested the idea of a registry but ethical and legal considerations have prevented widespread utilization of this approach. It is possible that the onset of managed care with the combination of designated primary physicians and improved data systems will allow for some of the benefits that earlier physicians sought with registries.

7.1 PHARMACOLOGICAL APPROACHES

Various clinicians have utilized medications for some patients with FPD. The earliest report was by Fras and Coughlin (1971). They described the use of a phenothiazine when psychotic thinking developed during psychotherapy with one patient. Similarly, Earle and Folks (1986) have suggested that since many patients with FPD have a borderline personality disorder, they may benefit from brief courses of neuroleptics to treat mini episodes of psychosis. These recommendations are quite comparable to those made by Van Moffaert (1989) in suggesting antipsychotic medications for self-mutilating "cutters".

A number of authors have noted the depressive and self destructive themes present in FPD. Because of this, various clinicians have utilized antidepressant medications for this population (Earle and Folks, 1986; Schwartz, 1993). Clinical experience suggests that when the patient is willing to take such an agent, it is often very effective. Moreover, my clinical experience with these patients suggests that selective serotonin agents may be particularly useful. This may be related to the possibility that FPD patients may fall somewhere on the spectrum of obsessive compulsive disorder. This spectrum includes compulsive behaviors (McElroy et al., 1994) that could be considered to include FPD. Certainly many FPD patients carry out their behaviors in a repetitive and compulsive fashion. Perhaps future studies could clarify the question of how well anti-obsessional agents work in the FPD population. Managed care environments, with continuity of caregivers may be particularly well suited for this type of investigation.

7.2 PSYCHOTHERAPEUTIC APPROACHES

Many patients with FPD are not receptive to the idea of medications for their condition. They are resistant to any attempt to give them a specifically psychotropic medication unless they are already involved in a strong alliance with a psychotherapist. Thus the primary approach to management of FPD requires a psychological intervention. There are two main approaches, the confontational and the nonconfrontational strategies.

After Asher's original article, physicians called for vigorous and occasionally punitive confrontations with the FPD patient. This technique met with little success and placed the physician in an adversarial role with the patient. Because of this, Hollender and Hersh (1970) developed another aspect to the confrontation. They advocated the physician and a consulting psychiatrist conjointly meet with the patient. In the meeting the primary physician would lay out the reasons for diagnosing the disorder as factitious. The behavior would be interpreted as the patient's a "cry for help". The psychiatrist would then offer the patient the opportunity to shift from pursuing medical treatments to more adaptive psychotherapy to understand and change his behavior.

In some instances this approach has been of benefit in enabling the FPD patient to enter psychiatric treatment. Usually this treatment takes place in the form of outpatient psychotherapy. Several authors have described the nuances of therapy with these patients (Hirsch, 1994; Mayo and Haggerty, 1984; Plassman, 1994; Schoenfel, 1987; Tucker et al., 1979). The therapy often utilizes an approach that looks at the patient's behaviors as metaphorical communications. Guziec et al. (1994) suggest to their patients that they shouldn't "let your body do your talking", while encouraging the patients to express their feelings. This approach may be quite useful in helping patients shift their focus from somatic to psychological factors. Unfortunately, the majority of FPD patients are either unwilling or unable to make such a shift. For these patients, nonconfrontational approaches are the treatment of choice.

Nonconfrontational strategies aim at shaping the patients behavior without forcing an acknowledgment that the origin of the problem was factitious. A number of authors have described this type of approach. Yassa (1978) was one of the first to illustrate such a technique in describing a patient in a state hospital type of setting who was treated with an operant conditioning model. The patient was rewarded with social approval for "healthy" behavior and denied hospital privileges for factitious seizures. This program was effective in diminishing the factitious behavior although its setting was obviously atypical for most FPD patients. Klonoff et al. (1983-4) described another behavioral strategy in an outpatient setting. In a patient with factitious seizures, positive reinforcement was given for success in a biofeedback program. The biofeedback was employed as a face-saving mechanism to offer a feasible rationale for why the patient could improve. Without such a mechanism, the patient would have been faced with recovering without any apparent "physical" reason for improvement; such an improvement was considered potentially humiliating since it would be an admission of the psychiatric origin of the problem.

In two patients with factitious paraplegia, Solyom and Solyom (1990) followed a different behavioral approach. After confirming the factitious origins of the patients' disorders, they specifically avoided overtly informing the patients of the origin. This tactic was followed in order to prevent the patients from having to increase their symptoms in order to "prove" the genuine nature of the paraplegia. The staff was given recommendations to positively reinforce healthy behaviors and to ignore maladaptive behaviors. In addition, the Solyoms added a negative reinforcer, faradic massage, for the factitious behavior. Electrodes were applied to the patients' legs to "increase circulation and stimulate nerve endings". The patients were told that if their legs did not respond to this painful treatment that the duration of treatments would be increased daily. Within two days, both patients responded by moving their legs and becoming ambulatory within a week. Once walking, the patients were videotaped in order to prove the ability to walk should either patient suffer an attempt at regression to paraplegia. The Solyoms' technique was effective over a follow-up period of several years.

In a different behavioral approach, Schwartz et al. (1993) treated a patient with factitious cellulitis. This condition had required 235 days in the hospital for the year prior to the intervention. The patient was regarded as having a strong dependency on the hospital so in an innovative maneuver, the patient was given a "permanent" bed on the medical floor with the freedom to enter and leave depending on the patient's own perceived need for inpatient treatment. There was no attempt at confrontation. The medical team encouraged self care with minimal radiology and laboratory testing or consultation. The patient was also given amitriptyline and weekly psychotherapy by one primary care provider. In the first year of treatment, because the hospital charges accrued even when the patient was not in the hospital, the cost of medical care increased 35%. Because of a low hospital census, these charges did not appear to represent a significant actual financial loss. Once the patient was finally discharged, moreover, the patient did not require any hospitalization during a 16 month period of follow-up. By granting the patient a sufficient period of dependency gratification, the patient apparently was able to sustain a prolonged recovery. Eisendrath (1989,1994) has described several behavioral approaches. The central element is to provide the patient a face-saving method to recover without the public admission of the origin of the factitious disorder. In one, the patient is offered self-hypnosis as a face-saving way to heal wounds that have not healed. In one young woman who maintained an abdominal wound for several years, self-hypnosis was provided as a way to improve blood circulation and promote healing. Using this approach, she was able to heal as well as begin discussing several painful emotional issues that she had been too guarded about to discuss without the cover of a medical hypnosis program.

Eisendrath also described the double bind approach to treating FPD (1989). In this technique, the patient is offered two options: one, be told that a full recovery will prove that the medical problem is genuine and not psychiatric; two, be told that less than full recovery means that the origin of the problem is factitious in origin. In essence, the patient is offered the opportunity to respond to medical treatment without having to admit the origin of the problem openly. The double bind also conveys to the patient that the caregiver has an idea of what factitious processes are occurring but does not want to force the patient to be humiliated. This approach often works best when the medical team can offer the patient a minor and harmless intervention that can be couple with the double bind.

For example, one young woman had a leg wound that had not healed despite several courses of antibiotics and skin grafts. After a psychiatric consultant suggested a double bind, the plastic surgeon told the patient that she should respond to the next graft or else it would mean that the problem was factitious in origin. The patient responded by healing the wound for the first time in several years.

Teasell and Shapiro (1994) utilized the double bind approach in helping three patients with factitious motor disorders. They told their patients that the full recovery would indicate an organic etiology and anything less would signify a psychiatric origin. They praised any improvements in functioning and encouraged these with physical and occupational therapies. They also predicted that any worsening prior to discharge would indicate the presence of a psychiatric disorder. This face-saving approach was highly successful improving the functioning of the all three patients.

Eisendrath (1989) has described the use of a specific psychotherapeutic technique with FPD patients. The technique, that of the inexact interpretation, was first described by Glover (1931) for patients in psychoanalysis. In using this approach with a FPD patient, the psychiatric consultant or primary caregiver who is providing psychotherapy, gives the patient an interpretation of the situation that is partially correct. The interpretation stops short of telling the patient that the therapist knows the disorder is factitious. For example, one patient with prominent guilt over any sexual relationship, appeared to be injecting herself in the abdominal wall to produce an abscess whenever she developed an intimate relationship. The psychiatric consultant suggested that whenever she had such a relationship, she might feel a need to hurt herself in some way to diminish her guilt. She responded quite affirmatively to this inexact interpretation. The following day she revealed that she had actually injected her abdomen to punish herself after sleeping with her boyfriend. The inexact interpretation may be useful for those patients who are able to form some psychotherapeutic alliance. As the above case illustrates, not forcing the patient to admit the factitious behavior initially, may allow her to bring forth the behavior's origin herself.

There are limits to the use of nonconfrontational techniques. When a patient is diagnosed with a FPD and the setting is one of medical crisis, there may be little time to implement the nonconfrontational intervention. For example, one woman had been discovered to be injecting herself with a chemotherapy medication to produce aplastic anemia. Because her bone marrow was still not recovering, she was requiring multiple transfusions. Since she was not recovering, she was considered to be potentially still injecting herself in her hospital room. The medical team decided that her situation was so urgent that she had to be confronted and her room searched. The patient was confronted because any delay might have missed finding ongoing causes of her critical condition.

7.3 SYSTEMS INTERVENTIONS

The above interventions are aimed at treating the individual with FPD. Perhaps just as importantly, a psychiatric consultant working with a case of FPD must also help the staff deal with their reactions (Eisendrath and Feder, 1996). In all cases of suspected FPD a psychiatric consultant should be called in as early as possible. It is quite natural for staff to feel anger and a sense of betrayal once a diagnosis of FPD is established. Physicians and nurses come to treat their patients with the belief that the patients are telling them the truth about their illnesses. As part of the contract with the patient, society allows a patient to be in the sick role, presuming they want to get out of it (Parsons, 1951). Patients with FPD operate in the opposite direction. It is important for the psychiatric consultant to help staff ventilate their anger over the factitious diagnosis. If this does not happen, the health care team may act out anger in inappropriate ways such as by prematurely discharging the patient or giving inappropriate medical treatments.

Usually a multidisciplinary meeting is the best place for physicians, nurses, and the psychiatric consultant to discuss a case of FPD. If this meeting can include social workers, ethicists, chaplains, and hospital attorneys, it is even more effective. The psychiatric consultant can help educate staff about FPD and why the patient is producing it. Ethical and legal questions can be discussed. These include questions like 1) can the patient's room be searched without her permission; 2) can the diagnosing physician tell a referring physician about the factitious diagnosis without the patient's permission; 3) should the patient be held on a psychiatric hold as a danger to herself; 4) should the patient be regarded as committing a crime such as fraud and therefore be held financially liable. A number of authors (Ford, in press; Ford and Abernethy, 1981; Sadler, 1987) have attempted to grapple with these complex legal and ethical issues.

8. CONCLUSION

Treating FPD is always a challenge. Yet certain concepts emerge from the work of many clinicians over the years. The patient with FPD is best treated when one physician coordinates all of the patient's medical care. Managed care settings may be in an ideal setting to carry out this foundation for treatment. The primary caregiver can prevent multiple invasive diagnostic procedures and iatrogenic complications. As with patients with other somatoform disorders (Kashner et al., 1992; Smith 1994), regular medical visits decrease the patient's need to invent new somatic complaints. The primary physician should praise and positively reinforce healthy behaviors and reassure the patient that the patient will not be abandoned because they are doing well. The goal of treatment, as well for the minority of FPD patients who enter psychotherapy, is a shift from maladaptive somatic complaints and iatrogenic intrusions, to more adaptive regular medical outpatient visits and/or psychotherapy. Of course, physicians must be alert to the presence of genuine organic diseases developing in patients with FPD and take appropriate steps to diagnose and treat these. As with many other illnesses, the physician should expect that FPD may flare into exacerbations from time to time. Such episodes can be treated supportively and in some instances offer both patient and physician new insights about the functions the FPD plays.

REFERENCES

Aduan RP, Fauci AS, Dale DD, et al. Factitious fever and self induced infection. Ann Intern Med 90:230-242, 1979

American Psychiatric Association: *Diagnostic and Statistical Manual of Mental Disorders, 4th Edition.* Washington, DC, American Psychiatric Association, 1994, p745

Apfelbaum JD, Williams HJ. Factitious simulation of systemic lupus erythematosus. West J Med 160:259-261, 1994

Asher R: Munchausen's syndrome. Lancet 1:339-341, 1951

Birch CA: Munchausen's syndrome. Lancet 1:412, 1951

Cohen LM, Shapiro E, Manson JE, et al. The high cost of treating a psychiatric disorder as a medical/surgical illness. Psychosomatics 26:453-455, 1985

Cramer B, Gershberg MR, Stern M. Munchausen syndrome. Its relationship to malingering, hysteria, and the physician-patient relationship. Arch Gen Psychiatry 24:573-578, 1971

Duffy TP: The Red Baron. N Engl J Med 327:408-411, 1992

Earle JR, Folks DG. Factitious disorder and coexisting depression: a report of successful psychiatric consultation and case management. Gen Hosp Psychiatry 8:448-450, 1986

Eisendrath SJ: Factitious illness: a clarification. Psychosomatics 25:110-117, 1984

Eisendrath SJ. Factitious physical disorders: treatment without confrontation. Psychosomatics 30:383-387, 1989

Eisendrath SJ. Factitious physical disorders, in *The Spectrum of Factitious Disorders*, Edited by Feldman MD, Eisendrath SJ, Washington D.C. American Psychiatric Press, 1996

Eisendrath SJ. Factitious physical disorders. West J Med 160:177-179, 1994

Eisendrath SJ. Factitious disorders and malingering, in *Treatment of Psychiatric Disorders*, 2nd Edition. Edited by Gabbard GO, Washington, D.C., American Psychiatric Press, 1995

Eisendrath SJ, Feder A. Management of factitious physical and psychological disorders, in *The Spectrum of Factitious Disorders*. Edited by Feldman MD, Eisendrath SJ, Washington, D.C. American Psychiatric Press, in press

Feldman MD. The costs of factitious disorders.
Psychosomatics 35:506-507, 1994

Folks DG, Freeman AM 3d. Munchausen's syndrome and other factitious illness.
Psychiatr Clin North Am 8:263-278, 1985

Ford CV. The Munchausen syndrome: a report of four new cases and a review of psychodynamic considerations.
Int J Psychiatry Med 4:31-45, 1973

Ford CV, Abernethy V. Factitious illness: a multidisciplinary consideration of ethical issues. Gen Hosp Psychiatry 3:329-336, 1981

Ford CV. Ethical and legal issues in factitious disorders: An overview, in *The Spectrum of Factitious Disorders,* Edited by Feldman MD, Eisendrath SJ, Washington, DC, American Psychiatric Press, 1996

Ford CV, King BH, Hollender MH. Lies and liars: psychiatric aspects of prevarication.
Am J Psychiatry 145:554-562, 1988

Fras I, Coughlin BE. The treatment of factitious disease.
Psychosomatics 12:117-122, 1971

Freyberger H, Nordmeyer JP, Freyberger HJ, et al. Patients suffering from factitious disorders in the clinico-psychosomatic consultation liaison service: psychodynamic processes, psychotherapeutic initial care and clinicointerdisciplinary cooperation.
Psychother Psychosom 62:108-122, 1994

Gavin H. Feigned and Factitious Diseases. London, J. and A. Churchill, 1843

Gault MH, Campbell NR, Aksu AE. Spurious stones.
Nephron 48:274-279, 1988

Geracioti TD, Van Dyke C, Mueller J, et al. The onset of Munchausen's syndrome. Gen Hosp Psychiatry 9:405-409, 1987

Glover E. Therapeutic effect of inexact interpretation: a contribution to the theory of suggestion. Int J Psychoanal 12:397-411, 1931

Guziec DO, Lazarus A, Harding JJ. Case of a 29-year-old nurse with factitious disorder: the utility of psychiatric intervention on a general medical floor. Gen Hosp Psychiatry 16:47-53, 1994

Herzberg JH, Wolff SM. Chronic factitious fever in puberty and adolescence. A diagnostic challenge to the family physician. Psychiatr Med 3:205-211, 1972

Hirsch M. The body as a transitional object. Psychother Psychosom 62:78-81, 1994

Hollender MD, Hersh SR. Impossible consultation made possible. Arch Gen Psychiatry 23:343-345, 1970

Ifudu O, Kolasinski SL, Friedman EA. Kidney-related Munchausen's syndrome. N Engl J Med 327:388-389, 1992

Kashner TM, Rost K, Smith GR, et al. An analysis of panel data. The impact of a psychiatric consultation letter on the expenditures and outcomes of care for patients with somatization disorder. Medical Care 30:811-821, 1992

Klonoff EA, Youngner SJ, Moore DJ, et al. Chronic factitious illness: a behavioral approach. Int J Psychiatry Med 13:73-83, 1983-4

Knockaert DC, Vanneste LJ, Vanneste SB, et al. Fever of unknown origin in the 1980's. An update of the diagnostic spectrum. Arch Intern Med 152:51-55, 1992

Mayo JP, Haggerty JJ. Long-term therapy of Munchausen syndrome. Am J Psychother 38:571-578, 1984

McElroy SL, Phillips KA, Keck PE Jr.. Obsessive compulsive spectrum disorder. J Clin Psychiatry 55:33-51, 1994

Menninger KA. Polysurgery and polysurgical addiction. Psychoanal Quarterly 3:173-199, 1934

Nadelson T. The Munchausen spectrum: borderline character features. Gen Hosp Psychiatry 1:11-17, 1979

Nickl P. *The Wonderful Travels and Adventures of Baron Munchhausen as Told by Himself in the Company of his Friends, and Washed Down by Many a Good Bottle of Wine.* New York, North-South Books, 1992

Nordmeyer JP. An internist's view of patients with factitious disorders and factitious clinical symptomatology. Psychother Psychosom 62:30-40, 1994

Overholser JC. Differential diagnosis of malingering and factitious disorder with physical symptoms. Behav Sci Law 8:55-65, 1990

Parsons T. *The Social System.* New York, The Free Press of Glencoe, 1951

Pilowsky I. A general classification of abnormal illness behaviours. Br J Med Psychol 51:131-137, 1978

Plassmann R. Inpatient and outpatient long-term psychotherapy of patients suffering from factitious disorders. Psychother Psychosom 62:96-107, 1994

Powell R, Boast N. The Million Dollar Man: resource implications for chronic Munchausen's syndrome. Br J Psychiatry 162:253-256, 1993

Reich P, Gottfried LA. Factitious disorders in a teaching hospital. Ann Intern Med 99:240-247, 1983

Sadler JZ. Ethical and management considerations in factitious illness: one and the same. Gen Hosp Psychiatry 9:31-39, 1987

Schoenfel H, Margolin J, Baum S. Munchausen syndrome as a suicide equivalent: abolition of syndrome by psychotherapy. Am J Psychother 41:604-612, 1987

Schwartz K, Harding R, Harrington D, et al. Hospital management of a patient with intractable factitious disorder. Psychosomatics 34:265-267, 1993

Smith GR: The course of somatization and its effects on utilization of health care resources. Psychosomatics 35:263-267, 1994

Solyom C, Solyom L. A treatment program for functional paraplegia/Munchausen syndrome. J Behav Ther Exp Psychiatry 21:225-230, 1990

Spivak H, Rodin G, Sutherland A. The psychology of factitious disorders: a reconsideration. Psychosomatics 35:25-34, 1994

Teasell RW, Shapiro AP. Strategic-behavioral intervention in the treatment of chronic nonorganic motor disorders. Am J Phys Med Rehabil 73:44-50, 1994

Tucker LE, Hayes JR. Factitial bleeding: successful management with psychotherapy. Dig Dis Sci 24:570-572, 1979

Van Moffaert M. Management of self-mutilation. Psychother Psychosom 51:180-186, 1989

Topazian M, Binder HJ. Brief report: factitious diarrhea detected by measurement of stool osmolality. N Engl J Med 330:1418-1419, 1994

Wallach J. Laboratory diagnosis of factitious disorders. Arch Intern Med 154: 1690-1696, 1994

Yassa R. Munchausen's syndrome: a successfully treated case. Psychosomatics 19:242-243, 1978

6

CHRONIC PAIN

Jon Streltzer, M.D.[1]

Professor of Psychiatry
Department of Psychiatry
University of Hawaii at Manoa

INTRODUCTION

Chronic pain is a clinical condition which is usually described as being multifactorial in origin. A common conception of chronic pain is that there is a physiological basis for the pain followed by a psychological reaction which can cause a "chronic pain syndrome."(1) This syndrome consists of a variety of behaviors, most of which are maladaptive. Treatment then typically takes into account the multifactorial theory of etiology. Physical and medical treatments are designed to address the underlying physiological basis for the pain. For the most part, this involves physical therapies designed to strengthen certain muscles and increase range of motion of joints in areas considered relevant to the individual's specific pains. It is generally believed that increasing strength, range of motion, and general fitness levels will lessen pain, although there is no evidence that the physically fit are less susceptible to developing chronic pain than less fit individuals.

Some theories suggest that chronic pain can be caused by misalignment of bones and other structures and pinching of nerves. This type of theory leads to the use of manipulative treatments such as chiropractic, massage, and passive physical therapies (2).

Other theories of chronic pain suggest that a chronic inflammatory process is occurring in the tissues located where the pain is felt. Anti-inflammatory medication thus becomes the basis for treatment. Rheumatoid arthritis is a clear example of an illness that involves chronic inflammation, for which anti-inflammatory medication is quite helpful. Although this can be a severe condition with a great deal of disability, chronic pain is not likely to become the major problem associated with this condition. Instead joint deformities, limitations of motion, and resulting disability are the major problems. Chronic pain clinics tend not to see these patients where the etiology of their disturbance is quite clear. Sometimes, however, patients are presumed to have a chronic inflammatory process where

---

[1]Correspondence: Department of Psychiatry, John A. Burns School of Medicine, University of Hawaii, Honolulu, Hawaii 96813

Biopsychosocial Approaches in Primary Care: State of the Art and Challenges for the 21st Century, Edited by H. Leigh, Plenum Press, New York, 1997

none can be demonstrated, i.e., myofascitis or fibrositis (3). These patients are likely to have great difficulty with chronic pain.

Many authorities tend to minimize the role of psychological factors in chronic pain. Pain is to be considered an indication of real suffering and taken at face value. While it is noted that pain is a subjective symptom, there is an emphasis on considering it as if it were objective. There have even been proposals to consider a patient's subjective rating of pain as a vital sign comparable to pulse or respiration, signs which can be counted or measured. Pain is thought to be vastly undertreated worldwide.

There has been a great reluctance to attribute etiology to psychological issues. Psychological factors are seen as important, but as complicating chronic pain rather than causing it (1). Chronic pain tends to be interpreted as follows: when the physiologically based pain does not go away, some patients become worn down by the pain. They become irritable and undergo personality changes. They might become dependent on medications or family members, and their dysfunction increases greater than need be on a physiological basis alone. Sensitivity to pain actually increases, leading to a vicious cycle of more pain, a greater reaction to pain and therefore more pain again. Depression is a common complication of chronic pain. Anti-depressant medication is considered good treatment in chronic pain not only because it treats the depression, but because it is thought to have a direct effect on the perception of pain itself (4,5).

Specialized multidisciplinary chronic pain centers have sprung up in numerous places(6). The first step in treatment is generally to eliminate addicting medications, most prominently narcotics and benzodiazepines. Frequently patients resist this and do not accept treatment. Other treatment tends to be nonspecific and multifocal. Multiple techniques for controlling chronic pain are available. In addition to the physical therapies, TENS (transcutaneous electrical nerve stimulation), biofeedback, and various types of manipulative techniques may be used. Antidepressant medication is used very liberally along with anti-inflammatory medication. Determinations about the patient's motivation are often made and used to explain any lack of progress.

From a psychiatric perspective, there has also been much less emphasis in recent years on the idea of psychologically based pain. It is no longer in vogue to consider that physical illnesses have psychological causes. The American Psychiatric Association's diagnostic manual DSM-III (1980) included a clear-cut diagnosis of a pain disorder with a psychological cause, "psychogenic pain disorder."(7) DSM-III-R (1987) removed the implication that there was a known psychological etiology and changed the diagnosis to "somatoform pain disorder."(8) The etiology was still presumed to be psychological, however, since the pain had to be grossly disproportionate to objective findings. DSM-IV (1994) took a further step away by allowing a diagnosis of "pain disorder associated with psychological factors and a general medical condition."(9) This allows the clinician to give a diagnosis more in fitting with the contention that chronic pain is multifactorial.

The diagnosis of a somatoform pain disorder can be a difficult one. There is no single test or series of tests that can measure or categorize chronic pain in such a way as to determine if the etiology is psychological or organic. A common solution to this dilemma is to view chronic pain as always having both psychological and organic features to it. Treatment of all chronic pain cases, therefore, involves both psychological support and medical management based on sound physiological principles. If the patient does not get better with the best efforts at treatment, then we accept that fact and support the patients' ability to cope with their chronic disability. The problem with this approach, however, occurs if indeed psychological factors are the most prominent part of the chronic pain condition. Attempts at medical treatments can lead to iatrogenic complications: failed operations, dependence on medications, and endless physical therapies which reinforce disability rather than improve functioning.

THESIS

Many chronic pain patients have predominantly psychologically based pain disorders whose medical or physiological component is relatively trivial. For these patients, the meaning of the pain and the meaning of treatment are more likely to determine outcome than any specific treatments that are rendered based on a particular etiological theory.

This contention is contrary to some of the trends and opinions described above. It is consistent with clinical practice, however, and with the results of new research.

CASE REPORT

Mr. A is a 41 year old married man with a five year history of chronic pain following an injury at work. He had been employed as a maintenance worker at a hotel for several years prior to his injury. He enjoyed his job a great deal and got along well with his supervisors and co-workers. When he went to work in the morning, he would cheer up his co-workers by making them laugh. He enjoyed the fringe benefits of his job and sometimes stayed at the hotel with his family at greatly reduced prices.

On the date of his injury, Mr. A was checking an outside light. He was on top of the ladder when a strong gust of wind caused him to lose his balance and he fell down landing on a 2-way radio that was strapped to his right hip. He recalled initially being very angry about the pain that he felt, and threw the radio away because he believed that it had caused his pain. He was taken to the emergency room of a nearby hospital where he was described as being in mild distress, and had tenderness in the middle of his low back and in the right hip area. He was diagnosed as having a contusion and was prescribed an anti-inflammatory medication and a mild codeine pain pill. Records from a family physician indicate the patient was seen the next day and complained primarily of a sore shoulder. It was expected the patient would return to work soon. Medical notes document that he did return to work one week later. The medical records revealed that the patient was seen for a checkup three months later and had some low back tenderness. An anti-inflammatory medication was prescribed. Five months after that the patient was seen again with low back pain. A CT scan was done which showed degenerative changes. The patient was given a back brace, and referred to physical therapy.

The patient did not recall this extended period of time when he received minimal medical care. As he reported it five years later, he believed that he saw his physician regularly after the accident, and was going to physical therapy shortly after the accident. Physical therapy appointments involved a long commute after work by bus. He did this three times per week. The therapy never helped, and, in fact, when he was given traction, he believed that it made his pain much worse.

The medical records revealed that after beginning physical therapy, his pain indeed did get worse and he was taken off work briefly. Electromyographic examination (EMG) of the legs was normal. The physical therapy provider was changed. The patient returned to work, but continued to complain that physical therapy caused increased pain. After two months of work with no letup in pain complaints, he was again taken off work in order to have complete bed rest in an attempt to effect improvement. An MRI was performed and revealed degenerative changes with "possible L4-5 disk herniation." The patient was referred for acupuncture. The patient complained that his pain was worsening and he did not want to return to work in that condition.

It was now more than a year since the original injury. A new orthopedic surgeon consulted on the patient and found several nonphysiological findings, including inconsistent areas of tenderness, "give way" weakness of muscle groups of the right leg, and nondermatomal sensory abnormalities. Review of the CT scan and MRI scan indicated unimpressive degenerative changes. A myelogram was recommended to clarify the diagnosis. The myelogram showed only bulging of L4-5 disk which was more significant on the asymptomatic left side than on the right side. A repeat physical exam again showed marked nonphysiologic findings. It was concluded that the patient should not have surgery and that he could return to light duty work.

Following this consultation, the patient reported to his primary care physician that he was somewhat better but had continued pain in the right hip and the right thigh. He was given an injection of a steroid solution in the right sacroiliac joint. The patient reported that he was 50 percent better following that, and wanted to return to work.

The patient did return to work, but again complained that the pain was worsening. He now had weakness in both legs. A repeat MRI was done which revealed spinal stenosis not noted on the initial study. An orthopedic surgeon, however, felt that the repeat of the MRI showed no changes from the initial one. There were no changes in the patient's physical examination. The patient indicated that he was content to continue to working but had received a notice that he was being laid off. This was one and a half years after his initial injury. An EMG was repeated, and was again normal. Another consultation was obtained with a neurosurgeon who confirmed there were no significant positive findings. The imaging studies were again reviewed and were felt to be completely inconsistent with the pain symptoms. He strongly felt the patient should not have surgery, and that the pain should be treated extremely conservatively.

Mr. A was not happy with this neurosurgeon. By this time, he had obtained an attorney to help him with his workers' compensation claim, and the attorney suggested another opinion from a different neurosurgeon. It was now more than three years since the initial injury. The new neurosurgeon elicited complaints of severe low back pain which would radiate to the right leg and to the upper back. There was also pain in the neck and the right side of the head. The patient also reported constant headaches. This neurosurgeon also discovered a history of pain in the right side of his jaw associated with chewing. It was noted that the patient chewed gum daily and was a constant nail biter. On physical exam, the patient had "total body pains," restricted range of motion in the lumbar and cervical spines and marked tenderness of the temporomandibular joint on the right. It was felt that the patient had a chronic lumbar strain and a "very significant temporomandibular disorder." The patient was ordered to stop chewing gum, and to keep to a strictly soft diet. This should result in definite improvement although a dental splint might be needed later. In a follow-up visit two weeks later, the neurosurgeon noted that the headaches had disappeared as well as the upper back and neck pains although the low back pain remained. The doctor concluded that the soft diet had relieved the temporomandibular disorder, resulting in great symptomatic improvement.

In reviewing this history with the patient, the patient noted that he actually had continued to chew his nails because it was a habit, and that he never stopped chewing gum because he wanted his mouth to smell better after smoking cigarettes and drinking coffee. Furthermore, he made no changes in his diet because most of the foods that he ate were fairly soft anyway.

The neurosurgeon referred the patient for another course of physical therapy for the low back pain. Physical therapy again resulted in greatly increased complaints of pain in many areas of the body. The neurosurgeon prescribed diazepam and a narcotic pain pill for the patient. Two and half months after his initial evaluation, this neurosurgeon noted that the pain had now narrowed down to be mostly in the area of the right hip. It was felt that previous physicians may have misinterpreted hip pain as being back pain. Physical therapy was stopped, and referral to an orthopedic surgeon was made to evaluate the hip.

The orthopedic consultant found no abnormality of the hip and the x-rays were normal. The patient complained that his entire right leg felt numb. The impression was chronic low back pain with no specific objective findings. Following this exam, the orthopedic surgeon then reviewed the MRI studies and noted that there was a degenerated disk at L5-S1. The orthopedic surgeon felt that the patient's complaints were consistent with a disk problem at this level. He noted the patient had not been working since the original injury, and, therefore, recommended surgery as offering a possibility to get better. The orthopedic surgeon did not realize that, in fact, the patient had been working most of the time since the injury, until his position was eliminated during financial cutbacks.

The patient was quite anxious about having surgery, but recalled that the orthopedic surgeon was quite confident that it would help him, and so he agreed. Surgery was performed four years after the initial injury. The orthopedic surgeon, in conjunction with the neurosurgeon, removed a degenerated L4-5 disk (not L5-S1), and did an interbody fusion with a bone graft.

On follow-up after surgery, the patient complained of severe pain which was worse than prior to surgery. The orthopedic surgeon indicated it would take a number of months for the bone graft to heal and felt that progress was satisfactory. The patient was angry that the orthopedic surgeon would not prescribe enough pain medication, and so he returned to the neurosurgeon two months after his surgery. He was able to obtain oxycodone and diazepam. After that, the neurosurgeon maintained the patient on narcotic pain medication. The patient was then sent for a new course of physical therapy. Again, the patient complained that physical therapy did not help.

Psychiatric evaluation occurred five years after the original injury and 13 months after surgery. The patient complained that his pain had continued to get worse following surgery. He had throbbing pain across his entire low back and in the whole of both legs. He also experienced a constant sharp pain all day long. He had burning in both feet. He also had constant pain in the back of his neck and in both shoulders. He also had great difficulty sleeping. He complained that his pain ranged from 8 to 10 on a 10 point scale all the time. He walked with the use of a cane.

The patient denied any emotional problems. He had a number of friends and got along well with his wife and three children. He enjoyed helping his children with their homework. He was able to work in his yard a little bit, which he enjoyed. He could take the bus everywhere and would come to town for his medical appointments and physical therapy, which was a one to two hour ride. He took a narcotic pain pill three times a day although he could not tell that it actually helped his pain. He was also given an antidepressant, venlafaxine, which he had taken for over a month. He was unable to tell any effect from the medication other than mild nausea. He also took a sleeping medication, temazepam, but this did not help his sleep.

With regard to background history, Mr. A was a middle child who grew up in a rural community. His father was a maintenance worker and his mother was a part-time dancer. In school, Mr. A had many friends, and was an excellent athlete. He was an average student who only got in trouble once for skipping school to go surfing with a friend. He graduated high school on time and then began working unskilled jobs after that. He had been married almost ten years, and had three children. His wife was a sweet, understanding woman who did not mind the fact that he had back problems. The children were doing well in school and the patient was devoted to them. The patient had never had any difficulty with drug or alcohol abuse.

Mr. A was optimistic about his future. He hoped that his pain would get better but indicated that he expected to be the same in five years. He wanted eventually to go back to fishing and teaching his children that skill. He was looking forward to having his workers' compensation case settled. After that he would not have to go to so many appointments and see so many doctors. Currently he believed that he was obligated to follow through on all medical appointments and recommendations,in order to get his pay (workers' compensation).

DISCUSSION OF THE CASE

The patient fits the DSM-IV diagnosis of Pain Disorder Associated with Both Psychological Factors and a General Medical Condition. No other axis 1 diagnosis seems applicable. Specifically, the patient does not have symptoms of depression, or an anxiety disorder, or a substance abuse disorder. The past history reveals essentially a good psychosocial history with regard to adjustment at work and with his family, and there is no evidence for a personality disorder.

There are clearly medical factors associated with the patient's pain since he had back surgery with a bone graft. It is not clear that medical factors were associated to a great extent with his pain prior to his surgery. The initial injury was considered to be only a contusion when evaluated in the emergency room. No significant objective findings appeared after that, although there was an extensive workup with EMG's, MRI, a CT scan and a myelogram. Nonphysiological findings on physical exam were documented on several occasions. Furthermore, the patient's complaints did not seem to be of much concern and did not affect work, until eight months after the initial injury.

One year following surgery, the patient's complaints also seemed greatly out of proportion. The patient rated his pain as 8 to 10 at all times every day with 10 being defined as the greatest pain imaginable. Furthermore, the patient stated that his pain had been worsening since surgery, although his activity level had greatly improved and he was walking longer distances every day. Furthermore, he was quite facile about taking the bus long distances.

It is striking that the interpretation of the patient's condition varied so much from one physician to another. The focal point of the pain symptoms seemed to shift from one location in the body to another from time to time (for example, from back to hip to back). It was as if the patient picked up cues from the examining physician and responded accordingly, in a manner that confirmed the physician's expectations. This seems most clear with regard to the neurosurgeon who diagnosed temporomandibular syndrome. This neurosurgeon was noted for frequently diagnosing this condition which he believed was often found in chronic back pain patients. Furthermore, this physician's notes indicated he believed that his instructions with regard to diet and gum chewing caused great improvement in the patient's symptoms; in contrast, the patient denied having changed anything at all, and was puzzled by the doctor's great interest in his jaw.

Of interest in the past history is the fact that Mr. A's father had chronic back problems, beginning when the patient was about nine years old. In fact, the father had back surgery twice, which did not improve his condition. The patient noted that his own back problem seemed to be worse than what his father had, however.

No treatment benefitted this patient. If anything, treatment seemed to make him worse. Several courses of physical therapy were attempted, which only increased complaints. Medication was used minimally in the beginning, but, eventually, the patient was using dependency-producing medications several times per day, with no improvement in symptoms. Most troubling, however, was surgical treatment, which greatly increased symptoms and disability. In fact, the patient ultimately settled in to a lifestyle of disability.

The availability of the medical records is critical in understanding this case. History from the patient without knowledge of the medical records would give a very different picture. The patient did not readily describe the fact that his symptoms were minimal for many months following his injury. The patient indicated that his understanding of the various tests that were performed was that they all showed major problems, which explained his pain. From the patient's perspective, he had a major injury which threw everything out of line in his back, pinching nerves, and causing pains in his legs. To a lesser degree this also occurred with his neck. Many trials of physical therapy failed to correct this problem and, ultimately, he was offered surgery. Thus far, surgery had also failed to correct the problem, and, perhaps, has made it worse. The patient had an attorney who was aware that the amount of permanent impairment that occurred following an injury was proportional to the amount of money that would ultimately be received when the compensation case was settled.

DIAGNOSIS OF PSYCHOLOGICALLY BASED CHRONIC PAIN

As the case above illustrates, the diagnosis of a pain disorder with psychological factors is not only possible, but seems readily apparent, when enough facts are known. Furthermore, there is increasing evidence that there are specific associated features which differentiate this type of chronic pain from conditions with a substantial organic basis. We are studying chronic pain patients in order to shed some light on the issues which have been so controversial. In a work in progress, we are comparing injured patients who have developed a somatoform pain disorder (SPD) with a control group of injured subjects(10). In all cases, subjects received extensive evaluations and extensive medical records were available for review.

Compared to the control group, somatoform pain disorder patients had much more treatment of all types but the pain was nonresponsive to all forms of treatment. Pain occurred in multiple sites, and it spread from the site of the original injury. Depression was common in both groups. Antidepressants were extensively used in the pain disorder patients. These were frequently helpful for depression but never for pain. Narcotic and benzodiazepine dependence were quite common in the pain disorder group but were rare in the controls. The pain disorder group was subject to many more tests and surgical procedures. In the pain disorder group, the majority of psychotherapists accepted the patients' pain as physically based, and the treatment was designed to help the patients adjust to their chronic pain.

A litigation/compensation scale was devised and tested for satisfactory reliability. Litigation/compensation was judged to be an important influence on symptoms in about half of the pain disorder cases, a significantly higher percentage than the control group who had equal access to compensation.

Diagnosis of a pain disorder requires not only a detailed medical and psychosocial history and mental status examination, but also an objective review of medical history and diagnostic tests, based on medical record review and/or direct contact with treating physicians. With somatoform pain disorder patients, medical records are typically filled with negative diagnostic evaluations and judgments from consultants that the symptoms are out of proportion to the objective findings.

The patient's description of pains and related symptoms should be explored in detail. The somatoform pain patient almost always describes more than one area of pain and headaches are a frequent concomitant. The description of the pains often have unusual characteristics. For example, the pain may be described as simultaneously sharp and dull. One patient claimed to have a constant "sore-numbness" in several areas of his body. The descriptions can be quite colorful. For example: "The pain is there 24 hours a day. It feels like I am being hit with a baseball bat." Commonly, the pain is described as extremely severe even though the patient does not appear to be in distress and sometimes even seems to be enjoying giving the description. When asked to rate the pain on a 10-point scale, some patients rate it as "10-1/2" or "12" to emphasize the severity. Most patients, however, rate the pain in the 7 to 10-point range, never going away, improving only slightly with treatments and medications and getting worse readily with most types of activity. Particularly striking is the high likelihood that there will be several distinct areas of pain. Also quite striking is the extremely common spread of pain from the original site of injury to new sites.

MEDICATION DEPENDENCE

Medications are frequently used for these patients. A minority of patients do not use any medications. Again, medications at best "take the edge off", but rarely make a substantial difference in the patient's condition. In our series, half of SPD patients were dependent upon narcotics and one-third upon benzodiazepines (10). Chronic pain patients are quite susceptible to narcotic and tranquilizer dependence. Patients sometimes have a long history of alcohol or other substance abuse, but more commonly not at all prior to their chronic pain. Physicians seem to vary greatly in their willingness to prescribe narcotics for chronic pain. Certain physicians tend to collect patients dependent on daily narcotics, while other physicians of the same specialty have them very rarely.

Iatrogenic drug dependence appears to be a real phenomenon and can maintain conditions of chronic pain (11). Patients' doses of narcotics escalate, until they are taking doses several times a day. They find that after taking the dose, they feel better for a little while until the medication wears off. They then take another dose. If they delay too long, they go through a period of irritability and discomfort which is invariably interpreted as increased pain. These patients commonly say that the pain is present all the time and that it is extremely severe but that the pain medications take the edge off and allow them to function. Our experience is that if patients can be detoxified from these medications, they tend to function better, and sometimes their pain improves greatly. At other times, pain complaints continue unchanged, in spite of improved activity and function. Personality changes, which have developed with the chronic pain often improve when the medication is eliminated. In one case, for example, a nurse with chronic pain had been using high doses of narcotic pain medications for several years. When these were eliminated, she complained that her pain, which had been previously rated as 9 to 10 on a 10-point scale, was now much worse. Her husband and her parents, however, expressed great appreciation for her treatment, because her activity level had greatly improved, and her personality had returned to normal, becoming pleasant with a good sense of humor.

DEPRESSION

Many pain disorder patients complain of depressive symptoms. The prevalence of a comorbid depressive disorder in chronic pain patients has been reported to range from 10% to 100% (5). In our study, we found almost half of SPD patients had a DSM-III-R depressive disorder, but this was no different from a control group of injured workers who did not develop SPD (10).

Most patients acknowledge feeling depressed and they attribute this depression to their chronic pain and associated disability. Chronic pain patients often have much to be depressed about, and, furthermore, pain medications may be central nervous system depressant drugs, which can contribute to depression. The diagnosis of a depressive disorder can be difficult, however. Some of these patients maintain an excellent appetite and interest in certain activities. Many of them work intensely, with remarkable concentration on the details of their associated litigation, all the while complaining of great depression. Collateral interviews with family members are often very helpful in the assessment of depression.

Many authors suggest that antidepressants can be helpful in chronic pain conditions (4,5). We have also found this to be the case, although we have never seen them helpful if the patient is also dependent on narcotics and/or benzodiazepines. Some medication-dependent patients like the sedating antidepressants, which can potentiate the effects of narcotics and benzodiazepines. They may claim benefit from their antidepressant even though their symptoms and functioning remain unchanged. Otherwise, antidepressants can be helpful for a depressive disorder that may be present, and they are also excellent antianxiety agents, and can be helpful for sleep. Since they are not addicting, antidepressants are often helpful medications to use as needed for pain complaints. It is impressive, however, that subjective complaints of pain almost never improve in somatoform pain disorder patients as a result of antidepressant medication. This is true even if there is a clinical depression which is effectively relieved.

PHYSICAL THERAPIES

In our study of somatoform pain patients, almost 90% had received physical therapy (10). Frequently, they had received multiple courses of physical therapy, sometimes with different providers utilizing varied techniques. Much of the time these therapies were primarily passive, utilizing such techniques as massage, heat, passive range of motion exercises, stretching and so forth.

We have observed two common responses to physical therapies. One response is typified by the patient who complains that physical therapy is painful and makes him/her worse. The other type of response is that the patient likes physical therapy, eagerly attends and is reluctant to stop. In particular, this type of patient likes massage. He/she describes the physical therapy as providing "temporary relief", although there is no acknowledgment of any sustained improvement in his/her condition. The patient insists that he/she will deteriorate if physical therapy stops. Many of these patients attend physical therapy three times per week. In addition, they may have other doctors' appointments, and possibly chiropractic treatments, to the extent that their rehabilitation is equivalent to a full-time job. Sometimes this can go on for years without any improvement in the patient's overall condition.

A transcutaneous electrical nerve stimulator (TENS) is sometimes prescribed. Some of the pain disorder patients complain that not only does this not help, but it makes their pain worse. Many patients, however, indicate that it is somewhat helpful. They, typically, say that whenever the stimulator stops, however, they are right back in the same place. Some patients wear their stimulators to all doctors' appointments and other public appearances as if it were a badge of disability. Long term follow-up, however, reveals that patients tend to abandon the unit, or use it only occasionally. Sometimes, when physicians are changed, it gets represcribed, and is used again for brief intervals.

RECOMMENDATIONS

1. Consider the diagnosis of a somatoform pain disorder in the patient with chronic benign pain. History from the patient alone is rarely sufficient to make this diagnosis. Access to medical records and contact with treating physicians will be required. First, it must be determined if a medical condition and physiological factors can explain the patient's pain complaints. If this is not clear-cut, there may well be the presence of associated features of a somatoform pain disorder. These will include multiple sites of pain, spread of pain from the initial site of injury, and lack of response to all treatments. The presence of medication dependence is a strong indicator of a pain disorder. Such patients are also likely to interpret common findings, such as the presence of a bulging disk, as indicative of severe pathology. They tend not to be reassured by negative findings on diagnostic studies, and they seem to delight more in positive findings.
2. Do no harm. Surgical procedures do not cure somatoform pain disorders. The lack

of response to conservative management is not an indication for surgery in these patients. Indeed, repeat diagnostic tests, as well as surgery, foster the idea of a chronic disabling condition. They help the patient adopt a role of being sick or permanently impaired.

3. Eliminate dependency producing medications. This may involve detoxification from narcotics, benzodiazepines and/or barbiturates. Since the patient is dependent on physicians for these prescriptions, it is much easier to wean him/her from these drugs than it would be an abuser of illicit drugs (12). Psychologically, however, the patient needs the medication to take whenever his/her complaints escalate. These medications must be benign, and can include small doses of antidepressants, antihistamines or very small doses of major tranquilizers.
4. Focus the treatment on function, not pain. Confronting the patient about nonphysiological findings or negative tests does not make the patient give up symptoms. Unless the patient is malingering, he or she is convinced that he/she has a painful disorder, and is indeed suffering. For whatever reason, the patient seems to need the pain. On the other hand, function can vary greatly among these patients, and encouraging activity, work, volunteer work, and family and social activities can be helpful. Including the spouse in treatment sessions can be particularly useful in this regard.

CONCLUSION

When a medical etiology appears clear-cut and understandable, chronic pain is rarely a difficult problem to manage. Psychologically-based chronic pain is common among chronic pain syndromes, however, and is known as a somatoform pain disorder. This disorder includes multiple sites of pain and nonphysiological findings on exam as well as negative or equivocal diagnostic tests. These patients should not be treated as if they have a chronic medical condition that they must learn to accept and with which they must learn to cope. Such an approach supports their dependency and disability. Rather the emphasis must be on minimizing iatrogenic complications and enhancing function.

REFERENCES

1.American Medical Association: *Guides to the Evaluation of Permanent Impairment, Fourth Edition.* Chicago. 1993. pp. 303-313.

2.Oths K.: Communication in a chiropractic clinic: How a D.C. treats his patients. Culture, Medicine and Psychiatry 18: 83-113, 1994.

3.Rosomoff HL, Fishbain D, Goldberg M, et. al.: Physical findings in patients with chronic intractable benign pain of the back and neck. Pain 37: 279-287, 1989.

4. Hendler H: Depression caused by chronic pain.
Journal of Clinical Psychiatry, 45: 30-36, 1984.

5. King SA, Stoudemire A: Pain Disorders, in Gabbard GO (Ed): *Treatments of Psychiatric Disorders, 2nd ed.*, Washington, D.C.
American Psychiatric Press, Inc., 1995, pp.1755-1782.

6.Aronoff. GM, McAlary PW: Pain centers: Treatment for intractable suffering and disability resulting from chronic pain. In Aronoff, GM (Ed): *Evaluation and Treatment of Chronic Pain. 2nd ed.*, Baltimore: Williams and Wilkins, 1992, pp. 416-429.

7.American Psychiatric Association: *Diagnostic and Statistical Manual of Mental Disorders (Third Edition).* Washington, D.C., 1980.

8.American Psychiatric Association: *Diagnostic and Statistical Manual of Mental Disorders (Third Edition - Revised).* Washington, D.C., 1987.

9.American Psychiatric Association: *Diagnostic and Statistical Manual of Mental Disorders (Fourth Edition).* Washington, D.C., 1994.

10. Streltzer J, Eliashof BA, Kline AE: Associated features of somatoform pain disorder. Psychosomatic Medicine 57:92, 1995.

11. Streltzer J: Chronic pain and addiction, in Leigh H (Ed): *Consultation-Liaison Psychiatry: 1990 and Beyond,* New York: Plenum Press, 1994, pp. 43-51.

12. Streltzer J: Treatment of iatrogenic drug dependence in the general hospital. General Hospital Psychiatry 2:262-266, 1980.

7

BIOPSYCHOSOCIAL APPROACHES TO MENTAL DISORDERS IN THE ELDERLY

Iqbal Ahmed, M.D.[1]

Associate Professor and Director of Residency Training,
Geriatric and General Psychiatry,
Department of Psychiatry, John A. Burns School of Medicine
University of Hawaii and Hawaii State Hospital

Junji Takeshita, M.D.

Assistant Professor and
Assistant Director of Residency Training, Geriatric Psychiatry,
Department of Psychiatry, John A. Burns School of Medicine
University of Hawaii and Hawaii State Hospital

INTRODUCTION

The elderly population is increasing rapidly in all developed countries (WHO, 1992). In the United States the elderly population is about 30 million or 12% of the total population and should increase to over 60 million or 20% of the total population by 2030. Indeed the very old (age 85+) are increasing rapidly and by 2050 should constitute 5% of Americans. Not surprisingly, older Americans have more chronic medical problems with twice the hospitalization rate and use of prescription medications compared to younger individuals. The elderly utilize a disproportionate amount of the health care dollar and are a significant proportion of the patients seen in primary care clinics as well as in the hospitals. The elderly account for one third of health care dollars (US Senate 1987; Fogel et al. 1990).

The elderly are not immune to mental disorders. 12% of the community elderly have a mental disorder (U.S. Senate Special Committee of Aging 1987-1988), with the percentage increasing in the medical hospital setting to about 40-50% (Small et al. 1988). In the

---

[1]Correspondence: Department of Psychiatry, John A. Burns School of Medicine,
University of Hawaii, Hawaii State Hospital,45-710 Keaahala Rd, Kaneohe, HI 96744

Biopsychosocial Approaches in Primary Care: State of the Art and Challenges for the 21st Century, Edited by H. Leigh, Plenum Press, New York, 1997

nursing home population the rate of mental illness may be as high as 80% (Rovner et al. 1990). Cognitive disorders are particularly common in the elderly compared with younger counterparts. Most elderly with psychiatric disorders are not seen in the mental health sector, but in the medical sector by primary care physicians (Goldstrum 1987; Yates 1986). This might be both due to lack of recognition of mental disorders by the elderly and their caregivers, reluctance to seek mental help due to cultural and age dependent attitudes and stigma toward mental illness and possibly an increased tendency to somatize. Therefore the recognition and treatment of mental disorders in the elderly in the medical setting by both primary care providers and consultation-liaison psychiatrists becomes particularly important. While detection and management of mental disorders in the elderly by primary care providers has been reported to be a problem, with appropriate education this could be rectified (German et al. 1987).

1. EPIDEMIOLOGY

Studies of the community incidence of psychiatric disorders indicate that the incidence of "functional psychiatric disorders" is probably either no different or about the same as in the non-elderly (Oxman 1987; Regier 1988). However, there appears to be a greater incidence of the "organic disorders" such as dementia, delirium, and disorders secondary to general medical conditions. This is especially so in medical populations (Rapp 1988; Small 1988). There are also unique social and developmental issues for the elderly which underscores the need to have a "biopsychosocial" understanding of the psychiatric disorders of the elderly.

1.1 Dementia

Although only 1% of 60-64 year old individuals have dementia, 30-40% are affected among those 85+. The rate of dementia shows a drastic increase, doubling every 5 years beginning at age 60. (Jorm et al. 1987) Although two-thirds of nursing home residents have dementia, only a minority of demented patients are cared for in a nursing home. Two to three individuals continue to reside in the community for every one in a nursing home (Katzman and Terry 1983).

1.2 Mood Disorders

Depressive symptoms are noted in about 10-15% of the community elderly although major depression is less than 1% (Blazer and Williams 1980). The incidence of depressive symptoms in outpatient medical clinics may be as high as 30-50% and 25% in nursing homes and other institutions (Katz et al. 1988). Coexisting depression is particularly common in Parkinson's disease, stroke, epilepsy and in the early stages of a dementia. Depression accounts for about 60% of hospital admissions to geriatric psychiatric units (Spar et al. 1980). Medically hospitalized patients were noted to have a depression rate of 40% (Koenig et al. 1991).

Mania and hypomania are noted in 5-10% of the geriatric population (Young and Klerman 1992). The incidence of late onset mania is not known although most cases of bipolar disorder present at a much younger age.

1.3 Psychoses

Chronic schizophrenia affects 0.3-1% of the community elderly. One third of the elderly in state hospitals are diagnosed with schizophrenia, most of whom are younger schizophrenic patients who have now aged (Katz et al. 1988). Harris and Jeste (1988) note that 13% of schizophrenic patients had onset of illness in 40s, 7% in 50s, 3% after age 60. Women constitute a higher percentage of patients with late-onset schizophrenia. Paranoia may be present in as many as 4% of the community elderly (Christenson and Blazer 1984).

1.4 Delirium

Delirium which frequently presents with psychotic symptoms may affect 30% of the hospitalized elderly (Gillick et al. 1982). Amongst patients admitted to a general hospital from a long term care facility the rate was 64.9% (Levkoff et al. 1991). Folstein (1991) noted the prevalence of delirium as 1.1% in a community population over age 55.

1.5 Anxiety Disorders

Anxiety disorders are common in older adults although prevalence is less compared with the general population. The prevalence of anxiety disorders for the elderly was noted in the Epidemiological Catchment Area (ECA) study as 5.5% with phobic disorders 4.8%, obsessive compulsive disorder 0.8% and panic disorder 0.1% (Regier et al. 1988). Data on generalized anxiety disorder were not determined. Female elderly had a slightly higher prevalence of anxiety disorders compared with the male counterpart.

1.6 Substance Abuse

Alcoholism is present in 5-10% of the community elderly, more than 10% in elderly seeking medical care and more than 20% of pateints in veterans and inner city hospitals (Fogel et al. 1990). Older men have alcoholism more frequently than women. Alcoholism typically starts as a young adult although a significant cohort of individuals develops a new alcohol problem after age 60. 1.6% of the elderly had a lifetime prevalence of illicit drug usage but current use was nearly zero (Anthony and Helzer 1991).

1.7 Elder Abuse

Like other forms of abuse, accurate statistics on elder abuse are difficult to obtain due to denial, under reporting and minimizing problems. Nonetheless, it has been estimated that 10% of Americans over age 65 have experienced some form of abuse (Clark 1984) with 4% as victims of moderate to severe abuse (U.S. Congress 1985). It has been estimated that only one out of five cases of elder abuse are reported. Elder abuse is recurrent in up to 80% of cases and a relative is involved in 86% of the cases (O'Malley et al. 1983), Thus, the magnitude of this problem is unfortunately very extensive.

2. DEVELOPMENTAL CHANGES WITH AGING

Before accurate psychiatric diagnosis can be made in elderly, normal age associated changes should be recognized and the psychological adaptation to these changes should be understood in the context of developmental needs and conflicts as well as changing social reality (Birren et al. 1992). These changes can be difficult especially for the oldest age group. This also has implications in the quality of life of the elderly and affects healthcare decisions.

Aging can be understood in the context of chronological, biological and sociological aging. Chronological aging can be further subdivided into young-old (65-75 years), middle-old (75-85 years) and old-old (85+years). The implication is that the old-old are more likely to have medical morbidity and functional limitations, and are more likely to fall into the category of "frail elderly." Biological aging can be further subdivided into primary aging (related to genetics of aging) and secondary aging (due to environmental factors and life-style factors such as pollution, exercise, smoking and diet with resultant tissue degeneration) (Vijg and Wei 1995). Psychological aging refers to changes in cognition and self-concept, and psychological adaptation to biological and sociological aspects of aging. Sociological aging is related to social attitudes and views of what is appropriate old age behavior i.e: disengagement or active engagement and mastery of one's life. An elderly person's concept of being impaired is presumed to be based on internalized societal biases towards the aged and the loss of social roles which might have played an important role in a positive self concept (Kuypers and Bengston 1973).

2.1 Biological Aging

With aging there are changes in multiple body systems, both external and internal, including the skin, musculo-skeletal system, special senses such as vision and hearing, cardiovascular and nervous system (both central and peripheral). These changes lead to co-morbid medical and cognitive symptoms and alteration in body image, ability to process and react to the environment, communication abilities, functional abilities, and ability to respond to treatments (Birren JE et al. 1992).

The biological changes in the brain include unreplaced neuronal loss in the central nervous system, diminished neurotransmitter synthesis, diminished neuromodulatory protein activity, altered receptor sensitivity, decreased receptor number and increased permeability of the blood-brain barrier. These changes occur in key neuronal systems affecting mood, cognition and behavior such as the norepinephrine, serotonin, acetylcholine and dopamine systems (Birren et al. 1992). The brain undergoes atrophy with resulting widening of sulci, increased ventricular size and an increase in the ventricular-brain ratio (VBR). There are also microscopic changes in brain such as changes in small vessels and microinfarcts in the subcortical periventricular areas which manifest themselves as areas of increased density on T2 weighted magnetic resonance images (MRI) (Ylikoski et al. 1995). These have also been described as "Unidentified Bright Objects" (UBOs).

2.2 Psychological Aging

The cognitive changes noted in the elderly appear to be related to the neuroanatomical changes in the brain including those seen on MRI scans (Schmidt 1993). These include decrements in "fluid intelligence" with no changes or an actual increase in "crystallized intelligence" (Albert and Moss 1988). "Fluid intelligence" refers to performance of novel tasks, speed of mental processing and perceptual-motor tasks. "Crystallized intelligence" refers to cognitive functions such as vocabulary, knowledge or acquired information, comprehension, reasoning and judgement. Other changes include a decrease in complex attention and retrieval of recent memory with the sparing of recognition memory.

Psychological adaptation in aging can be understood in terms of Erikson's developmental construct of the final stage of the "eight ages of man," namely "ego integration versus despair" (Erikson 1950). During this stage the elderly have to come to terms with their life so far and move on to a different level of adaptation. This would include coping with losses which could potentially make them vulnerable to psychiatric disorders. This would include resolution of conflicts with family, grieving over losses including the one over the sense of disappointment of not achieving expectations of one's own life. New relationships are formed and old relationships are negotiated. Issues of dependency and anxiety about death, disability, social isolation and abandonment have to be dealt by the elderly. They must deal with the challenges of physical and cognitive limitations, and develop new interests and activities. Issues of preparation for death, such as leaving a legacy behind, saying goodbye to loved ones, become more important with increasing age or illness (Birren et al. 1992). The elderly, especially those who may lack other social supports, could discuss these issues with their primary care physician. This would ensure a reduction of demoralization and an increased sense of well being.

2.3 Sociological Aging

The process of aging occurs in a larger sociocultural context. The sociocultural milieu affects attitudes toward aging and mental health, and can be stressful or supportive. Ethnicity, immigration, minority status, and socioeconomic status can be a source of stress through the mediating effects of discrimination and decreased availability of resources (Ahmed, in press, 1996). As the elderly tend to have a smaller social network, the family (including the extended family) is of particular importance to the elderly. Intergenerational issues related to dependency and role reversals become more prominent.

3. ASSESSMENT ISSUES AND CLINICAL SYNDROMES

Vulnerability to Psychiatric Disorders

The elderly appear to have vulnerability to psychiatric disorders due to a unique set of biopsychosocial changes associated with aging such as:

1. Increased losses such as job, status, health, functioning, financial and relationships (there could be an alteration in the nature of the relationship instead of actual loss) with spouse, children, siblings and friends through death or relocation.
2. Decreased adaptive capacity, both physical and psychological.
3. Neurotransmitter and receptor changes in the brain.
4. Increased incidence of physical illness and concomitant medication use.
5. Increased incidence of cognitive impairment, including dementia and delirium.

It appears that themes of loss in various domains predominate. It speaks to the resilience of the elderly that there does not appear to be an increase in the incidence of psychiatric disorders such as depression. This is in spite of the apparent "homeostenosis" or decreased physiological and psychological reserve and capacity for homeostasis in the elderly.

Distinctive features of psychiatric disorders:

1. These disorders are more likely to be etiologically related to or co-exist with physical disorders and their treatments.
2. The elderly are more likely to have concomitant dementia or delirium and a functional psychiatric disorder.
3. The elderly are more likely to have cognitive symptoms as part of the presenting clinical picture e.g: dementia of depression.
4. Patients with these disorders are also more likely to present with somatic complaints disproportionate to any underlying physical problems.

3.1 Dementia

Dementia presents as memory impairment along with impairment of other cognitive functions such as language, visuospatial functions and executive functions such as judgement, planning and organizing and alteration in personality, mood and reality testing with resulting inability to function (American Psychiatric Association, DSM IV 1994). These impairments occur in a setting of clear sensorium unlike delirium. Cognitive impairment including dementia in primary care and hospital settings can lead to increases in need for nursing care and other healthcare services and increased mortality (Erkinjutti 1986; Callahan 1995). It can also lead to impairment in the decisional capacity of patients thereby affecting their competency to make medical, self care and placement decisions. These can lead to prolonged hospitalization.

Alzheimer's dementia is the most common cause of dementia in the elderly, accounting for 50-60% of cases of late-onset cognitive deterioration (Cummings 1995). Other causes of dementia include other degenerative disorders (such as Pick's, Parkinson's, Huntington's and Creutzfeldt-Jakob's disease) and vascular, traumatic, demyelinating, infectious, inflammatory, hydrocephalic, neoplastic, metabolic,endocrine, nutritional (vitamin B12 deficiency) and toxic (including from prescription drugs) conditions.

Since up to 25% of patients with dementia have conditions that are reversible or arrestable (Fogel et al. 1990), early intervention is important. However, families often do not recognize the early symptoms and signs of dementia and these patients may not come to medical attention until secondary or co-morbid conditions develop. In addition to history and mental status, cognitive screening tests such as the Mini-Mental State Exam (Folstein et al. 1975) can be helpful in diagnosis of dementia. Appropriate workup including necessary blood tests for cell counts, metabolic, endocrine, toxic, infective and nutritional problems should be done. Structural brain imaging such as CT scan or MRI should be done to look for intracranial pathology if history, mental status or other routine investigations do not establish a diagnosis (Cummings 1995). Other tests such as electroencephalography (EEG), lumbar puncture (LP), single photon emission computerized tomography (SPECT) and neuropsychological testing should be ordered if indications are that they would provide additional diagnostic information.

Older patients with psychiatric disorders, such as depression can present with cognitive disturbances. This syndrome has been referred to as "pseudodementia" (Wells 1979). More accurately, this is now considered to be a true dementia (Emery and Oxman 1992). This dementia is believed to be secondary to neurochemical changes in the brain which occur during depression. These patients may be at increased risk of developing an irreversible dementia over the ensuing years (Alexopoulos et al. 1993). Recognition of dementia of depression is helpful in the identification of depression with its attendant risk of suicide. It is eminently treatable and it should be distinguished from other dementias such as Alzheimer's dementia. Some of the distinguishing features are presented in Table 1.

Patients with Alzheimer's dementia can also have depression manifesting as irritability, passivity and somatic preoccupation or as dysthymia early in the course of the dementia (Duffy and Coffey 1996). Over half of the patients with Alzheimer's dementia have behavioral problems (Schneider and Sobin 1992). These are primarily agitation and aggression (with or without psychosis), mood disorders, anxiety, wandering and inappropriate social behaviors (Reisberg et al. 1987).

These symptoms are particularly likely to occur in moderate to severe Alzheimer's dementia. These behaviors add to the disability of the cognitive symptoms such as memory and language problems. This is of importance because, in addition to problems in activities of daily living (ADL) such as toileting and feeding, these symptoms lead to inability of families to care for patients at home. This leads to institutionalization, loss of autonomy, loss of function because of physical and chemical restraint, and withdrawal of emotional support (Schneider 1993). As many as half of caregivers such patients will suffer will suffer from significant depressive symptoms that are likely to have an adverse impact on both their health and the person for whom they are caring (Drinka et al. 1987).

Table 1

Dementia	Dementia of Depression
No prior history of depression	History of depression
Gradual onset with slow worsening	Rapid worsening
Long duration	Short duration
Mood changes with or after cognitive dysfunction	Mood changes predate cognitive dysfunction
Awareness of deficits minimal or absent	High awareness
Wrong answers to testing questions	"I don't know" responses
Cognitive impairment is stable	Cognitive impairment fluctuates

3.2 Mood Disorders

As the epidemiology of depression suggests, the estimates of depression in elderly people vary widely as a function of setting, threshold of diagnosis, and definition of depression. There appear to be a number of differences in the presentation of depression in the elderly as compared to the depression in the younger population (Caine et al. 1994; NIH Consensus Development Panel on Depression in Late Life 1992). Older depressed patients:

1. Are less likely to have ideational symptoms (guilt and suicidal ideation), co-morbid personality disorder and family history of depression.
2. Are more likely to have psychotic depressive and melancholic symptoms, anorexia and weight loss, psychomotor abnormalities, cognitive impairment ("dementia of depression"), hypochondriasis ("masked depression"), medical co-morbidity, and mortality from both medical causes and suicides.

Recognition of depression may be more difficult in the elderly due to the heterogeneity of symptoms. Both patients and clinicians may attribute depressive symptoms to the aging process. Concomitant presence of dementia may further compromise the recognition and reporting of depression. This leads to undertreatment of a very treatable disorder.

Associated neuroimaging findings in the depressed elderly include evidence on CT and MRI scans of cortical atrophy (Caine et al. 1994). There are also numerous reports of diffuse high-signal subcortical hyperintensities on T2-weighted MRI images in elderly patients with unipolar depression with somewhat greater frequency than in healthy elderly. These findings are suggestive of small vessel cerebrovascular disease and are associated with neuropsychological impairment. SPECT scan studies have shown both a pattern of decreased frontal (left frontal) and basal ganglia activity as well as a pattern of more widespread regional dysfunctions (Caine et al. 1994).

There can be numerous co-morbid chronic diseases and disabilities in the depressed elderly such as cardiovascular disease, neurological disorders, malignancies, arthritis, and sensory loss (including vision and hearing). These conditions create psychosocial stress, physiological burdens, and functional disabilities that may contribute to the pathogenesis of depression as well as complicate treatment (NIH Consensus Development Panel on Depression in Late Life 1992). This is particularly so when there is no ameliorating psychosocial support such as a confiding relationship (Evans and Katona 1993). Patients with physical illness and disability who are also depressed are less likely to regain function and have poorer functional outcomes than those without depression (Fogel et al. 1990). Current data indicate that depressive symptoms respond to treatment in many of these patients.

In case of bipolar disorder, late-onset mania with or without antecedent depressive symptoms, may differ from bipolar disorder in young adulthood (Young and Klerman 1992). It may be more heterogeneous. It appears less directly genetically determined. It may in part be due to changes in the aging brain and disorders associated with aging. Late-onset manic symptoms should be evaluated for mania secondary to a general medical condition such as brain tumors, epilepsy and strokes, or due to medications such as corticosteroids. On the other hand, age associated brain changes may also modify early-onset bipolar disorder. These patients may have a "burning out" or reduction in manic symptoms, but more often the frequency and duration of manic symptoms tends to increase over the life cycle. Also anger rather than euphoria may be the predominant mood, and the delusions more likely being paranoid than grandiose. The response to treatment is less robust or less likely.

3.3 Psychoses

This group of disorders in the elderly include schizophrenia, delusional disorder, dementia with psychosis, mood disorder with psychotic features, psychosis secondary to general medical conditions, and other disorders with psychotic conditions. In general, late life schizophrenia is considered to be the prototypical chronic psychosis (Jeste et al. 1996). Patients with this disorder include both the patients with late-onset schizophrenia (LOS) and the patients with the more prevalent early-onset schizophrenia (EOS) who live into middle and old age.

Clinically LOS is similar to EOS in terms of positive symptoms such as hallucinations and delusions, and family history of schizophrenia (Jeste et al. 1995). LOS is more common in women than in men and presents with fewer negative symptoms such as social withdrawal and emotional blunting. The type of cognitive impairment while comparable, is somewhat less severe in LOS.

Possible risk factors in the development of late life psychoses include premorbid cluster A personality disorders or traits, social isolation, sensory impairment including vision and hearing loss, cerebral abnormalities (both specific disorders and nonspecific changes such as cortical atrophy), immigrant status, lower socioeconomic status, female gender, early physical and sexual trauma and failure to produce progeny (Lacro et al. 1993). Some of these risk factors can be reduced by appropriate interventions such as correction of hearing, vision, social support and psychotherapeutic interventions. This is important as even mild psychotic symptoms can become problematic when the elderly have to be hospitalized or treated for acute medical illness. In these situations paranoia can become a major barrier to cooperation with care.

3.4 Delirium

This disorder has also been referred to as "acute confusional state" and "encephalopathy." It is characterized by acute onset, global cognitive impairment, attentional abnormalities, altered level of consciousness, increased or decreased psychomotor activity and altered sleep-wake cycle. Although delirium can affect a person of any age, the elderly, particularly those with some degree of baseline brain damage or dementia, are more likely to develop delirium as a result of an acute or chronic physical illness or drug toxicity (Lipowski 1989). This might be as a result of decreased functional reserve and reduced homeostatic capacity with resultant increased vulnerability to both biological and psychosocial stressors. They may also have multiple medical problems, be taking multiple medications with CNS effects, and have a higher prevalence of hearing and visual problems. The aging brain also has decreased amounts of neurotransmitters, particularly acetylcholine. About half the patients with dementia appear to develop delirium during hospitalization for medical illness (Francis et al. 1990).

Clinically delirium may be the only or the most conspicuous feature of serious medical illnesses such as CNS or cardiovascular disorders, other organ failures and infections such as pneumonia, and hip fractures (Lipowski 1989). The underlying etiology of delirium is usually multifactorial. Patients may present in a hypoalert-hypoactive state and the patient may look depressed ("pseudodepression"). Others may present in a hyperalert-hyperactive state with agitated behavior and prominent hallucinations and other perceptual disturbances or in a mixed state of the above two clinical pictures. In the elderly delirium tends to last longer, weeks rather than days. Delirium in the elderly is considered as a true medical emergency as it is associated with an increase morbidity and mortality (Gustafson and Berggren 1988; Francis and Kapoor 1992; Lipowski 1989). The elderly are more likely to have an adverse outcome after delirium as a result of its underlying etiology. Delirium can progress to death or dementia.

3.5 Anxiety

Old age can be a time of intense anxiety related to unresolved developmental issues, feelings of loneliness, fear of isolation, chronic illness, financial problems, functional limitations and fear of death, disability and abandonment. The real life problems challenge an older person's sense of security and self-esteem, and thereby predispose that individual to increased risks of experiencing symptoms of anxiety. There appears to be a direct relationship between anxiety and depression, life stress and medical co-morbidity and an inverse association with age and general health measures in a primary care population (Smith et al. 1994). Anxiety disorders appear to be associated with multiple, expensive, unproductive, medical work-ups and ineffective treatment for functional somatic symptoms, and patients fail to receive effective treatments for the anxiety disorder (Lish et al. 1995). However, a variety of medical disorders (thyroid disorders) and substance-related conditions (stimulants, steroids and decongestants) can cause anxiety symptoms or exacerbate an anxiety disorder.

3.6 Substance Abuse and Dependence

Substance abuse disorders are an under-recognized but treatable cause of disability, morbidity, mortality, and excess medical costs in the elderly, especially those who are medically ill (Lish et al. 1995). This is particularly so with alcoholism (both abuse and dependence) which decreases with increasing age, but remains a prevalent condition among the elderly (Callahan and Tierney 1995; Council on Scientific Affairs 1996). A majority of the elderly alcoholics are those whose alcoholism occurred relatively early in life, with the rest developing problems with their drinking at or after 60 years of age. Late onset alcoholism appears to be precipitated by, or made more manifest by, situational factors such as age associated losses and social isolation than to family history or genetic influences.

Problem drinking tends to occur later in elderly women than in men.

The elderly alcoholics are less likely to present with social consequences of alcoholism and comorbid personality disorders and more likely to present with adverse medical consequences of alcoholism. These include toxic effects of alcohol on the heart, liver and nervous system as well as trauma and accidents (with resultant hip fractures and subdural hematomas), poor nutrition, sleep impairment, cognitive impairment, depression and suicide. The elderly alcoholics are more likely to have drug interactions and be non-compliant with medications and other treatment recommendations. Use of prescription drugs is common in the elderly, with abuse of these drugs likely by those abusing alcohol. Even when abuse of medications does not occur, the elderly are more prone to the adverse effects of both prescribed as well as over the counter medications such as cold, sleep and arthritis medications. A number of all these medications have anticholinergic and sedative properties and cause drug interactions with resultant problems such as falls, delirium and other medical consequences.

3.7 Elder Abuse

Elder abuse, neglect and exploitation are considered to be under-recognized major public health problems (Council on Scientific Affairs 1987). Of these neglect is probably the most common. Abuse may take the form of physical assault, emotional abuse, denial of rights, withholding of basic life resources and sexual abuse. Emotional abuse is often linked with physical abuse. Emotional abuse includes threats, insults, harassment, harsh orders, infantilization, lack of safe environment and restriction of social and religious activity (Council on Aging 1995). Both physical and emotional abuse can result in disorders caused by stress. Psychiatric symptoms seen in abused elderly include resignation, ambivalence, fear, anger, cognitive impairment, depressed mood, insomnia, substance abuse, delirium, agitation, lethargy and self neglect.

The overwhelming abused elderly are women. The typical abused patient is a white, widowed, female, over age 75, who is financially, physically, or mentally unable to live alone. The caregiver at risk of becoming an abuser is a daughter or daughter-in-law, white, and over age 45. Risk factors for elder abuse include increasing caregiver burden and stress, increasing cognitive impairment and dependency of the frail elderly patient, lack of close family ties, history of family violence, lack of financial resources, and substance abuse and psychopathology in the abuser. Often there is denial of abuse by both the abuser and the abused. However detection of abuse can be improved by observing for the risk factors of abuse and telltale signs of physical abuse such as signs of trauma, signs of neglect such as poor nutrition and skin care, and signs of emotional abuse such as fear, anger and resignation.

4. GENERAL TREATMENT ISSUES

Aging results in a number of biological changes in organ systems including increased sensitivity to medication side effects, complex interplay of medical and psychiatric illness and increased susceptibility to delirium. Age-related changes in physiology such as decreased renal function may not be evident until the onset of acute illness. Inappropriate medical treatment as well as non-compliance by the patient results in additional morbidity and mortality.

Psychosocial treatments are important in managing psychiatric illness in the elderly. Indeed, although medications can target specific symptoms, other problems such as problems in social support, changing roles in the family, coping with death, and caregiver stress require psychosocial interventions. The elderly often have negative views about mental illness and may refuse to see a mental health professional. The patient and family may assume that symptoms like depression are a part of growing old and deny the need for treatment. Although a full discussion of various forms of psychotherapies and psychosocial intervention is well beyond the scope of this chapter, some general guidelines can be helpful.

Commonly used individual therapies in the elderly include cognitive behavior therapy, behavioral therapy, interpersonal therapy, supportive and psychodynamic therapy. Group therapies which include reminiscence, music, recreational and sensory stimulation can be of considerable benefit by encouraging socialization, providing stimulation and increasing self-esteem. The goals and pace of treatment may need to be slowed down due to cognitive and physical impairments in the elderly.

Family therapies are an important part of psychosocial treatment. Treatment should be geared to the patient and caregiver rather than the patient alone. Old unresolved conflicts frequently emerge as an elderly relative has a decline in health. Families experience difficulty coping with institutionalization, the financial stressor of paying for medical care, along with feelings of hopelessness and helpless in the face of increasing deterioration of a relative. Finally, community based programs such as senior centers, volunteer organizations, and adult day care agencies can become a vital part of the psychosocial treatment.

5. PRINCIPLES OF PHARMACOLOGIC TREATMENT

5.1 Pharmacokinetics

Pharmacokinetics refers to the effect of a patient on a drug and involves absorption, distribution, metabolism, and excretion. On the other hand, pharmacodynamics refers to the action of a drug on the patient. Physiological changes, disease states and drug mediated effects can result in changes in pharmacokinetics which have clinical significance and have been well reviewed (Young and Meyers 1991; Spar and La Rue 1990; Leipzig and Saltz 1992; Abernethy 1992).

5.1.1 Absorption: Absorption is not significantly affected despite changes in gastrointestinal mucosa and pH. Systemic absorption of topical medications such as steroids and beta-blocker eye drops can result in central nervous system (CNS) side effects and need to be used with caution.

5.1.2 Distribution: Increase in the fat/lean body mass ratio results in decreased concentration and increased half life of fat-soluble medications such as diazepam. A relative decrease in body water results in increased concentration of medications distributed in free water such as lithium. Most psychiatric drugs are protein bound with the exception of lithium. The free fraction is defined as that part of the drug not bound to protein. For benzodiazepines and neuroleptics protein binding depends primarily on albumen which decreases with age. As a result, benzodiazepine and neuroleptics levels can be increased in the elderly. For tricyclic antidepressants, alpha1-acid glycoprotein which increases with age can cause changes in free fraction.

5.1.3 Metabolism: Drugs are primarily metabolized by the liver through a two phase metabolism, the first phase involving oxidation, reduction or hydrolysis and the second step acetylation or conjugation. Conjugation is unchanged with aging. As a result, benzodiazepines such as lorazepam and oxazepam which are metabolized through a single step conjugation are unaffected by aging whereas other benzodiazepines such as diazepam and chlordiazepoxide which require both steps for metabolism tend to have accumulation of intermediate metabolites resulting in a significantly increased half life. Furthermore, many of these metabolites are active resulting in an even longer duration of action.

5.1.4 Excretion: Aging results in decreased renal function as evidenced by decreased glomerular filtration rate, reduced renal plasma flow and tubular function in the elderly. This change can result in clinically significant increase in blood levels of medications which are renally excreted such as lithium. Desipramine metabolites which are water soluble and may be cardiotoxic can accumulate in an elderly patient with decreased renal function.

5.2 Pharmacodynamics

Pharmacodynamics refers to the response of the patient at the receptor or tissue level after exposure to a drug. Alterations in the blood-brain barrier and decrease in neurotransmitters make the elderly patient's brain more sensitive to CNS effects such as increased risk of cognitive dysfunction due to benzodiazepines. Medical disorders such as Alzheimer's disease and Parkinson's disease further increase sensitivity to anticholinergics and antipsychotics, respectively resulting in the clinically significant effects. On the other hand, elderly patients respond to tricyclic antidepressants at similar blood levels compared with the younger counterparts despite increasing sensitivity to drug side effects. Polypharmacy can result in pharmacodynamic changes at the drug-drug level, for example, the interference of tricyclics with the antihypertensive effect of clonidine due to competition at the alpha-2 receptor level.

5.3 Problems of Pharmacotherapy

The improper use of psychoactive medications has been well documented in the literature (Beers et al. 1988). One fourth of patients on antidepressants were treated with amitriptyline, a sedating and anticholinergic medication. 40% were treated with sedative/hypnotics, with extensive usage of diphenhydramine, an anticholinergic agent. Long acting benzodiazepines were widely used. No clear documentation was indicated for the use of psychotropics. He concluded that inappropriate and incorrect usage of medications was widespread. Unfortunately, a later study (Beers et al. 1992) continued to show serious problems in pharmacotherapy with 40% of patients at a skilled nursing facility having one inappropriate medication and 10%, two medications used incorrectly. Unfortunately, benzodiazepines are frequently prescribed inappropriately for long term use in the elderly. Mellinger et al. (1984) noted that 1.6% of elderly had taken benzodiazpines daily for more than one year.

The problem of incorrect medication usage in the elderly is further compounded by the practice of polypharmacy. The elderly already have more medical illness and not surprisingly use a significantly greater number of medications compared with the younger population. Excessive medications combined with increased sensitivity to side effects frequently can precipitate a serious drug toxicity. For example, the use of low potency neuroleptics and anti-Parkinsonian agents can result in an anticholinergic delirium from the additive effect. This problem is compounded when a patient sees a number of different physicians who may each prescribe a different medication unbeknownst to each other.

It is not surprising that polypharmacy results in poor compliance. The use of complicated drug schedules or excessive number of medications is problematic for any elderly patient but is especially difficult for a patient with even mild cognitive deficits. Poor compliance usually results in under utilization of drugs although excessive usage can occur.

Other impairments in vision, hearing, motor and swallowing may further contribute to age-specific problems in medications.

5.4.4 Practical Suggestions for Pharmacotherapy

1. Psychosocial interventions should be utilized as much as possible such as the use of night lights, well lit rooms, clocks to assist with orientation and frequent checks by nursing staff prior to instituting pharmacotherapy.

2. Carefully review current medications and try to minimize the number of medications. Remember to ask about non-prescription as well as prescription medications. Many patients with complicated drug regimens can actually improve as medications are discontinued. Try to maximize existing medications prior to adding a new medication.

3. If medications are indicated, determine target symptoms and confirm appropriate functioning of organ system, e.g. renal function for lithium.

4. Start with low doses, generally one third to one half of the usual dose of a younger patient and increase slowly at half the usual rate.

5. Change only one medication at a time. Maintain adequate dose for a adequate duration before considering treatment a failure. Blood levels can be particularly helpful in checking compliance and adequacy of treatment. At the same time, use the least anticholinergic medication and the lowest effective dose to minimize side effects.

6. Anticipate side effects. Monitor orthostasis, check for falls, confusion, constipation, urinary retention, incontinence, stiffness or syncope. Ask about sexual dysfunction which is common in many classes of medications. The elderly may be hesitant or embarrassed to report these side effects. Be aware of the pharmacodynamic profile of psychotropics in choosing a medication. For example one should avoid an antidepressant with anticholinergic properties in a patient who already has urinary retention.

7. Always continue to think about medical causes for behavioral changes even if the patient has an obvious primary psychiatric diagnosis.

8. A trial off psychiatric medications can often be helpful in instances where iatrogenic factors are high on the differential diagnosis.

9. Do not hesitate to obtain a consultation in cases where symptoms are serious such as suicidality, psychotic depressions, and severe agitation/dangerousness.

6. TREATMENT OF CLINICAL SYNDROMES

6.1 Dementia

Agitation or other behavioral disturbances due to dementia is a common reason for a psychiatric consultation in the elderly. Treatment with any pharmacologic agent should be carried out only after coexisting treatable conditions have been ruled out such as medical illness, delirium and depression. Psychosocial interventions such as the use of orienting stimuli, for example, using a calendar and a clock, minimizing isolation, and occupational/recreational therapies should be maximized prior to usage. Education of family and caregivers is also critical. Then at that point pharmacotherapy should be considered. A number of reviews have been published for the treatment of agitation in the elderly (Devanand and Levy 1995; Tariot et al. 1995; Ahmed 1995; Salzman et al. 1995; Sakauye 1995; Schneider 1993; Flint 1994).

6.1.1 Neuroleptics

Neuroleptics have long been used for the treatment of agitation in the elderly. Unfortunately, prior excessive and inappropriate use of neuroleptics in nursing homes as chemical restraints resulted in the Nursing Home Reform Amendments of the Omnibus Budget Reconciliation Act (OBRA) of 1987 which has limited use of neuroleptics and sedative hypnotics as well as mandated appropriate treatment. The OBRA regulations have resulted in significantly curtailment of the use of neuroleptics in the elderly, by some reports as much as 45% (Sakauye 1995). Nonetheless, neuroleptics remain the most commonly used and studied class of drugs for the treatment of agitation. Antipsychotics are particularly effective and indicated in patients where agitation in dementia is associated with clear psychotic symptoms or with schizophrenia. Unfortunately, the neuroleptics are less effective for chronic non-psychotic agitation which is quite common with dementia. In fact, some patients become worse with neuroleptics and improve when antipsychotics were discontinued.

Typical neuroleptics are believed to be generally equal in efficacy and selection involves efforts to minimize side effects. Unfortunately, the elderly are particularly prone to orthostatic hypotension, sedation, tardive dyskinesia and drug-induced Parkinsonian symptoms although dystonia may be less common.

The low potency antipsychotics such as thioridazine and chlorpromazine have a greater incidence of sedation, orthostasis, confusion, constipation and other anticholinergic side effects and are generally not preferred despite a lower risk of Parkinsonian symptoms. High potency medications such as haloperidol and fluphenazine are more likely to produce extrapyramidal symptoms but preferred due to minimal anticholinergic side effects. Typically, in low doses such as 0.5 mg two or three times per day, such Parkinsonian side effects tend to be minimal. Drug-induced Parkinsonism should be treated by lowering the dose if possible rather than the addition of anticholinergic medications. Neuroleptic-induced akathisia can present as worsening of agitation in a demented patient and neuroleptic should be decreased. Therefore, one should be very cautious in increasing antipsychotic dosages.

Risperidone, an atypical antipsychotic, may possibly have a lower risk of tardive dyskinesia and extrapyramidal symptoms compared to standard neuroleptics and does not require weekly blood monitoring. These features make risperidone a useful antipsychotic for the elderly. Preliminary data from an open trial in elderly with agitation are quite positive (Raheja 1994).

6.1.2 Non-neuroleptic Treatment for Agitation

Due to partial efficacy, serious side effects and efforts to comply with OBRA regulations, researchers have extensively sought effective non-neuroleptic alternatives. Although there are many case reports of efficacy, unfortunately, controlled studies are lacking (Devanand and Levy 1995; Tariot et al. 1995; Ahmed 1995; Salzman et al. 1995; Sakauye 1995; Schneider 1993; Flint 1994; Lake and Grossberg 1996).

Benzodiazepines have not been extensively used in dementia due to general ineffectiveness for chronic agitation and serious side effects which include sedation, ataxia, worsening of cognition, habituation, and disinhibition. Short acting benzodiazepines such as lorazepam may have some use for acute episodes of agitation on an as needed basis.

Beta blockers such as propranolol in doses of 60-520 mg/day and pindolol to 60 mg/day have been used. The selective beta blockers such as pindolol have less systemic side effects and are preferred. Unfortunately, results using beta blockers have been mixed.

Trazodone has been used in the belief that its serotonergic effect may decrease agitation. Doses of 150-400 mg/day have been used with some efficacy. Hypotension is a common side effect.

Buspirone is believed to have anti-aggressive effect through its serotonergic action. Daily doses of 20-80 mg in divided doses has been effective in some patients with minimal side effects.

Selective serotonin reuptake inhibitors (SSRIs) show significant promise in treating agitation due to its tolerability in the geriatric population. A double-blind study showed improvement using citalopram in Alzheimer's dementia but not vascular dementia (Nyth and Gottries 1990).

Selegiline (deprenyl) a selective monoamine oxidase inhibitor type B (MAO-B) has been used for Alzheimer's dementia due to the finding of increased MAO-B activity in aging and Alzheimer's dementia. Selegiline has shown some efficacy at 10 mg/day although other studies have been less positive.

Lithium has shown some efficacy in some studies. However due its toxicity, it is difficult to justify without a diagnosis of bipolar disorder or at least a mood disorder.

The anticonvulsants carbamazepine and valproic acid has shown considerable promise in the treatment of agitation. They may be particularly useful in agitation associated with affective symptoms. Both medications require monitoring for blood levels and for hematological side effects (leukopenia with carbamazepine, thrombocytopenia with valproic acid). Liver function tests are important in using valproic acid. Carbamazepine has a number of clinically relevant drug interactions including lowering of antipsychotic levels.

Medications to improve cognition have also been extensively studied. Tacrine is an acetylcholinesterase inhibitor which raises acetylcholine levels which are believed to be low in Alzheimer's disease and as treatment for Alzheimer's dementia. Tacrine has been moderately effective in the earlier stages of the illness. Side effects such as nausea, vomiting, and liver toxicity are noted and limit use. Selegiline, vitamin E, nimodipine, anti-inflammatory medications, physostigmine, hydergine and lecithin have been investigated without significant results in improving cognition. Deprenyl and vitamin E are being investigated to see if the rate of progression of Alzheimer's dementia can be decreased. Fluvoxamine, an SSRI did not improve cognitive status (Olafsson et al. 1992).

6.1.3 Recommendations for treatment

There are no clear guidelines for using medications although some strategies have been suggested (Ahmed 1995; Sakauye 1995). Data on dose and duration for an adequate trial are lacking.

- Try non-pharmacologic treatment first.
- Use medications with less serious side effects first.
- Anticonvulsants are promising and have the advantage of being able to check blood levels for toxicity.
- Neuroleptics are modestly useful and their use is supported by most data. OBRA 1987 encourages the use of non-neuroleptics.

6.2 Mood Disorders

The pharmacotherapy of depression includes numerous antidepressants with differing side effect profiles and has been extensively reviewed (Salzman 1994; Reynolds et al. 1994; Salzman et al. 1995). Indeed, Gerson et al. (1988) in his review of 25 double-blind studies noted that all antidepressants were of comparable efficacy and concluded that side effect and drug interaction should be the aim of rational pharmacotherapy. Antidepressants have a slow onset of action and often require a minimum of 4-6 weeks at a therapeutic dosage.

Antidepressants should be continued for at least 9-12 months as part of acute treatment after resolution of depressive symptoms. Patients with many previous episodes of depression are at particular risk for relapse and may need even longer treatment. Some patients may require maintenance antidepressants after acute treatment; the dosage of antidepressant for maintenance treatment is equal to that for acute therapy. Maintenance electroconvulsive therapy (ECT) may be needed for refractory patients who respond to ECT. Psychotic depression needs to be treated with both an antidepressant and antipsychotic.

6.2.1 Tricyclic antidepressants

Tricyclic antidepressants (TCA) have been widely used for the treatment of depression and may be more effective than the selective serotonin reuptake inhibitors (SSRIs) in older patients with severe depression and medical illness (Roose et al. 1994). Secondary amines such as desipramine and nortriptyline have less risk of orthostatic hypotension, sedation, and anticholinergic symptoms. Conduction abnormalities need to be carefully evaluated with an electrocardiogram (EKG) due to the quinidine-like effect of TCA. Nortriptyline which is the most studied antidepressant among the elderly has a therapeutic window similar to younger patients.

Tricyclics should be started at a low dose such as 10-25 mg per day and increased upward slowly. Desipramine and nortriptyline have the further advantage of accepted therapeutic levels allowing for monitoring of an adequate dose. Unfortunately, some patients may be unable to tolerate an adequate trial of tricyclics due to side effects.

6.2.2 Trazodone

Although trazodone has minimal anticholinergic effect, its use for depression is limited by sedation and orthostasis. More recently, it has gained a resurgence of use in treating insomnia or agitation due to depression or concurrent treatment with SSRIs. Typical doses for sleep are 25-50 mg po q hs.

6.2.3 Buproprion

Minimal cardiac effects and anticholinergic effect make buproprion a good choice in the pharmacotherapy of depression. Side effects include activation, seizure risk, confusion and nausea.

6.2.4 Selective serotonin reuptake inhibitors (SSRIs)

The SSRIs have come into widespread use due minimal side effects of cardiotoxicity, anticholinergic activity and orthostatic hypotension. Unfortunately, other problems such as nausea, nervousness, insomnia, sexual dysfunction and headache are common. Dosages need to be frequently decreased by as much as 1/2 or 1/4 for the elderly patient to minimize side effects. Weight loss can be particularly a problem with the elderly with fluoxetine, nausea and vomiting with fluvoxamine and insomnia or sedation with paroxetine or sertraline.

6.2.5 Monoamine oxidase inhibitors

Monoamine oxidase inhibitors (MAOIs) have been shown to be effective with minimal side effects. The nonselective, irreversible MAOIs require a special diet free of tyramine to prevent a hypertensive crisis and have a potentially dangerous interaction with common medications such as phenylephrine, SSRIs and meperidine. As a result, MAOIs have fallen into disfavor. MAO-B inhibitors such as deprenyl may be of particular interest in treating depression superimposed on dementia or Parkinson's disease. Selegiline in doses higher than 10 mg becomes nonselective in its MAO inhibition and would require dietary and medication restriction. Reversible, selective MAO-A inhibitors such as moclobemide which do not require the special restrictionS are available outside of the United States.

6.2.6 Electroconvulsive Treatment (ECT)

Electroconvulsive treatment is probably the single most effective treatment for depression with high efficacy even in a refractory population. In the past, the stigma of use has curtained the use of ECT. There is now a resurgence of interest due to improved anesthetic agents and brief pulse machines with less cognitive side effects. Indications include severe depressive disorders, concurrent medical illness or inability to tolerate standard pharmacotherapy. ECT is also used for mania and psychosis. Age is not a contraindication and in fact, elderly patients may have a better response compared with younger patients.

6.2.7 Stimulants and newer antidepressants

The use of stimulants such as dextroamphetamine and pemoline can be effective in the elderly population, particularly for the medically ill depressed patient. Stimulants have the advantage of safety and quick onset of action. Newer antidepressants such as venlafaxine and nefazodone show considerable promise for the elderly due to a favorable side effect profile but there is little data.

6.2.8 Suggestions for pharmacotherapy for depression and mania

Depression:

1. No individual antidepressant is optimal
2. SSRIs, nefazodone and venlafaxine hold promise but there is less data on usage and plasma levels.
3. Nortriptyline and desipramine have substantial data regarding efficacy as well as plasma levels allowing more confidence in treatment. Side effects may be more marked.
4. Guidelines for the old-old patients (over 85 years) are unclear.

Mania:

Lithium remains the mainstay of treatment of mania. Unfortunately the low therapeutic index of lithium, decreased renal capacity, central nervous side effects and decreased free water make the use of lithium in the elderly rather complicated necessitating the need for frequent drug monitoring, lowering of doses by 1/2 or 1/3 as well as possibly a lower effective drug level. The anticonvulsants are now being widely used for mania and may be better tolerated than lithium. Antipsychotics and ECT can be of value in treating mania.

6.3 Psychosis

Antipsychotics are the most effective treatment for both early and late onset schizophrenia in the elderly. Delusional disorders may be less responsive to antipsychotics. Unfortunately, serious side effects such as tardive dyskinesia which may be particularly a problem in the elderly have complicated the use of antipsychotics. The elderly are also prone to other problems such as sedation, anticholinergic effects and extrapyramidal symptoms and thus, dosages of antipsychotic should be kept at a minimum. Among the typical antipsychotics, higher potency medications such as haloperidol are generally preferred to minimize anticholinergic effects. Jeste et al. (1996) conclude that the newer agents such as risperidone and clozapine show considerable promise in treatment but that the data are limited.

Clozapine and risperidone are atypical antipsychotics which are believed to have efficacy through both the serotonin and dopamine systems. Clozapine has little risks of extrapyramidal symptoms and tardive dyskinesia but has other serious side effects such as agranulocytosis which requires weekly blood monitoring. Other problems include sedation and anticholinergic side effects. Nonetheless Frankenberg and Kalunian (1994) report efficacy with refractory psychotic geriatric patients using clozapine. Clozapine can be particularly useful in psychosis complicated by idiopathic Parkinsonism (Factor et al. 1994)

6.4 Delirium

The treatment of delirium first involves the diagnosis of delirium. Unfortunately many cases of delirium are missed due to ignoring symptoms or attributing symptoms to a functional basis. After the diagnosis is made, treatment involves trying to correct the underlying cause. The causes of delirium are many including infection, metabolic abnormalities, drug intoxication/withdrawal. Occasionally delirium is the only symptom evident in an elderly patient with a serious medical illness such as a pneumonia or a urinary tract infection (UTI). Treatment of delirium primarily involves correcting the underlying causes.

Frequent pharmacologic interventions involves efforts to minimize the dose and numbers of drugs. In fact, all psychotropics should generally be discontinued as such agents can be contributory to delirium. Low doses of high potency neuroleptics (doses of haloperidol 1-2 mg/day) can be used in cases of severe behavioral problems. Unfortunately, even such doses should be used with caution as there is some risk of worsening delirium. Delirium due to anticholinergic medications can usually be treated with discontinuation of the offending drugs although physostigmine is sometimes used.

6.5 Anxiety

Anxiety is commonly treated with benzodiazepines. Benzodiazepines with a short half life which are only metabolized through conjugation are preferred. The dose needed for the elderly is frequently decreased. Unfortunately, benzodiazepines have side effects of toxicity, sedation, falls, ataxia and cognitive impairment. Buspirone may be useful for the treatment of anxiety as it is a non-benzodiazepine.

6.6 Substance Abuse

Substance abuse treatment will focus on managing alcoholism, the predominant drug problem in the elderly. The elderly alcoholic first needs to undergo a safe detoxification by the use of short and intermediate acting benzodiazepines, thiamine, folate, minerals, and multivitamins, and the institution of hydration, along with close medical supervision including monitoring of electrolytes. Compared with the younger counterpart, withdrawal in the elderly may be more severe due to medical complications and even with abstinence improvement in health and cognition tends to be slower.

Treatment after detoxification can involve medications as well as psychosocial treatment to maintain sobriety. Disulfuram, an aversive agent which causes unpleasant side effects upon ingestion of alcohol can be of benefit to a particularly motivated individual who has no medical contraindications and fully understands the potential serious risks. Naltrexone, a non-aversive agent can also be beneficial (O'Malley et al. 1995). Psychosocial treatment involves both the patient and family. The elderly may resist efforts at referral to a self-help group such as Alcoholics Anonymous, but may benefit from such a group with an older membership. Families of alcoholics can benefit from groups such as Al Anon. Both family and patient need to be educated on the possible medical complications of alcoholism (Council on Scientific Affairs 1996).

6.7 Elder Abuse

Treatment should involve a multidisciplinary team to look at a comprehensive treatment plan for both the abuser and the abused patient. Management might involve psychotherapy to assist the abuser in identifying stressors and using alternative coping strategies, and treatment of underlying psychiatric and substance abuse problems. Social services and community resources should be utilized to provide assistance to the caregiver in the care of the dependent elderly family member. This might include ways for the elderly patient to have a different living arrangement including respite care, legal assistance from attorneys as well as the police along with medical and psychiatric treatment for the abused victim (Council on Scientific Affairs 1987).

REFERENCES

Abernethy DR: Psychotropic drugs and the aging process: pharmacokinetics and pharmacodynamics, in *Clinical Geriatric Psychopharmacology*. Edited by Salzman C. Williams and Wilkins, Baltimore, 1992

Addonzio G, Alexopoulos GS: Affective disorders in the elderly. Intl J Psychiatry 8:41-47, 1993

Ahmed I: Geriatric Psychopathology, in *Culture and Psychopathology: A guide to clinical assessment*. Edited by Tseng WS, Streltzer J, New York, Brunner/Mazel (In Press)

Ahmed I: Pharmacologic treatment of behavioral symptoms of Alzheimer's dementia - a review and a possible strategy. Clinical Gerontologist 16:3-16, 1995

Albert MS, Moss MB: *Geriatric Neuropsychology*. New York, Guilford, 1988

Alexopoulos GS, Meyers B, Young RS et al. The course of geriatric depression with "reversible dementia": a controlled study.
Am J Psychiatry 150: 1693-1699, 1993

American Psychiatric Association: *Diagnostic and Statistical Manual of Mental Disorders, 4th Edition.* Washington DC, American Psychiatric Association, 1994

Anthony JC, Helzer JE: Syndromes of drug abuse and dependence, in *Psychiatric Disorders in America: The Epidemiologic Catchment Area Study.*
Edited by Robins LN, Regier DA. New York, Free Press, 1991

Beers MH, Avon J, Soumerai SB, et al.: Psychoactive medication use in intermediate-care facility residents. JAMA 260:3016-3020, 1988

Beers MH, Ouslander JG, Fingold SF, et al. Inappropriate medication prescribing in skilled-nursing facilities. Ann Intern Med 117(8):684-689, 1992

Birren JE, Sloane BR, Cohen GD (eds): *Handbook of Mental Health and Aging, 2nd Edition.* San Diego, 1992

Blazer D, Williams C: Epidemiology of dysphoria and depression in an elderly population. Am J Psychiatry 137:439-444, 1980

Caine ED, Lyness JM, King DA et al. Clinical and etiological heterogeneity of mood disorders in elderly patients, in *Diagnosis and Treatment of Depression in Late Life: Results of the NIH Consensus Development Conference.* Edited by LS Schneider, CF Reynolds, BD Lebowitz, AJ Friedhoff, Washington DC,
American Psychiatric Press, 1994

Callahan CM, Hendrie HC, Tierney WT: Documentation and evaluation of cognitive impairment in elderly primary care patients. Ann Intern Med 122:422-429, 1995

Callahan CM, Tierney WM: Health services use and mortality among older primary care patients with alcoholism. J Am Geriatr Soc 43:1378-1383, 1995

Christenson R, Blazer D: Epidemiology of persecutory ideation in an elderly population in the community. Am J Psychiatry 141:1088-1091, 1984

Clark GB: Geriatric abuse -- out of the closet. J Tenn Med Assoc 77:470-471, 1984

Council on Aging: Position statement on elder abuse, neglect, and exploitation.
Am J Psychiatry 152: 820, 1995

Council on Scientific Affairs: Abuse and neglect.
JAMA 257:966-971, 1987

Council on Scientific Affairs: Alcoholism in the elderly.
JAMA 275:797-801, 1996

Cummings JL: Dementia: the failing brain. Lancet 345:1481-1485, 1995

Devanand DP, Levy SR: Neuroleptic treatment of agitation and psychosis in dementia. Journal of Geriatric Psychiatry and Neurology 8 (suppl 1): S18-27, 1995

Drinka JR, Smith JC, Drinka PJ: Correlates of depression and burden for informal caregivers of patients in a geriatric referral clinic. J Am Geriatr Soc 35: 522-525, 1987

Duffy JD, Coffey CE: Depression in Alzheimer's disease. Psych Annals 26:269-273, 1996

Emery VO, Oxman TE: Update on the dementia spectrum of depression. Am J Psychiatry 149: 305-317, 1992

Erikson E: *Childhood and Society*. New York, WW Norton, 1950

Erkinjuntti T, Wilkstrom J, Palo J, et al. Dementia among medical inpatients: evaluation of 2000 consecutive admissions. Arch Intern Med 146:1923-1926, 1986

Evans S, Katona C: Epidemiology of depressive symptoms in elderly primary care attenders. Dementia 4:327-333, 1993

Factor SA, Brown D, Molho ES, et al. Clozapine: a 2-year open trial in Parkinson's disease patients with psychosis. Neurology 44:544-546, 1994

Flint, AJ: Recent Developments in Geriatric Psychopharmacotherapy. Can J Psychiatry 39(8) Suppl 1:S9-18, 1994

Fogel BS, Gottlief GL, Furino A: in *Mental Health Policy for Older Americans-Protecting Minds At Risk*. Edited by Fogel BS, Gottlieb GL, Furino A. Washington, DC, American Psychiatric Press, 1990

Folstein MF, Bassett SS, Romanoski AJ, et al. The epidemiology of delirium in the community: the Eastern Baltimore Mental Health Survey. International Psychogeriatrics 3:169-176, 1991

Folstein MF, Folstein SE, McHugh PR: "Mini-Mental State": a practical method for grading the cognitive state of patients for the clinician. J Psychiatr Res 12: 189-198, 1975

Francis J, Kapoor WN: Prognosis after hospital discharge of older patients with delirium. J Am Geriatr Soc 40:601-606, 1992

Francis J, Martin D, Kapoor WN: A prospective study of delirium in hospitalized elderly. JAMA 263:1097-1101, 1990

Frankenburg FR, Kalunian D: Clozapine in the elderly. Journal of Geriatric Psychiatry and Neurology 7:129-132, 1994

Furino A, Fogel BS: The economic perspective, in *Mental Health Policy for Older Americans - Protecting Minds at Risk.* Edited by Fogel BS, Furino A, Gottlieb GL. Washington, DC, American Psychiatric Press, 1990

German PS, Shapiro S, Skinner EA, et al. Detection and management of mental health problems of older patients by primary care providers. JAMA 257:489-493, 1987

Gerson SC, Plotkin DA, Jarvik LF: Antidepressant drug studies, 1964 to 1986: empirical evidence for aging patients J Clin Psychopharmacology 8(5):311-322, 1988

Gillick MR, Serrell NA, Gillick LS: Adverse consequences of hospitalization in the elderly. Social Science and Medicine 16:1033-1038, 1982.

Goldstrum ID, Burns BJ, Kessler LG et al. Mental health services use by elderly adults in a primary care setting. J Gerontol 42:147-153, 1987

Gustafson Y, Berggren D, Brannstrom B et al: Acute confusional states in the elderly patients treated for femoral neck fracture. J Am Geriatr Soc 36:525-530, 1988

Harris MJ, Jeste DV: Late-onset schizophrenia: an overview. Schizophr Bull 14:39-55, 1988

Jeste DV, Eastham JH, Lacro JP, et al: Management of late-life psychosis. J Clin Psychiatry 57:(suppl 3):39-45. 1996

Jeste DV, Harris MJ, Krull A, et al. Clinical and neuropsychological characteristics of patients with late-onset schizophrenia. Am J Psychiatry 152: 722-730, 1995

Jorm AF, Korten AE, Henderson AS. The prevalence of dementia: a quantitative integration of the literature. Acta Psychiatr Scand 76:464-479, 1987

Katz IR, Curlik S, Nemetz P: Functional psychiatric disorders in the elderly, in *Essentials of Geriatric Psychiatry*. Edited by Lazarus LW. New York, Springer, 1988

Katzman R., Terry R: *The Neurology of Aging*. Philadelphia, F.A. Davis, 1983

Koenig HG, Meador KG, Shelp F, et al. Depressive disorders n hospitalized medically ill patients: a comparison of young and elderly men. J Am Geriatr Soc 39:881-890, 1991

Kuypers JA, Bengston VL: Social breakdown and competence: a model of normal aging. Human Development 16: 181-201, 1973

Lacro JP, Harris MJ, Jeste DV: Late life psychosis. Int J Geriatr Psychiat 8:49-57, 1993

Lake JT, Grossberg GT: Management of psychosis, agitation and other behavioral problems in Alzheimer's disease. Psych Annals 26:274-279, 1996

Leipzig RM, Saltz B: Adverse reactions to psychotropics in geriatric patients, in *Adverse Effects of Psychotropic Drugs*. Edited by Kane JM and Lieberman JA. Guilford, New York, 1992.

Levkoff SE, Cleary PD, Liptzin B, et al. Epidemiology of delirium: an overview of research issues and findings. International Psychogeriatrics 3:149-167, 1991

Lipowski ZJ: Delirium in the elderly patient. N Engl J Med 320:578-581, 1989

Lish JD, Zimmerman M, Farber NJ et al. Psychiatric screening in geriatric primary care: Should it be for depression alone? J Geriatr Psychiatry Neurol 8: 141-153, 1995

Mellinger GD, Balter MB, Uhlenhuth EH: Prevalence and correlates of the long-term regular use of anxiolytics. JAMA 251:375-379, 1984

National Institutes of Health Consensus Development Panel on Depression in Late Life: Diagnosis and treatment of depression in late life. JAMA 268:1018-1024, 1992

Nyth AL, Gottfries CG: The clinical efficacy of citalopram in treatment of emotional disturbances in dementia disorders. A Nordic multicentre study.
Br J Psychiatry 157:894-901, 1990

O'Malley SS, Croop RS, Wroblewski JM: Naltrexone in the treatment of alcohol dependence: a combined analysis of two trials. Psych Annals 25:681-688, 1995

O'Malley TA, Everitt DE, O'Malley HC, et al. Identifying and preventing family-mediated abuse and neglect of elderly persons. Ann Intern Med 99:998-1005, 1983

Olafson K, Jorgenson S, Jensen HV et al. Fluvoxamine in the treatment of demented elderly patients: a double-blind placebo-controlled study.
Acta Psychiatry Scan 85:453-456, 1992

Oxman TE, Barrett JE, Barrett J et al. Psychiatric symptoms in the elderly in a primary care practice. Gen Hosp Psychiatry 9: 167-173, 1987

Raheja RK, Bharwani I, Penetrante AE: Efficacy of risperidone for behavioral disorders in the elderly: a clinical observation.
Journal of Geriatric Psychiatry and Neurology 8:159-161, 1995

Rapp SR, Parisi SA, Walsh DA: Psychological dysfunction and physical health among elderly medical inpatients. J Consult Clin Psychol 56: 851-855, 1988

Regier DA, Boyd JH, Burke JD et al. One month prevalence of mental disorders in the United States. Arch Gen Psychiatry 45: 977-986, 1988

Reisberg B, Borenstein J , Salob SP, et al. Behavioral symptoms of Alzheimer's disease: Phenomenology and treatment. J Clin Psych 48 (Suppl):9-15, 1987

Reynolds CF, Schneider LS, Lebowitz BD, Kupfer DJ: Treatment of Depression in Elderly Patients: Guidelines for Primary Care in *Diagnosis and Treatment of Depression in Late Life* Results of the NIH Consensus Development conference. Edited by LS Schneider, CF Reynolds, BD Lebowitz, AJ Friedhoff, Washington DC,
American Psychiatric Press, 1994

Roose SP, Glassman AH, Attia E, Woodring S: Comparative efficacy of selective serotonin reuptake inhibitors and tricyclics in the treatment of melancholia.
Am J Psychiatry 151:1735-1739, 1994

Rovner BW, German PS, Broadhead J, et al. The prevalence and management of dementia and other psychiatric disorders in nursing homes. Int Psychogeriatr 1990:2:13-24

Sakauye K: Behavioral disturbances: pharmacologic therapies.
Psychiatric Annals 25:425-431, 1995

Salzman C: Pharmacological Treatment of Depression in Elderly Patients, in *Diagnosis and Treatment of Depression in Late Life* Results of the NIH Consensus development conference. Edited by LS Schneider, CF Reynolds, BD Lebowitz, AJ Friedhoff, Washington DC, American Psychiatric Press, 1994

Salzman C, Satlin A, Burrows AB: Geriatric Psychopharmacology, in *The American Psychiatric Press Textbook of Psychopharmacology*. Edited by Schatzberg AF, Nemeroff CB. Washington DC, American Psychiatric Press, 1995

Salzman C, Schneider LS, Alexopoulos GS: Pharmacological Treatment of Depression in Late Life, in *Psychopharmacology: The Fourth Generation of Progress*, Edited by FE Bloom, DJ Kupfer, Raven Press, New York, 1995

Schmidt R, Fazekas F, Offenbacher H et al. Neuropsychologic correlates of MRI white matter hyperintensities: a study of 150 normal volunteers. Neurology 43:2490-4, 1993

Schneider LS: Efficacy of treatment for geropsychiatric patients with severe mental illness. Psychopharmacology Bulletin 29(4):501-524, 1993

Schneider LS, Sobin P: Non-neuroleptic treatment of behavioral symptoms and agitation in Alzheimer's disease and other dementia. Psychopharmacol Bull 28:71-79,1992

Small GW, Fawzy FI: Psychiatric consultation for the medically ill elderly in the general hospital: need for a collaborative model of care. Psychosomatics 29:94-103, 1988

Spar J, Ford CV, Liston EH: Hospital treatment of elderly neuropsychiatric patients, II: statistical profile of the first 122 patients in a new teaching ward.
J Am Geriatr Soc 28:539-543, 1980.

Spar JE, La Rue A: *Concise Guide to Geriatric Psychiatry*, Washington DC, American Psychiatric Press, 1990

Tariot PN, Schneider LS, Katz IR: Anticonvulsant and other non-neuroleptic treatment of agitation in dementia.
Journal of Geriatric Psychiatry and Neurology 8 (suppl 1): S28-39, 1995

U.S. Congress: *Elder Abuse: A National Disgrace: Report by the Subcommittee on Health and Long-Term Care of the Select Committee on Aging* (Committee Publication No. 99-502). U.S. House of Representative, 1985

U.S. Senate Special Committee of Aging: *Aging America -- Trends and Projections*. Washington, DC, U.S. Department of Health and Human Services 1987-1988

Vijg J, Wei JY: Understanding the biology of aging: The key to prevention and therapy J Am Geriatric Assoc 43:426-434, 1995

Wells CE: Pseudodementia. Am J Psychiatry 136: 895-900, 1979

World Health Organization: World Health Statistics: *Demographic Trends, Aging and Noncommunicable Disease*. Geneva, Switzerland, World Health Organization, 1992

Yates WR: The National Institute of Mental Health epidemiologic study: Implications for family practice. J Fam Pract 22:251-255, 1986

Ylikoski A, Erkinjuntti T, Raininko R et al. White matter hyperintensities on MRI in the neurologically nondiseased elderly. Analysis of cohorts of consecutive subjects aged 55 to 85 years living at home. Stroke 26:1171-7, 1995

Young RC, Klerman GL: Mania in late life: focus on age of onset.
Am J Psychiatry 149:867-876, 1992

Young RC, Meyers BS: Psychopharmacology, in *Comprehensive Review of Geriatric Psychiatry*. Edited by Sadavoy J, Lazarus LW, Jarvik LF. Washington, DC, American Psychiatric Press, 1991

8

AGGRESSIVE NUTRITIONAL PROGRAM FOR THE INSTITUTIONALIZED ALZHEIMER'S PATIENT[1]

Vincenta M. Leigh, M.S.N.

Assistant Clinical Professor of Psychiatry
University of California, San Francisco, and
Fresno Community Alzheimer's Living Center, and

A. Knudsen, R.D.
M.S. Franklin
A. Rauch
S. Leiby

Fresno Community Alzheimer's Living Center
Community Hospitals of Central California

INTRODUCTION

It is generally recognized that patients with Alzheimer's Disease (AD) lose weight during the course of the illness (Gray, 1989). Patients with AD weigh an average of 21% less than non-demented institutionalized geriatric patients (Singh et al., 1988). In addition to the memory problems associated with this devastating illness, there are changes in olfaction and eating habits that contribute to this weight loss. Patients with AD usually develop a preference for sweet and salty foods (Gray, 1989; Mungas et al., 1990). Energy requirements may be increased as much as 1600 kcal/ day with pacing and agitation. Patients lose their ability to use utensils, and may no longer recognize food or may just refuse to eat. They lose the ability to recognize hunger or thirst and certainly cannot communicate these needs. Others may forget how to chew or swallow. The nutritional consequences of these changes with Alzheimer's and multi-infarct dementia is an average weight loss of 5 kg/year (11 pounds) once the patients are institutionalized (Gray, 1989). In addition, they are at risk for dehydration and malnutrition (Sandman et al., 1987).

Institutionalized patients seem to be more severely affected than those living in the community (Burns et al., 1989) and body weight was significantly negatively correlated with

[1]Correspondence: Vincenta Leigh, MSN, Program coordinator, Intensive Outpatient Program, Mental Health Department, Kaiser Permanente Medical Center, 4785 North First Street, Fresno, CA 93726-0513

length of hospitalization. It is a management issue in nursing homes as the complications resulting from weight loss are costly to treat and often take more professional staff time. These complications range from increased infection rates and other medical problems, increased cognitive impairment, skin breakdown, physical deterioration and overall debilitation (Morris et al., 1989). In one study, malnutrition, manifested as low body weight, was present in 50% of the institutionalized, demented patients. These malnourished patients had four times as many infectious periods treated by antibiotics as patients with no malnutrition (Sandman et al., 1987). Furthermore, acute illness is a major cause of weight loss in the institutionalized elderly (Wright, 1993). In our clinical observations, we found that both physical and psychosocial stress (i.e, illness, admission) resulted in change in eating habit or food refusal resulting in weight loss. We decided to study the effectiveness of a multifaceted aggressive nutritional program to minimize weight loss in an Alzheimer facility.

SETTING AND METHODS

The setting was a 99 bed long term care facility for patients with Alzheimer's and related dementias. The facility was part of a larger medical center located in Fresno, California. Patients were admitted with symptoms that would be considered middle early-stage to terminal stage of the illness. Some patients required assistance with eating, some were independent and others were totally dependent on staff to feed them. Weight was monitored on the first day of each month on an electronic scale (Acme) by the same clinician for all the patients in the facility from February 1991 to February 1993. From February 1992 to February 1993, all of the patients who lived at the facility over the course of the entire year (72 patients) were included in this intervention study. Fifty-three of the patients were females, and 19 were males.

BASELINE PERIOD

Since the geriatric Alzheimer patient always needs nutritional monitoring and intervention, there was already a nutritional program in place at the facility from February 1991 to February 1992. The available options of this pre-existing program included:

1) Large or double portions of foods from established menus which met established nutritional guidelines for major and micro nutrient.

2) Between-meal or with-meal nourishments of liquid supplements supplying 1-1.5 Kcal/cc.

3) "Hidden Calories" - addition of melted margarine to hot foods supplying up to 400 Kcal/day.

4) Monthly weights and occasional weekly weights for those patients who were losing a significant amount of weight, initiated after the weight loss was discovered. A 5 pound loss or gain in one month was reported to the physician.

5) Between-meal snacks were offered to all patients, mid morning, mid afternoon and late evening.

Despite our best efforts, average weight loss per resident was 0.2 pounds from February 1991 to February 1992.

INTERVENTION

We launched an intense aggressive nutritional program from February 1992 to February 1993, increasing the amount and variety of food offered to patients, while expanding the time frame over which the food was provided. This was in addition to the pre-existing program. There were eight components of this new program:

1) "Early Bird" Continental Breakfast
At least ten patients /day took part in this optional early (6 a.m.) meal consisting of sweet rolls, Danish, donuts, diet cookies for diabetic diets, juices and milk and occasional fresh fruit. Average caloric intake was about 200-500 Kcal/day. This early morning meal was created after discussions with nursing staff who noted that there were some patients who were early risers, who walked around looking for something to do and who had a long wait before breakfast. None of the patients were coerced to eat this meal and all those who were up and about seemed to be pleased when offered food from this early bird cart.

2) Enhanced Breakfasts
Extra meat and fruit was added to the breakfasts. From our clinical observations, patients with AD seem to have a bigger appetite for breakfasts than for other meals. This segment began shortly after the aggressive nutritional program started.

3) Extra Mealtime Sweets
Approximately 40 patients a day received extra sweet items at the lunch and supper meals including extra desserts, puddings, ice cream and chocolate milk. Those patients who did not seem to get enough calories or who often did not eat all the food from their tray and liked sweets were offered this. Approximately 150-300 Kcal/tray.

4) Pureed Diets Enhanced
"Puree Appeal" was used to thicken pureed foods for visual pleasure and texture as well as to increase calorie/protein content of these diets. Approximately 120-240 Kcal/ day.

5) Between-Meal Nourishments
Reports came from nursing staff that only a few patients consumed the late evening snacks. This was reviewed, and it was found that many patients fell asleep for the night after supper and those that were up were too tired to eat. We eliminated the late evening snack and instead doubled the calorie content of the mid-afternoon snack which consisted of baked cakes, cookies, bar cookies and tarts as well as cold snacks including ice cream. Average 200-300 Kcal/day.

6) Sweetened Foods Program
Ten sugar packets were added to the tray and sprinkled over all the food as one would sprinkle salt and pepper. Ten patients were selected and participated in this part of the program. We were careful to exclude diabetics and to monitor blood sugar levels, as well as behavior. Over the years, we observed that most patients with AD love sweets. The biological mechanisms accounting for this is unclear, but it has been suggested that the craving for sweet food may be a significant part of the clinical syndrome of dementia (Mungas et al., 1990). In fact, very often our patients ate dessert first and then sampled the rest of the foods on the tray. Some ate desserts to the exclusion of other food. Those patients who had sugar sprinkled on all their food, ate a greater percentage of the protein and vegetables from the meal. Average 160 Kcal/ tray.

7) Weekly Weight on New Admission and Change in Status

We monitored weights more closely for at least one month after admission since this required a period of adjustment for the patient, and usual eating habits were disrupted. It is the time of getting to know the patient in whom significant weight loss could occur. Otherwise the weight loss could be overlooked until the patient becomes significantly thinner. Weekly weights were also ordered on any change in status - physical illness, emotional disruption or stress since this often resulted in food refusal, change in eating habit resulting in weight loss.

8) Using "Feeder Aides" During Key Hours

Two 8-hour nursing assistant positions were divided and turned into four 4-hour feeder aide positions. The main responsibilities of these staff were to assist the patients with meals. One was placed on days and helped with breakfast and lunch, and the others assisted with the evening meal, when general staffing was less, daily structure decreased and patients were more confused and"agitated".

RESULTS

Patients gained a mean increase of 3.472 pounds at the end of one year following the aggressive nutritional program, p =0.007. Forty-two patients gained weight, twenty-seven lost weight and three remained the same.

Weight Change for One Year

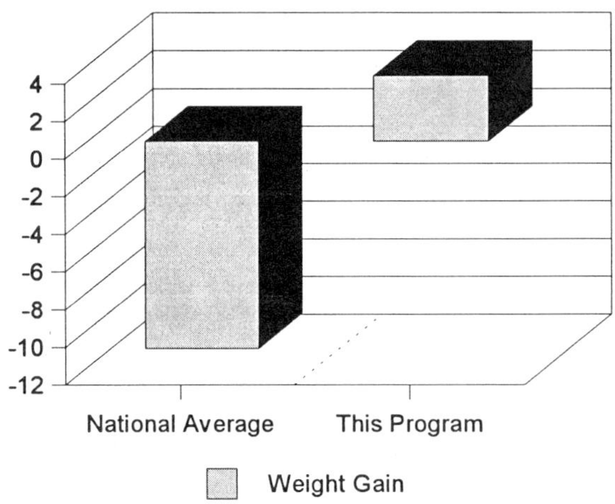

DISCUSSION

The national expected weight loss of 11 pounds per year for institutionalized patients with Alzheimer's and multi-infarct dementia dramatizes our remarkable results of over 3 pounds average weight gain. Remarkable, also, was the patients' response to this intervention. They loved the increased mealtimes and the wider variety of foods offered to them. They enjoyed their food. We found that the patients did not like the commercially prepared food supplements, which were expensive and were often thrown away because of refusal. Instead they loved the chocolate milk, ice cream, milk shakes, the "early bird" breakfast and the sweetened food. There was some concern, in our umbrella medical center, that the increase in sweets might cause more behavioral "incidents",- fights or altercations. A review of *incidents reports*, where patient fights, outbursts, falls, etc. are documented showed no change in this behavior over two years (from February 1991 to February 1993).

Patient infection rate from February 1992 to 1993 decreased by 19%, and continues to remain low. This might be the result of good nutritional status of the patients. However, other factors might have contributed to this, such as the virulence of the flu outbreaks that season.

This was a multi-level program that involved the cooperation of dietary, nursing services, and the administration. The program's cost of providing the wide variety of interventions offered, including high calorie, large portions, milkshake-type supplements, are offset by eliminating expensive, commercial, canned formulas. Administration's commitment to the program was crucial as the expenses wavered and then began to even out. The program's success was dependent on the commitment and good communication between nursing and dietary staff. There is unquestionably more work involved due to increased time in preparing and dispensing food as well as encouraging or assisting patients to eat it. Over time, problems occurred which necessitated some reevaluation and adjustment of the program. For example, when the dietary supervisor noticed an increased plate waste after the 6 am "early bird" continental breakfast, it was discovered that donuts were being left at the bedside of sleeping patients. This particular program had been intended for the approximately thirty people who were early risers and were up and about. Changes in the nursing staff had resulted in a misunderstanding of the reason for this early snack, calling for an inservice education. At another point, dietary staff discovered many of the sugar packets coming back to the kitchen. It turned out that some of the nursing staff were not aware of why the sugar packets were on the tray! Others said, "I thought too much sugar was not good for you." Ongoing staff inservice education by the director of staff development and the registered dietician was an essential part of its success and continuation.

This aggressive nutritional program was conceived to give the patients a more gratifying quality of life at mealtime. Patients' verbal responses as well as big smiles told us that we had accomplished this goal.

SUMMARY

Weight loss in the institutionalized geriatric patient with Alzheimer's Disease is a major factor in rapid decline, increased medical problems, physical deterioration and overall debilitation of these patients. Malnutrition is a common complication of Alzheimer's, and weight loss of 11 pounds per year is considered average in the United States. Minimizing patients' weight loss becomes a treatment challenge in nursing home care. Weight loss in a 99 bed Alzheimer facility with an existing nutritional program was monitored over the course of a year. There was an average weight loss of 0.2 pounds per patient. Then, we launched an intense, aggressive nutritional program over the following year, increasing the amount and variety of food offered to patients, while expanding the time frame over which the food was provided. There were 8 components of this program: 1) early bird continental breakfast; 2) enhanced breakfasts; 3) extra mealtime sweets; 4) enhanced pureed diets; 5) increased variety of between-meal nourishments; 6) sweetened foods program; 7) closer monitoring of weight upon admission and upon any significant change in status; 8) using "feeder aides" during key hours. Results: Our patients gained an average of 3.472 pounds following this intervention over the study period. They responded positively to the increased mealtimes and the wide variety of food choices offered, therefore, improving the quality of life provided to them by the facility.

REFERENCES

Burns A, Marsh A, Bender D: Dietary intake and clinical, anthropometric and biochemical indices of malnutrition in elderly demented patients and non-demented subjects Psychological Medicine 19:383-391, 1989

Gray GE: Nutrition and dementia Journal of American Dietary Association 89:1795-1802, 1989

Morris CH, Hope RA, Fairburn CG: Eating habits in dementia British Journal of Psychiatry 154:801-806, 1989

Mungas D, Cooper JK, Weiler PG, Gietzen D, Franzi C, Bernick C: Dietary preference for sweet foods in patients with dementia Journal of American Geriatric Society 38:999-1007, 1990

Sandman PO, Adolfsson R, Nygren C, Hallmans G, Winblad B: Nutritional status and dietary intake in institutionalized patients with Alzheimer's disease and multiinfarct dementia Journal of American Geriatric Society 35:31-38, 1987

Singh S, Mulley GP, Losowsky MS: Why are Alzheimer patients thin? Age and Ageing 17:21-28, 1988

Wright BA: Weight loss and weight gain in a nursing home: A prospective study Geriatric Nursing 14:156-159, 1993

9

THE EXPANDED BIOPSYCHOSOCIAL MODEL IN CHILD PSYCHIATRY

David A. Fox, M.D.[1]

Associate Clinical Professor of Psychiatry
University of California, San Francisco
Fresno, California

INTRODUCTION

George Engel's biopsychosocial model {BPSM} (1977, 1980) of medical evaluation and treatment has provided a clear and comprehensible picture of the clinical encounter. Medical students and residents in primary care, instead of approaching psychiatric issues with "fear and loathing", delight in the diagrammatic approach of a non-reductionistic system. The BPSM is readily applicable to the domain of child psychiatry and pediatrics. The model lends itself well to multivariate research on a variety of childhood illnesses and diseases. Thoughtful investigations in childhood asthma, juvenile chronic arthritis, and eating disorders have drawn on the BPSM as an organizing principle (Miller and Wood, 1991; Miller and Wood, 1994; Vandvik et al . 1991; Vandvik and Eckblad, 1991; Vandvik and Hoyeraal, 1993; Conners and Morse. 1993). In the realm of clinical practice, the BPSM becomes an informal guide to the "Willie Sutton principle" (going where the money is), in the choice of interventions. This strategy is highly useful in an era when the search for efficiency gets utmost priority.

Within child psychiatry the response to the BPSM has been slight. Two of the most prominent current textbooks (Rutter & Hersov, 1985; Lewis, 1991) and a current review of consultation-liaison psychiatry with children and adolescents (Lask, 1994) make no reference to the BPSM. The major journals in child psychiatry are similarly devoid of reference: the Journal of Child Psychology and Psychiatry has not a single citation between 1979 and 1992. The Journal of the American Academy of Child and Adolescent Psychiatry has only a single reference to the BPSM between 1989 and 1994 (Combrinck-Graham, 1990), and in this article there is no mention of George Engel.

---

[1]Correspondence: Department of Psychiatry, UCSF-Fresno, 2615 E. Clinton Ave, Fresno, CA 93703

Biopsychosocial Approaches in Primary Care: State of the Art and Challenges for the 21st Century, Edited by H. Leigh, Plenum Press, New York, 1997

The indifference to the BPSM within child psychiatry is in sharp contrast to the enthusiastic reception in journals of primary care, psychosomatic medicine, and consultation-liaison psychiatry (Burkett,1991; Elias et al, 1994; Eshet et al, 1993; Gallagher et al, 1990; Goldberg, 1992; Smith et al, 1993). Within the adult psychiatric literature there have been numerous thoughtful articles exploring clinical and political aspects of the model as well as offering theoretical extensions and modifications (Beigel, 1995; Gordon, 1992; Justice, 1994; Wise, 1993). I attribute some of this neglect by child psychiatrists to their sense that "what's new? we think this way all the time", and to the general isolation of child psychiatrists from adult psychiatry. It is striking, however, that heuristic models of similar degree of abstraction, such as Anna Freud's concept of developmental lines (1965), or Stella Chess's (1990) explorations of temperament have generated a wealth of clinical and research literature within child psychiatry.

The absence of an explicit developmental framework within the BPSM may explain part of this communication gap, although transaction analysis (Sameroff and Chandler, 1975) and path analysis (Rutter, 1989) provide strategies for addressing the intersection of temporal dimensions with biopsychosocial variables. Transactional analysis addresses the interplay between the environment and the developing child as a series of reciprocal influences resulting in permanent structural modifications in both child and environment. When transactional analysis is combined with the statistical methodology of path analysis, a temporal dimension is added to the BPSM. Interactions between hierarchical levels across time can then be conceptualized and investigated.

The analysis of influences on development has always been a central focus of investigation in child psychiatry. With growing attention to biological determinants of development, the question of bidirectional influences within a family system has acquired greater importance (Friedman and Downey, 1993; Matorin and Greenberg, 1992; Minde, 1994). In this respect the perspective of the BPSM is of great help, for instance, in defining research questions such as, "what family environment is optimal for a developing autistic child?" or "how do gender-specific patterns of abuse occur in children with attentional disorders?" The perspective of multiple non-reducible levels within the BPSM offers researchers a model for the investigation of the role of early experience in shaping intrapsychic structures, which will manifest themselves in later behavior (Hughes et al, 1991; Paris, 1994).

RECENT MODIFICATIONS OF THE BIOPSYCHOSOCIAL MODEL

Several other attempts at expansion and revision of the BPSM hold promise for increasing its relevance and applicability to child psychiatry. Jasnoski and his colleagues (1985, 1991) have proposed a synchronous systems model in which physical, physiological, psychological, and social systems are explicitly interconnected. Within each system, subspheres are arranged hierarchically, as in Engel's model. Jasnoski asserts that his synthesis of the BPSM and ecosystems model allows for more explicit consideration of exchanges of energy and information between domains. The concepts of synchrony and dysynchrony between spheres are described as models of health, adaptation, and disease. Negative feedback loops of energy and information between spheres provide stability, while positive feedback permits flexible integration of new inputs allowing for novel steady state adaptations.

Goodman (1991) has taken issue with the objectivist bias in Engel's approach and has dissected the "person" level in the BPSM into separate conceptual networks of physical data (behavior) and mental data (experience). His proposed organic unity theory addresses the non-interchangability of the two sets of data and avoids dualism and reductionism in the relationship between brain and mind. These considerations are of particular relevance to child psychiatry because of the importance of the development and maldevelopment of symbolic systems of representation and expression.

Sadler and Hulgus (1990, 1992) have proposed adding ethical and pragmatic aspects of medicine to what they call the epistemic aspect of the BPSM. They note that the actual practice of medicine extends beyond the "knowing" aspect of diagnosis and clinical intervention, and must include a consideration of the value systems of each of the participants and principles for translating understanding into effective action in a complex environment. This reformulation provides the crucial link between the conceptual framework of the BPSM and the current political-financial climate of medicine in the United States. Sadler and Hulgus assert that for the practicing clinician, awareness of his or her own value hierarchies as well as those of others in the system is essential for both analysis and effective action.

The ethics and pragmatics of clinical medicine are in fact the greatest challenges of the current health care environment. In the remainder of this paper I will elaborate on these challenges, with special application to child psychiatry, and will suggest the role of the BPSM and George Engel's contributions as particularly helpful in the current system crisis.

IMPACT OF THE CURRENT HEALTH CARE REVOLUTION ON CHILD PSYCHIATRY

In the past five years the pace of change in health care systems in the United States has been dramatic. During this period the proportion of "externally regulated" transactions between patient and health care provider has grown from less than 25% to over 60%. Rapid shifts of control, corporate mergers, and the capitalization of medical enterprises (Schreter, 1993) have occurred at ten times the speed of the English Industrial Revolution. As in the eighteenth century, the threatened change of identity for the physician from independent artisan to managed factory worker has been fiercely resisted. In addition to the confusion and distress caused by the rapidity of change, there have been specific outcomes for patient and health care provider as a consequence of the values and procedures of the new systems, whether described as Health Maintenance Organizations or Managed Care Organizations (Lazarus, 1994).

The most dramatic of these changes is the loss of autonomy of the patient/physician dyad. Whereas previously there was an acknowledgment that external factors, ranging from geographic to political, social, and financial, needed to be considered in clinical decision-making, the decisions themselves were seen as under the control of the dyad. Clinicians experience this shift as a loss of potency and self-esteem, with corresponding demoralization, shared negative identification with patients as victims, and loss of creativity. Alternatively, aggressive responses by psychiatrists directed at managed care reviewers temporarily improve the psychiatrist's self-esteem, but have little impact on policy.

Specific restrictions on diagnosis and treatment have produced formidable obstacles within clinical child psychiatry. Many developmental disorders, including attention deficit disorder and conduct disorder are excluded from treatment. Chronic disorders and "behavior disorders", frequently defined capriciously, are excluded. Specific modalities of treatment are required or excluded, in the absence of clinical justification, such as treatment only being authorized if medication is given, or family therapy being non-reimbursable. Standards of care appropriate to adult patients are applied indiscriminately to child and adolescent patients. The ideology of "crisis resolution", particularly inappropriate for many child psychiatric disorders, has become a method of restricting interventions to three or four visits.

Child psychiatrists, in some instances, have been restricted to consultations and medication management. Long-term treatment relationships have frequently been disrupted.

The shift from a three-party (psychiatrist-patient-family) relationship to a four-party relationship, including the managed care reviewer, has created new ethical conflicts. There have been attempts at restriction of freedom of speech of the clinician (e.g. not to speak unfavorably of the managed care plan restrictions) and propositions such as individual case capitation which produce direct conflicts between the interests of patient and therapist. A resulting atmosphere of mistrust among all four parties has been highly anti-therapeutic. Generally, managed care reviewers present the perception that clinicians are self-serving, either for individual greed or the preservation of institutional systems (hospitals, clinics, academic departments). Psychiatrists have had difficulty in differentiating between responsible and corrupt managed care entities.

Case Examples

S.R. is a bright, artistic 17 year old who had become depressed and oppositional in the midst of interminable parental conflict. He was barely managing to get through school and was losing enthusiasm for long-sustained interests. His long-term therapeutic relationship with a psychiatrist was interrupted by the managed care company, who insisted that he been seen by a social worker. The preexisting therapeutic relationship was later restored at the insistence of the patient who became depressed enough to warrant medication.

C.G. is a 14 y.o. diabetic admitted to a psychiatric unit following a suicide attempt with insulin. The patient and family were willing to seek help; the managed care company was unwilling to pay for hospitalization if the patient's status was converted from involuntary to voluntary, despite the fact that state law required a voluntary status to be offered.

A.B. is a 15 year old with a history of two years of drug use. Shortly after his admission for substance abuse treatment it was discovered that the patient and his family were fighting as a means to avoid grieving over his brother's unexpected death from leukemia, after surviving osteogenic sarcoma. The representative of his insurance carrier insisted that, because his policy only covers substance abuse treatment, other family issues central to his treatment not be addressed during hospitalization.

S.C. is a 16 year old with extensive acting out behavior and rage at her father which developed after she learned that she had been conceived while her father was still married to his first wife. Despite attempts at family therapy, the patient remained too angry to return home. Placement was arranged with her aunt while she and her parents were to undertake out-patient individual and family therapy. The managed care company was unwilling to cover therapy by an out-of-area provider (in the aunt's city of residence) in order to facilitate the patient's return home. After six weeks the patient resumed her drug use and was re-hospitalized.

D.W. is an 8 year old exposed to abuse and neglect while in custody of her substance abusing and psychotic mother. She exhibited explosive tantrums and severe oppositional and aggressive behavior. Her insurance carrier excluded her from psychotherapy because of a concomitant diagnosis of ADHD.

System Hierarchy of Physician-Patient Relationship

Conceptual Network of Physical Terms (Patient)	Conceptual Network of Mental Terms	Conceptual Network of Physical Terms (Doctor)
biosphere		biosphere
society-nation		society-nation
culture-subculture		culture-subculture
community		community
financial-economic		**financial-economic**
family		family
two person	**experience of self and other in dyad**	two person
(self experience)	**-------------------**	**(self experience)**
observable person		**observable person**
organ systems (including nervous system)		organ systems (including nervous system)
organs		organs
tissues		tissues
cells		cells
organelles		organelles
molecules		molecules
atoms		atoms
subatomic particles		subatomic particles

THE EXPANDED BPSM AS A WORKING MODEL FOR CURRENT CLINICAL PRACTICE

The current climate of the health care system in the United States has lead to a rude awakening for the participants. The invalidation of previous practices has resulted in a heightened consciousness of system influences. It is as if the fish, who had been blissfully unaware of their watery surroundings, became painfully conscious as the water became too hot and too polluted with toxins. The "protected space" of the clinical encounter has been invaded. But awareness of the impact of economic and political systems is only part of the necessary response to these changes. The other part can be found in Engel's writings on the BPSM, and in particular his 1992 clinical and autobiographical essay, in which he describes his own evolution in the practice of medicine.

Engel's clinical writings convey an extraordinary sense of human relatedness and intuitive understanding. He states (1992), "the requirement to be human in order to be scientific is evident at many levels." It is his understanding of himself as a person, his relinquishment of invulnerability, and his reaching out which create the genuine clinical encounter. In allying and aligning himself with his patient, Engel creates a shared space, and indirectly, a shared context of experience. Implicit in this work is the assumption that the contact of patient and clinician is much more than the interpersonal dyad, with its accompanying transference and countertransference manifestations. Instead, it is the entire biopsychosocial reality of *both* participants which becomes relevant to their mutual understanding. Self-awareness by the clinician of his or her own values, perceptions, and representations of multiple system levels accompanied by a dialogue which makes explicit the patient's values, perceptions, and representations is thus a prerequisite for effective clinical action. The accompanying diagram of an expanded BPSM outlines the elements potentially addressed in this dialogue. Levels of the BPSM closest to the dyadic interaction are addressed initially.

Like all developmental processes the equilibration to the new model requires a decentering on the part of the clinician, and a recognition that the "splendid isolation" of the consulting room is a self-defeating illusion. The resulting narcissistic loss is more than compensated by the increased power of the clinical model. The value of the expanded BPSM becomes a guide to interventions, locating the appropriate system level from the physician side of the matrix from which resources must be drawn for effective actions.

Case Example

A.V., a mildly retarded 15 year old male, with pickwickian syndrome and congestive heart failure, became combative when hospitalization was recommended because of increasing edema, secondary to non-compliance with medication and diet. A.V. comes from a family of multiple children with developmental disabilities and acting out behaviors. He has a history of depression and aggressive outbursts following previous placement. His mother has been unable to set limits with him because of her chronic depression, in part related to her unresolved loss of patient's twin at birth, which she has attributed to abduction by hospital staff. A.V. was terrified of hospitals and distraught about separation from his family. The hospital staff expressed hopelessness about the possibility of effective intervention, and requested psychiatric hospitalization for the patient.

After first establishing that this intervention was not only financially unrealistic, but also likely to be detrimental to the patient and family, I initiated a systems analysis. While the patient's congestive heart failure was being treated, I helped the hospital staff coordinate multiple system levels of intervention. The nursing and dietary staff simplified diet and medication regimes to be congruent with the patient's cognitive level and the family's organizational skills. I engaged a neighbor and her family of six children to provide ongoing supervision and support. Social service staff obtained supportive funding for the neighbor to assist. I initiated an educational assessment to assist the patient's return to school, and the hospital psychologist alerted the school system to the patient's requirements. The patient and family were given an opportunity to "self-manage" while still in the hospital and demonstrate their competence. Social service staff assisted the mother in locating the hospital records of the patient's and twin's births and in working through her grief. The hospital staff and family established rewards for the patient for achieving goals. During this clinical process, staff perceptions of the patient and family changed dramatically for the better, and there was general enthusiasm when the patient could be discharged in time to attend the wedding of his runaway sixteen year old sister.

As can be seen in this case example, both patient and physician are embedded within a biopsychosocial matrix. The crucial step in generating effective change is the self-awareness of the physician (and ultimately of the patient) of the possibilities and limitations inherent in the matrix as it impacts on shared goals. Rather than the clinical encounter representing a conflict between individual and institutional values, the patient-physician dyad remains the center of energy and locus of action. Financial or managed care restrictions are placed in the proper context as one of many challenges within the matrix.

The discomfort and malaise caused by the disequilibration of the current health care system can in fact be a stimulus for the development and incorporation of this new clinical model, in which the social, economic, and political realities of patient and clinician become not distractions from the clinical process, but an integral part of understanding and action. The expanded BPSM provides a conceptual framework for the human miracle of medicine.

REFERENCES

Beigel, A., 1995, A proposed vision of psychatry at the turn of the century.
Comprehensive Psychiatry 36:31-39.

Burkett, G., 1991, Culture, illness, and the biopsychosocial model.
Family Medicine 23:287-291.

Chess, S., 1990, Studies in temperament: a paradigm of psychosocial research.
Yale J. Biology and Medicine 63:313-324.

Combrinck-Graham, L., 1990, Developments in family systems theory and research.
J. Am Acad. Child Adolesc. Psychiatry 29:501-512.

Connors, M. and Morse, W., 1993, Sexual abuse and eating disorders: a review.
International J. Eating Disorders 13:1-11.

Elias, M. et al. 1994, Adolescent health promotion and risk reduction: cementing the social contract between pediatricians and the schools.
Bull. N.Y. Acad. Medicine 71:87-110.

Engel, G., 1977, The need for a new medical model: a challenge for biomedicine.
Science 196:129-136.

Engel, G., 1980, The clinical application of the biopsychosocial model.
Am. J. Psychiatry 137:535-544.

Engel, G., 1992, How much longer must medicine's science be bound by a seventeenth century world view?
Psychother. Psychosom. 57:3-17.

Eshet, I. et al. 1993, SFAT-AM: short family therapy in ambulatory medicine. Treatment apporach in 10-15 minute encounters.
Family Practice 10:178-187.

Friedman, R. and Downey, J., 1993, Neurobiology and sexual orientation: current relationships. J. Neuropsychiatry 5:131-153.

Freud, A., 1965, *Normality and Pathology in Childhood,*
New York, International Universities Press.

Gallagher, R. et al. 1990, The behavioral medicine service: an administrative model for biopsychosocial medical care, teaching, and research.
General Hospital Psychiatry 12:283-295.

Goldberg, R. et al. 1992, The recognition and management of somatization: what is needed in primary care training.
Psychosomatics 33:55-61.

Goodman, A., 1991, Organic unity theory: the mind-body problem revisited.
Am. J. Psychiatry 148:553-563.

Gordon, J., 1992, Holistic medicine and mental heatlh practice: toward a new synthesis.
Amer. J. Orthopsychiat. 60:357-370.

Hughes, J. et al. 1991, Medical, family, and scholastic conditions in urban delinquents
J. Clin. Psychology 47:448-464.

Jasnoski, M. and Schwartz, G., 1985, A synchronous systems model for health.
American Behavioral Scientist 28:468-485.

Jasnoski, M. and Warner, R., 1991, Graduate and post-graduate medical education with the synchronous systems model.
Behavioral Science 36:253-273.

Justice, B., 1994, Critical life events and the onset of illness.
Comprehensive Therapy 20:232-238.

Lask, B., 1994, Paediatric liaison work. *In:* Rutter, M. et al. *Child and adolescent psychiatry, 3rd edition.*
Oxford: Blackwell Scientific Publications.

Lazarus, A., 1994, A proposal for psychiatric collaboration in managed care.
Am. J. Psychotherapy 48:600-609

Lewis, M., ed., 1991, "Child and Adolescent Psychiatry".
Williams and Wilkins, Baltimore.

Matorin, S. and Greenberg, L., 1992, Family therapy in the treatment of adolescents.
Hosp. Comm. Psychiatry 43:625-629.

Miller, B. and Wood, B., 1991, Childhood asthma in interaction with family, school, and peer systems: a developmental model for primary care.
J. Asthma 28:405-414.

Miller, B. and Wood, B., 1994, Psychophysiologic reactivity in asthmatic children: a cholinergically mediated confluence of pathways.
J. Am Acad. Child Adolesc. Psychiatry 33:1236-1245.

Miller, W., 1992, Routine, ceremony, or drama: an exploratroy field study of the primary care clinical encounter.
J. Family Practice 34:289-296.

Minde, K., 1994, Future of child psychiatry: models and guiding principles.
Can. J. Psychiatry 39:321-325.

Paris, J., 1994, The etiology of borderline personality disorder: a biopsychosocial approach.
Psychiatry 57:316-325.

Rutter, M., 1989, Pathways from childhood to adult life.
J. Child Psychology and Psychiatry 30:23-52.

Rutter, M. and Hersov, L. (eds), 1987, *Child and Adolescent Psychiatry, 2nd Edition.*
Oxford: Blackwell Scientific Publications.

Sadler, J. and Hulgus, Y., 1990, Knowing, valuing, acting: clues to revising the biopsychosocial model.
Comprehensive Psychiatry 31:185-195.

Sadler, J. and Hulgus, Y., 1992, Clinical problem solving and the biopsychosocial model.
Am. J. Psychiatry 149:1315-1323.

Sameroff, A. and Chandler, M., 1975, Reproductive risk and the continuum of caretaking casualty. In: Horowitz, F. et al.(eds.) *Review of Child Development Research, Volume 4*
Chicago: University of Chicago Press.

Schreter, R., 1993, Ten trends in managed care and their impact on the biopsychosocial model.
Hospital Comm. Psychiatry 44:325-327.

Smith, G. et al. 1993, Consultation-liaison psychiatry in Australia.
General Hospital Psychiatry 15:121-124.

Vandvik, I. et al. 1991, Prediction of short term prognosis by biopsychosocial variables in pateints with juvenile rheumatic diseases.
J. Rheumatol. 18:125-132.

Vandvik, I. and Eckblad, G., 1991, Mothers of children with recent onset of rheumatic disease: associations between maternal distress, psychosocial variables, and the disease of the children.
Devel. Beh. Pediatrics 12:84-91.

Vandvik, I. and Hoyeraal, H., 1993, Juvenile chronic arthritis: a biobehavioral disease. Some unsolved questions.
Clin. Exp. Rheumatology 11:669-680.

Wise, T., 1993, Teaching psychosomatic medicine: utilizing concurrent perspectives.
Psychother. Psychosom. 53:99-106.

PART II. CHALLENGES FOR THE 21ST CENTURY

10

FROM BIOPSYCHOSOCIAL MODEL TO PATIENTOLOGY

Hoyle Leigh, M.D.[1]

Professor of Psychiatry
University of California, San Francisco, and
Fresno VA Medical Center

BIOPSYCHOSOCIAL MODEL : THE MUDDLE

George Engel coined the term, "biopsychosocial model" (1977), as an alternative to the prevailing disease model that he called the "biomedical model". While recognizing the contributions that the biomedical model made to the development of modern medicine, Engel objected to the "dogma" of biomedical model on the grounds that it is reductionistic, mechanistic, and dualistic. In its stead, Engel proposed the biopsychosocial model that takes into account the psychological and social variables as well as the biological in the experience of the patient of the disease, the *illness*. In addition, he also proposed that conditions of life constitute significant variables in *influencing a disease process*.

The biopsychosocial model has found wide acceptance among psychiatrists and medical educators, but has been criticized as being too time consuming (Joynt, 1980), and often not very practical (Sadler & Hulgus, 1990). There is evidence that medical students and residents clearly prefer the scientific elegance of the biomedical rather than biopsychosocial notions of illness (Silverman et al, 1983). What are the reasons that biopsychosocial model is seen to be more time consuming, less practical, and less appealing than the biomedical model?

I believe that the reasons include: (1) conceptual confusion about the role of grand-theories, particularly about the mind-body problem and the role of general systems theory in the model, (2) conceptual confusion about what the biopsychosocial model is a model of, leading to (3) conceptual confusion about whom the biopsychosocial model is for, and (4) a lack of an operational technique of applying the model crisply. In this essay, I shall discuss each of these problems and describe a more systematic operational approach in implementing a practical biopsychosocial model for the patient.

Engel's biopsychosocial model implicitly has two components, a model of the disease

---

[1]Correspondence: Department of Psychiatry, UCSF-Fresno, 2615 E. Clinton Ave, Fresno, CA 93703

and a model of the illness. Disease in this sense denotes the abnormality at the biological level, and illness is the distressing experience of the person together with the symptoms emanating from the disease (Feinstein, 1974; Leigh & Reiser, 1992). There has been much confusion because of the ambiguity concerning whether biopsychosocial model is a model of disease or of illness.

The theoretical underpinning of Engel's model is Bertalanffy's general systems theory (1968). General systems theory posits that the universe is made up of various levels of systems and subsystems, and each level interacts with other levels of organization. Therefore, disease processes in the cellular level are affected by processes in the person level events (psychological events), which are in turn affected by social events. Of course, the arrow of interaction in the other direction, i.e., cellular changes affecting psychological events is the familiar biomedical model.

Long before George Engel, Hippocrates wrote, " The visiting physician must consider the attitude, wind direction, purity of water supply, and the season of the year before making diagnosis. In order to cure the human body, it is necessary to have a knowledge of the whole of things". The idea that the personality system and the environment affect disease processes long antedates the advent of the biopsychosocial model. Wise physicians have always practiced a form of biopsychosocial model, whether it is called that or not. Psychosomatic medicine developed as a field of scientific enquiry concerning this interface between psychological states (personality system) and biologic pathogenesis. Consultation-liaison psychiatry evolved as a specialized area of the application of psychiatric concepts and skills in treating medical patients with emotional problems (Leigh & Reiser, 1977). Consultation-liaison psychiatrists have attempted to practice the biopsychosocial model in treating patients with varying degrees of success. For example, by emphasizing the personality dimension of the patient (such as the need for attention, splitting, idealization, etc) as requiring attention on its own, consultation-liaison psychiatrists have helped their medical colleagues manage difficult borderline patients, regardless of their disease.

While both psychosomatic medicine and consultation-liaison psychiatry contributed much to our understanding of the interface between the mind (personality system) and the body (biological system), I believe they also contributed to the conceptual confusion concerning the biopsychosocial model. George Engel, an internist and psychosomaticist, espoused a general systems interaction between the biological system and the personality system in all disease processes (1980), essentially an expansion of the psychosomatic concept in the tradition of Franz Alexander (1950). It should be noted, however, that psychosomatic concepts in the form of "psychological factors participating in the pathogenesis of a physical disease" apply only *for some but not all diseases*. Even in those diseases, understanding the psychological factors responsible does not necessarily result in an effective management plan. For example, even if it were true that conflicts over dependency needs and striving toward independence may play a role in the pathogenesis of peptic ulcer, the treatment of the ulcer is more efficacious through a course of antibiotics and histamine blockers, rather than the psychiatric remake of the personality which may take decades. And no psychological understanding or treatment would be more effective in a patient with ventricular fibrillation (even if it may be caused by anger and frustration mobilizing a fight/flight reaction resulting in circulatory changes causing myocardial infarction and electrical instability, as in the case of famous Mr. Glover[2]) than a defibrillator.

I call the notion that problems originating in the personality system can best be treated through a technique directed at that system *isodimensional fallacy*. In fact, general

---

[2]Engel, 1980

systems theory would predict that intervention at any dimension might be as efficacious as one in another dimension if one only knew how to do it effectively. It is in the area of prevention that identifying the origin of a problem finds the best use.

GENERAL SYSTEMS THEORY, QUANTUM THEORY, AND THE MIND-BODY PROBLEM

Is the general systems theory necessary for the biopsychosocial model, as Engel implies? It may be useful to consider which aspect of the biopsychosocial model requires general systems theory. One aspect of Engel's biopsychosocial model is that psychological factors affect a physical state. This is at the level of observation, hypothesis generation, and hypothesis testing. Just as the observation that the presence of lead in the environment is associated with certain neurologic conditions led to the determination of lead poisoning as a disease, so can a psychosomatic sequence be established without a grand theory. How about the notion that the subjective experience of illness must be considered together with disease? The concept of illness behavior (Mechanic, 1962) antedates Bertalanffy by six years.

Does the general systems theory necessarily debunk the "dogma" of the biomedical model? Engel argues that the biomedical model is reductionistic and dualistic. General systems theory does offer the concept of emergence. *Emergence* involves the notion that there are certain properties that characterize the system as a whole and which no system component has (Bunge, 1977); such properties cannot be predicted by studying the components alone. Many adherents of the biopsychosocial model believe that the mind (or the meaning system) is an emergent phenomenon, and therefore cannot be fully understood by studying the brain alone.

According to Sperry (1969, 1980), mental phenomena have dynamic emergent properties arising from cerebral excitation, which are different from and more than material brain processes. Once generated from neural events, the higher order mental patterns and programs are proposed to have their own subjective qualities and progress, operate and interact by their own causal laws that cannot be reduced to neurophysiology. Popper and Eccles (1977) maintain that mental processes are emergent relative to physical processes but believe in a dualism where the relationship of the brain to the body is that of computer to programmer, with the self-conscious mind playing a superior interpretive role. Suffice it to say that general systems theory does not necessarily lead to psychobiological monism. It should be obvious, also, that biomedical reductionism is not dualism. In fact, reductionism is, in a true sense, always monistic.

Mind-body identity theory, historically formulated by Spinoza, Leibnitz, Russell, and others, has gained considerable acceptance. This theory postulates that the nature of an event (or phenomenon) is neither mental nor physical, but the event referred to by any given mental term is identical to the event referred to by some physical term. It is the way of experiencing conceptualizing, and describing it that belongs to one or the other of the mind-body dichotomy. Goodman (1991) proposed the organic unity theory as a synthesis of the biopsychosocial model and the mind-body identity theory by describing corresponding general systems equivalent levels between the "conceptual network of physical terms (e.g, atoms-organ-nervous system-person behavior-society)" and the "conceptual network of mental terms (e.g. person experience). According to this theory, each event involved in the etiology, pathogenesis, symptoms, and treatment of disorders is both biological and psychological.

What is the nature of awareness in psychophysical unity? Software written by binary language is both patterns of magnetic or optical properties as well as information, as defined with the interacting entity (without interaction, no communication, and no information). How do these entities become interactional (communicational)? Such interaction may be inherent in nature, as matter and antimatter "know" to annihilate each other upon encounter. Psychological awareness, although a subset of communication (interaction), might arise as an emergent phenomenon in a complex system of lower level interactions. Perhaps, as a critical mass of uranium will start a chain reaction, a "critical mass" of "proto-awareness" might result in a series of events leading to what we call awareness. To the extent that humans can hardly guess at the experience of "awareness" of beings such as photons, electrons, or, for that matter, dogs and chimpanzees, a true description of others' awareness may be an impossible task. Nevertheless, whether mental or physical, it appears to me that information is exchanged at all levels of organization in the cosmos.

Modern quantum theory presents us some intriguing notions of the mind. Quantum mechanics places the conscious observer at the center of reality. It is a quantum theory maxim that "No phenomenon is a phenomenon unless it is an observed (or recorded - resulting in some irreversible change) phenomenon". Until observation has occurred, reality exists only as potentials or probabilistic waves. At the instant of observation, however, the wave function collapses into a reality according to the orthodox Copenhagen interpretation (Bohr, 1958), or the universe splits into a number of possible universes according to the many worlds hypothesis (Everett,1973; Wolf, 1988). Consciousness, though arising as a result of brain processes, may be regarded as a cosmic process of creation (as the choices it makes are not locally determined but cosmically inherent) that produces events or reality (Stapp, 1993). Such events, or the observation-induced collapse of the wave function into particles, seem to supercede the barriers of space-time. Einstein proposed an experiment which tried to show what he considered to be a failing in quantum theory: Suppose two particles arising from an interaction are flying apart at the speed of light. According to quantum theory, if one quality of the particle is observed at a later time (say, particular spin - left), at one place by observer A, another observer B, observing the other particle (say, 20 light years away from observer A) must observe the complementary quality that is being observed by A. As it is purely by chance that A would observe the spin of "left", until the moment of observation of A, the spin of B is indeterminate. But once A is observed, B's spin can be nothing but "right", which Einstein considered to be "spooky action at a distance" at speeds faster than light (The Einstein-Podolsky-Rosen Paradox, 1935). Later reformulation of the EPR experiment (Bell's Inequality, 1964) that was carried out by Aspect (1982) proved the quantum theory predictions over Einstein's objections. It should be pointed out, however, that the quantum theory predictions do not presuppose "communication faster than light". It simply shows a cosmic connectedness or unity beyond spacetime separation. One way of looking at this is to consider the two particles not to be separate at all, but a part of a whole (a single wave). Some consider the universe to be a single wave.

The conscious mind may be equated with the universal creative process that invents new realities de novo through the collapse of the wave function that selects one reality out of many potential realities, or through the participation in the one universe among many other universes in the many worlds interpretation of quantum mechanics. In the latter, of course, there would be individual consciousnesses in each of the many universes that would be aware of the realities of the split-off universe. In any case, modern quantum theory revives the notion of the "free will" as an important player in our realities. In playing a role as to when and how observation is done, free will (or an illusion thereof) influences the way reality occurs (wave function collapses), or it may choose (for this time) the universe in which awareness occurs among the many possible universes at any juncture of its exercise.

In this regard, it may be useful to ponder about the role of the *observing physician* in the diagnosis and treatment of disease, and in patient care. What is the role of a patient's *will to live*, that may arise out of an interaction between the patient and the physician and/or the family and friends? The practice of medicine may truly be a creative process. The interaction between the physician and the patient creates new paths of reality for both participants.

It may be that epistemology is inevitably reduced to psychology or linguistics for the only way for humans to "know" is through the "mind" and to communicate the knowledge is through language (Gregory,1988). Perhaps, for humans, knowledge has to begin with the notion that "mind" is inherent in all things, just as the history of an intimate contact with photons and/or energy is inherent for any object that exists in a photograph.

At a more practical level, a systems concept that is useful in medical practice is the distinction between the matter-energy processing system and the information processing system. In a computer, the former represents the hardware, the latter the software. In humans, the body is the matter-energy processing system; the mind, the information processing system. Of course, there is great overlap between the systems - each system is made of the same "stuff", obeys the same physical laws, and, indeed, some hardware in computers are also information processing components, and in humans, DNA's are certainly both packets of chemicals as well as information, just as the magnetism on a computer disk is both a physical property as well as packets of information. Diagnosing which system is awry is an important step in repairing the problem.

Then, what about the notion of emergence? Emergence would be an important subject of research if we can show that certain degrees of complexity or kinds of interaction of components predictably produces "emergent" phenomena, as might be the case with the famed computer program, "life". If this term were to be used to attempt to close the door to investigating the components of a phenomenon (reductionistic research), it would find scientific company with the words, "divine" and "sacred".

LEVELS OF ORGANIZATION

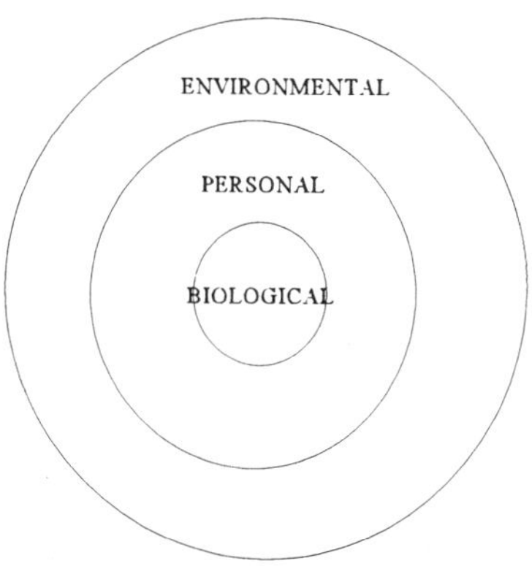

A GENERAL SYSTEMS ANALYSIS OF THE BIOPSYCHOSOCIAL MODEL: WHAT IS BIOPSYCHOSOCIAL MODEL A MODEL OF?

The term, biopsychosocial model, gave rise to much conceptual confusion because it failed to follow its own implicit basic thrust - levels of organization. Thus the model was at times used to indicate that psychosocial factors such as stress may participate in the pathogenesis of disease (biological level), and at other times to state that an understanding of the experience of the patient including sociocultural factors are important in his/her reaction to disease (person level). What is the biopsychosocial model a model of ?

Biopsychosocial approach in medicine can be used for three different entities - the disease, the illness, and the patient. A general biopsychosocial approach could be used for two additional entities - the person, and the society/environment.

Biopsychosocial Model of Disease

The crux of this model is the disease, the biological abnormality, which may be caused/influenced significantly by events occurring at a higher level, such as psychological conflicts (person level) and environmental stress (environmental level). This is the only biopsychosocial model that may seem to be in conflict with the reductionistic biomedical model in that the disease may not be completely understood by studying the subsystems alone. Nevertheless, if reductionistic studies can identify the subsystem changes (such as immunosuppression) associated with a more macrosystem change (such as stress), the conflict may be more apparent than real. This field is the subject matter of classical psychosomatic medicine. It is important to note that this model is *not necessarily useful for all diseases.* In fact, a major task for the investigator is to define the diseases and pathogenetic mechanisms for which the biopsychosocial model would be useful.

LEVEL SPECIFIC DYSFUNCTIONS

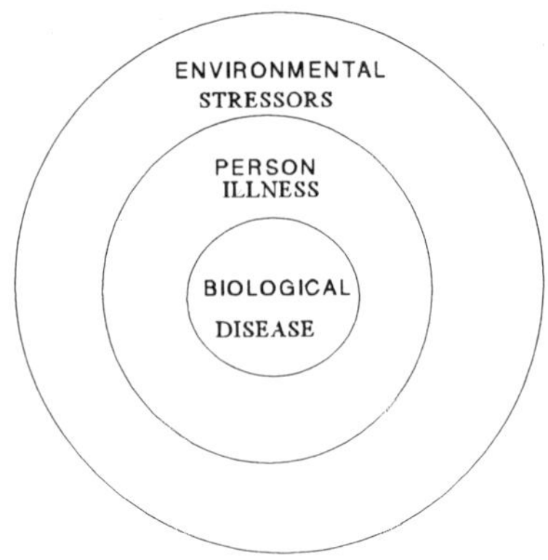

Biopsychosocial Model of Psychiatric Illness

The central point of this model is the illness or disorders at the level of the person. This includes abnormalities in behavior, mood, cognition and perception. These disorders, usually categorized as psychiatric or mental, are almost always a result of interactions among the three levels (dimensions) of the person - biological components, personal (psychological) level, and the environmental (social) level. Anxiety, depression, substance use problems, and psychosis are examples. The task of the investigator is to tease out the various pathways for illness in each of the levels and the patterns of interaction among levels.

Biopsychosocial Model of Patient

This is the biopsychosocial approach to the person who has one or more of the entities described in the previous two models - disease and illness. It is important to note that this is a model of a person, as opposed to the previous two models which are models of disorders. The main area of understanding for this model is the experience of the person who is the patient, given a disease and/or an illness.

THE PATIENT

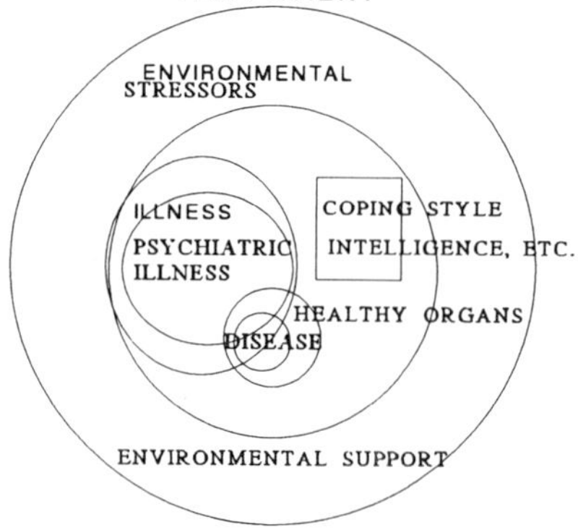

The main area of concern is *not* whether the disease or illness is biopsychosocial in pathogenesis, but what *is to be understood biopsychosocially* in better *understanding and managing the person* who is the patient. A whole gamut of concepts now become relevant in this approach, including the patient's cultural background and expectations, habitual ways of dealing with pain and stress, personality and coping styles, intelligence, genetic endowments for resilience, etc. Successful management of any patient may hinge on a successful application of this model.

Non-medical Extensions of the Biopsychosocial Model: Person and Society
Biopsychosocial approaches can be used for a comprehensive understanding of normal events such as the person and the society. As an understanding of normal physiology is essential in understanding pathology and pathophysiology, a biopsychosocial understanding of the normal person and society, which might be represented in the broad fields of psychology and sociology, would greatly enrich the science and practice of psychiatry and medicine (Schwartz, 1982).

WHAT IS THE BIOPSYCHOSOCIAL MODEL FOR ?

Who should use biopsychosocial model at what level? Engel proposed the biopsychosocial model as a reaction to the biomedical model that he considered to be dehumanizing. He argued, "Medicine's crisis stems from the logical inference that since 'disease' is defined in terms of somatic parameters, physicians need not be concerned with psychosocial issues which lie outside medicine's responsibility and authority". He states, "...one authority urged that medicine concentrate on the 'real' diseases and not get lost in the psychosociological underbrush" (Engel, 1977). Engel, therefore, seems to have expanded the notion of 'disease' in his biopsychosocial model to include all disorders, from cellular diseases to psychiatric illness to (probably) social ills.

I have concluded, in the above section, that the biopsychosocial model has varying degrees of usefulness depending on whether it is a model of disease, illness, or the patient. This analysis is also helpful in defining the scope of the physician's role regarding each level of organization.

The biopsychosocial model of *disease* calls for the diagnosis and treatment of the somatic conditions underlying the illness (or distress). At this level, the biomedical model has had excellent success, and the biopsychosocial model is a complement to the biomedical model to the extent that environmental and symbolic factors may be contributing to the pathogenesis and/or maintenance of the biological disorder. The primary care physician plays the role of the primary diagnostician and treater, with the essential participation of the medical scientist. The medical specialist functions as consultant and referral resource. *The biopsychosocial model of disease, then, is primarily for the student of psychosomatic medicine.*

The biopsychosocial model of *psychiatric illness* calls for the diagnosis and treatment of the disorder (or psychiatric syndrome) that is almost always a final common pathway phenomenon primarily resulting in an experience of distress at the person level, which is determined by known and/or suspected factors in the biological, psychological, and environmental dimensions. At this level, the primary care physician plays an essential role in the recognition of the disorder and initial diagnosis and treatment or referral. The physician with expertise in biopsychosocial analysis and treatment of these disorders, the psychiatrist, plays the role of consultant and specialist. *The biopsychosocial model of psychiatric illness, then, is for the psychiatrist and the primary care physician.*

The biopsychosocial model of *patient* calls for an understanding of the person who is the patient and the experience of the person with the disease or psychiatric illness. An understanding of the patient's personality needs, his/her strengths as well as vulnerabilities in all biological, psychological, and environmental dimensions, and a formulation of a management approach that will be efficacious and acceptable both to the patient, family, and the medical care establishment, are important aspects of this model. This model, then, encompasses what has been called *the art of medicine*, but it is far more comprehensive than that. It strives to develop a systematic approach to the patient, a science for the art of medicine. Biopsychosocial model, advocated as a pragmatic pluralism of sciences (Sadler & Hulgus, 1990), is most applicable at this level. The primary care physician, the front-line clinical practitioner who tends to treat patients longitudinally, often including family members, almost by default utilize some aspects of this model. The challenge is how to systematize it so that the practice of this model is no longer a haphazard creation of art but a systematically learned skill. The psychiatrist, as an expert in biopsychosocial analysis and integration, would play a consulting role at this level.
The biopsychosocial model of the patient, then, is primarily for the primary care physician and the psychiatrist.

OPERATIONALIZING THE BIOPSYCHOSOCIAL MODEL

In spite of the apparent popularity of the term, biopsychosocial, there is little evidence that the advent of the model has had much impact in the practice of medicine. Even in psychiatry, there is controversy as to how useful the biopsychosocial model actually is (Fink, 1988). The diagnostic and statistical manual (DSM) of the American Psychiatric Association since its third edition clearly adopted the multidimensional approach of the biopsychosocial model in diagnostics. Nevertheless, the "axes" of the DSM often seem incoherent to our medical colleagues (Leigh et al, 1982). Axis I and II are psychiatric disorders, Axis III is medical disorder, and Axis IV and V are not disorders at all but stressors and levels of functioning. A much more coherent approach would be to specify disorders in the biological, psychological, and social dimensions as implied by the biopsychosocial model.

Another reason the biopsychosocial model has not achieved much practical use has to do with the conceptual confusion already mentioned, i.e., what it is a model of. Biopsychosocial model of the disease has only limited application, whereas that of the psychiatric illness and the patient are necessary part of clinical practice.

As long as biopsychosocial model remains a purely conceptual desideratum, it is unlikely to be useful in medical practice, especially with the present-day emphasis on efficiency. The usefulness of the model may nevertheless be demonstrated in terms of patient satisfaction and efficacy of management if the model of the patient could be operationalized in such a way that it could be used easily in busy clinical practice.

Defining the level of the biopsychosocial approach as being the person level is the first step in operationalizing the model. Leigh, Feinstein, and Reiser developed an operational technique for the model at the person level, which they call *The Patient Evaluation Grid* (Leigh, Feinstein, & Reiser, 1980; Leigh & Reiser, 1992). The Patient Evaluation Grid (PEG) consists of the three dimensions (levels) of the patient (biological, personal, and environmental) intersected by three time contexts (current, recent, and background). The nine squares formed by this grid represent the areas of investigation and understanding for the whole patient.

The Patient Evaluation Grid has been computerized (Leigh, 1994) - a clinician can input into a database the items requested by the computer, then the computer will print out

THE PATIENT EVALUATION GRID (PEG)

	CURRENT CONTEXT	RECENT CONTEXT	BACKGROUND CONTEXT
BIOLOGICAL DIMENSION	PHYSICAL EXAM, LAB DATA CURRENT SYMPTOMS & SIGNS	ONSET OF SYMPTOMS, SIGNS, LAB TESTS, CHANGES IN PHYSICAL STATUS	CONSTITUTION, GENETIC ENDOWMENT, EARLY DISEASES
PERSONAL DIMENSION	MENTAL STATUS, CURRENT MOOD, CURRENT EXPECTATIONS	PRESENT ILLNESS, CHANGES IN MOOD, ADAPTATION TO ILLNESS	COPING STYLES, PERSONALITY, INTELLIGENCE, EDUCATION
ENVIRONMENTAL DIMENSION	SIGNIFICANT OTHER, SUPPORTIVE FIGURES, STRESSORS, PHYSICAL ENVIRONMENT	LIFE CHANGES, STRESSORS, CONTACT WITH HEALTH CARE SYSTEM	CULTURAL HERITAGE, EARLY FAMILY ENVIRONMENT

PATIENT EVALUATION GRID - MANAGEMENT FORM

	IMMEDIATE MANAGEMENT	LONG-TERM MANAGEMENT
BIOLOGICAL DIMENSION	TREATMENT OF DISEASE DRUG Rx OF DISTRESS (E.G. ANXIETY)	CHANGE IN DIET, PROPHYLACTIC DRUGS, ETC.
PERSONAL DIMENSION	PSYCHOTHERAPY OF DISTRESS, RELAXATION TECHNIQUES, EDUCATION, EXPLANATION	HEALTH PROMOTION MEASURES (E.G. EXERCISE, RELAXATION, HABIT CONTROL, ETC.)
ENVIRONMENTAL DIMENSION	HOSPITALIZATION, FAMILY EDUCATION, SOCIAL SUPPORT, VACATION, ENVIRONMENTAL CHANGE	ENHANCING SOCIAL SUPPORT, FURTHER EDUCATION, ENVIRONMENTAL CHANGE

both a narrative summary and a PEG[3]. On the basis of the PEG, the clinician can then generate a biopsychosocial management form in the same format. This leads to a truly operationalized biopsychosocial practice of medicine for the patient.

PATIENTOLOGY: TOWARD AN INTEGRATIVE STUDY OF THE PATIENT

A cursory perusal of the Patient Evaluation Grid would show that the state of our systematic understanding is the highest in the biological dimension, followed by those items in the personal dimension, with the environmental dimension factors being least systematically understood. Furthermore, attempting to find relevant literature and information in each dimension to construct a PEG is often a frustrating affair because much of the information assigned to the psychological and environmental dimension are not readily available to the primary physician.

An important task for medical science is to develop a systematic method of integrating and relating information in all of the three dimensions of the patient for optimal diagnosis and

[3] This software is available from the author directly. For inquiries, write to Hoyle Leigh, MD, Department of Psychiatry, UCSF-Fresno, 2615 E. Clinton Ave, Fresno, CA 93703

management of the illness and disease. I believe that this integration would be best achieved through the development of an interdisciplinary discipline within medicine that might be called *patientology* (Leigh, 1980, 1981). Such a discipline would encompass within it consultation-liaison psychiatry, psychosomatic medicine, medical psychology, health psychology, medical sociology, medical social work, clinical nutrition, epidemiology, clinical diagnosis, medical anthropology, and even esthetics. The purpose of this discipline would be to integrate new information arising from dimension-specific disciplines (e.g., molecular biology and sociology) so that the information can be used in helping the patient, and to generate new questions concerning interdimensional relationships and influences. This integrative approach would not be an alternative to the reductionistic approach of the biomedical model, but a true complement to it. In teaching the physician how to best help the patient, patientology should be omnivorous and atheoretical, pluralistic and pragmatic-optimizing what is best of the science and art of medicine.

CONCLUSIONS

Biopsychosocial model as proposed by Engel suffers from conceptual confusion because of unnecessary grand-theorizing and lack of sharp focus on what it is a model of, and for whom it is useful. General systems theory is not essential for biopsychosocial model but provides potentially useful concepts such as levels of organization and "emergence". Quantum theory provides insights about the central role of consciousness and observation in the creation of reality as well as of cosmic connectedness. Biopsychosocial model is not an alternative to the biomedical model but a complement to it, with varying degrees of usefulness depending upon at what level it is focused. Biopsychosocial model of *disease* is of limited usefulness, while that of *psychiatric illness* and of *the patient* are indispensable for the primary care physician and the psychiatrist. For optimal patient care, biopsychosocial approaches at the person level should be systematized, operationalized, and computerized. The Patient Evaluation Grid, presented in this paper, is one such attempt.

I propose the designation of a new field of medicine, which I call *patientology*, that integrates knowledge and skills in the three dimensions of the patient. Patientology will make essential contributions in making medical science more comprehensive, medical practice more efficient *and* gratifying, and consumers more satisfied. In patientology, the art of medicine would find union with the science of medicine.

REFERENCES

Alexander F: *Psychosomatic Medicine*, Norton, New York, 1950

Aspect A, Dalibard J, Roger G: Experimental test of Bell's inequalities using time-varying analyzers
Physical Review Letters 49:1804, 1982

Bell JS: On the Einstein-Podolsky-Rosen paradox
Physics Vol 1, 1964

Bohr N: *Atomic Physics and Human Knowledge*
Wiley, New York, 1958

Bunge M: Emergence and the mind.
Neuroscience 2:501-509, 1977

Einstein A, Podolsky B, Rosen N: Can the quantum mechanical description of physical reality be considered complete?
Physiological Reviews 47:777, 1935

Engel GL: The need for a new medical model: a challenge for biomedicine
Science 196:129-136, 1977

Engel GL: The clinical application of the biopsychosocial model.
American Journal of Psychiatry 137:535-544, 1980

Everett III H: The theory of the universal wave function, in DeWitt B, Graham N (eds): *The Many Worlds Interpretation of Quantum Mechanics*
Princeton University Press, Princeton, 1973, pp 3-140

Feinstein AR: *Clinical Judgment*
Huntington, New York, Robert E Krieger Publishing Co, 1974

Fink PJ: Response to the presidential address: Is "biopsychosocial" the psychiatric shibboleth?
American Journal of Psychiatry 145:1061-1067, 1988

Goodman A: Organic unity theory: The mind-body problem revisited
American Journal of Psychiatry 148:553-563, 1991

Gregory B: *Inventing Reality: Physics As Language*
John Wiley & Sons, New York, 1988

Joynt RJ: Introduction to the challenge of the biopsychosocial model
Psychosomatic Medicine 42:77, 1980 (supplement)

Leigh H, Feinstein AR, Reiser MF: The Patient Evaluation Grid: A Systematic Approach to Comprehensive Care
General Hospital Psychiatry. 2:3-9, 1980.

Leigh H, Reiser MF: *The Patient: Biological, Psychological, and Social Dimensions of Medical Practice, 3rd Edition*
Plenum Publishing Company, New York, 1992

Leigh H: Doctors, Patients, and Medicine (Editorial).
Archives of Internal Medicine 140:1277, 1980.

Leigh H: "Patientology" Exists (letter)
Archives of Internal Medicine 141:1101, 1981.

Leigh H, Price L, Ciarcia J, Mirassou MM: DSM III and Consultation-Liaison Psychiatry: Toward a Comprehensive Medical Model of the Patient.
General Hospital Psychiatry. 4:283-289, 1982.

Leigh H, Reiser MF: Major Trends in Psychosomatic Medicine:

The Psychiatrist's Evolving Role in Medicine.
Annals of Internal Medicine. 87:233-239, 1977.

Mechanic D: The concept of illness behavior
Journal of Chronic Disease 15:189-194, 1962

Popper KR, Eccles JC: *The Self and Its Brain - An Argument for Interactionism*
Springer International, Berlin, 1980

Sadler JZ, Hulgus YF: Knowing, valuing, acting: Clues to revising the biopsychosocial model
Comprehensive Psychiatry 31:185-195, 1990

Schwartz, GE: Testing the biopsychosocial model: The ultimate challenge facing behavioral medicine?
Journal of Consulting & Clinical Psychology 50:1040-1053, 1982

Schwartz MA, Wiggins O: Science, humanism, and the nature of medical practice: a phenomenological view
Perspectives in Biology and Medicine 28:331-361, 1985

Schwartz MA, Wiggins OP: Systems and the structuring of meaning: contributions to a biopsychosocial medicine
American Journal of Psychiatry 143:1213-1221, 1986

Silverman D, Gartrell N, Aronson, M, et al: In search of the biopsychosocial perspective: An experiment with beginning medical students
American Journal of Psychiatry 140:1154-1158, 1983

Sperry RW: the modified concept of consciousness
Psychological Review 76:532-536, 1969

Sperry RW: Mind-brain interactionism; mentalism,yes;dualism,no.
Neuroscience 5:195-206, 1980

Stapp HP: *Mind, Matter and Quantum Mechanics*
Springer Verlag, Berlin, 1993

von Bertalanffy L: *General Systems Theory*
George Braziller, New York, 1968

Wolf FA: *Parallel Universes*
Simon & Schuster, New York, 1988

11

TEACHING PSYCHIATRY TO PRIMARY CARE PHYSICIANS

Don R. Lipsitt, M.D.[1]

Clinical Professor of Psychiatry
Harvard Medical School
Chairman, Department of Psychiatry
Mount Auburn Hospital

INTRODUCTION

In another five years, psychiatry will have had approximately a one-hundred year history of trying to reintegrate physical medicine with psychological medicine. If one were to graph the course of this history, one would quickly see the oscillations that Freedman[1] called the "to and fro" of trends in psychiatry toward medicalization, demedicalization and remedicalization. In almost a century of persevering efforts, we have come not very far in achieving the objective of teaching nonpsychiatrist physicians to synthesize psyche-medicine and soma-medicine. The first part of this chapter will examine some of the many efforts which have been made over time to overcome the barriers to biopsychosocial practice. The second part will offer some speculative reasons for their degree of success or failure.

1. ATTEMPTS TO BRIDGE THE GAP

It is a rare physician who will deny the impact of stress and emotional factors on the existence and course of physical illness. Yet this acknowledgment is made more a promise than a real practical application to patients seen in the physician's office. The literature abounds with references to the continuing failure of physicians to recognize affect in the doctor-patient relationship, to diagnose or treat bona fide psychiatric illness, let alone a wide variety of subsyndromal states requiring attention to emotional issues in the patient's life.[2-4] While physicians attest to the prevalence of somatization in their practices, they generally continue to treat presenting physical complaints as though they have a pathophysiological basis.

---

[1]Correspondence: Department of Psychiatry, Mount Auburn Hospital, 330 Mount Auburn Street, Cambridge, MA 02238

1.1 Freud's Early Attempt

How do we explain this state of affairs? Have all of the attempts to bridge the gap been flawed or is there something inherently oppositional to the integrating of psychological medicine? One is reminded of Freud's earliest attempts to explain emotional disorders through scientific knowledge of the nervous system of his day. Although his Scientific Project exhibited brilliant insights in this effort, he ultimately abandoned the effort because of what he considered the impossibility of the venture, ultimately inventing an entirely new theory of emotional life which could be accessed through the technique of psychoanalysis; curiously, he never abandoned the belief that one day there would be biochemical and physical explanations for the conditions he treated in his office.

Perhaps it is these impressive achievements in neuroscience and biological psychiatry which have now diminished interest and curiosity in the nature and effects of those psychosocial factors which they have sought to explain.

1.1.1 Psychoanalytic and Psychosomatic Efforts

Between the first and second world wars, American psychiatry was strongly influenced by a wave of psychoanalysis and psychosomatic medicine.[5] Relatively large numbers of psychiatrists and psychoanalysts, many of whom had studied with Freud, sought refuge and freedom in the United States. New ideas about the etiology of some physical illnesses were creative and perhaps even fanciful. The term "psychosomatic" was embraced by the professional as well as lay communities as a description of some conditions whose onset seemed clearly related to emotional trauma as well as some which seemed mysterious in their origins. Unfortunately, the term itself was not only embraced, but also at times promiscuously and pejoratively used to describe someone who seemed a bit on the fringe of acceptable illness behavior. Negative attitudes towards emotional illness continue today in the use of words like "supratentorial," "psychological overlay," or "difficult patient."

1.1.1 General Hospital Psychiatry

Prior to the second world war, general physicians remained fairly dubious about psychoanalysis and psychosomatic medicine. But the war infused a new respect for psychiatry into what otherwise seemed magical and elusive. Psychiatrists in the war worked side-by-side with nonpsychiatrists who were able to witness first-hand the impressive results of psychiatric and psychoanalytic interventions, especially with traumatized soldiers who could quickly be returned to active duty after brief psychiatric treatment. The public was also newly informed of the widespread emotional disability which kept many recruits from entering military service. After the war was over, psychiatry had gained a level of prestige not previously seen. Many generalists sought postwar training in psychiatry through continuing education in what was described as office psychiatry. Government and other resources for training, education and treatment reached a new zenith in the history of psychiatry. All of this gave a great boost to the development of general hospital psychiatry and consultation-liaison services, although they had modest beginnings in the late 1920's and throughout the 1930's.[6]

1.1 Courses in "Office Psychiatry"

A course called "Psychotherapeutic Medicine,"[7] considered a model of such courses, was taught in two weeks in 1946 at the University of Minnesota. The introduction to the course stated that the general physician had always had his share of depressed and anxious patients presented in a wide variety of physical complaints, but "it took the war and its psychiatric casualties to spotlight their need." It was said of this experience that "it challenged the doctors' ability to hold the two aspects of medicine in balance." Although this course was said to have enhanced the attitude of physician-participants toward the importance of physician-patient relationships and the impact of emotional factors on disease, there were no follow-up data or outcome studies to substantiate the results. In the intervening fifty years, many such courses have been offered, some with attempts at measurement of results, but for the most part with disappointing findings, in that most physicians continue to show low levels of recognition and diagnosis and poor therapeutic outcomes.

1.1 Consultation-Liaison Psychiatry

Another venue of rapprochement between psychiatry and medicine existed in the development of consultation-liaison psychiatry[8]. It was felt that the important teaching arm of this psychiatric subspecialty (i.e., liaison) would provide the thrust required to train scores of medical students, house officers and attending physicians in the importance of a holistic approach to the patient. For many years, liaison was provided without concern for a source of financial support, but as this aspect became more urgent, the focus shifted considerably to only the reimbursable aspect of psychiatric collaboration, namely the consultation itself. The tradition of unpaid voluntary teaching by psychiatrists in clinical settings of general hospitals has become virtually a thing of the past. And although psychiatrists working in general hospital settings appear to have won a degree of respect and prestige, the pressures of modern medicine have seemingly encouraged their use in consultation as more operational and less pedagogical. That is, psychiatrists are asked for consultations to help hasten treatment and disposition of patients rather than for the inherent educational benefits of such interaction. In 1982, Dr. Steven Cole and colleagues[9] reported that training in liaison and consultation both improved physicians' knowledge of psychiatric and psychosocial factors in medical treatment, but that structured teaching with skills rehearsal is much more effective for improving skills and changing physician behaviors.

In Cole's review of the literature[10], there were 67 reports since 1970 of educational programs for primary care physicians, but only 22 attempted to evaluate the impact of such training and half of those showed no impact at all. In spite of the demonstration of improved knowledge and skills in psychosocial medicine with longitudinal training on consultation-liaison services, few primary care residency training programs in the U.S. have this as a formal part of postgraduate education.

1.1 The Primary Care Movement

The 1970's saw the first wave of the "primary care movement," which, once again, seemed to promise a new opportunity for psychiatry to have a pivotal teaching role with nonpsychiatrist physicians.[11] However, many family practices and primary care training programs turned toward nonpsychiatrist mental health professionals because of economic restrictions and, very likely, increased competition amongst physicians for patients. Experience with community health centers had also incorrectly taught physicians that there was no difference between different mental health disciplines, that psychologists and social workers could provide the same interventions as psychiatrists. George Engel,[12] who had made the word "biopsychosocial" virtually a household word, said disappointedly in 1979 that "as long as physicians are imbued with the reductionism and dualism of western science, there is no way in which the conflict between psychiatry and the rest of medicine can be resolved."

1.1.1 Balint Groups

In the past several decades, another important but relatively unrecognized means of teaching psychiatry and psychosomatic medicine to primary care physicians has quietly taken place in what are known as Balint Groups.[13] An innovation of Michael Balint, a Hungarian (and later English) psychoanalyst, practicing physicians would meet in non-therapy groups on a regular basis to present and discuss cases from everyday practice that posed a challenge to the treating physician. The process of discussion would elicit emotional aspects of the patient's presenting complaint as well as attitudes, reactions and behavioral responses in the physician. Such groups, embraced early on by family practice residencies, offered a continuous (sometimes for years) exposure of participants to the emotional repercussions of both patient and physician in their efforts to find solutions to the patients' presenting problems. Over time, much seemed to be learned about aspects of transference and counter transference that would influence outcome of treatment. Although Balint insisted that the purpose of such groups was not individually therapeutic, he did acknowledge that changes would occur over time that were the equivalent of what one might expect in treatment.

Balint groups appear to be enjoying an upsurge in popularity amongst physicians. The relatively small numbers of self-selected physicians who participate and the paucity of outcome studies, however, continue to limit the educational impact of this sophisticated approach to teaching psychiatric principles of medical practice.

1.1.1 Managed Care Movement

The latest phase of medical care which has influenced the opportunities for teaching psychiatry to primary care physicians is the "managed care movement." Because of the economic restraints exerted by this approach to health care delivery, most educators feel that it has had a pernicious effect on all of medical education and perhaps most especially on mental health aspects. Because days in hospital have been drastically reduced and approved treatments have been curtailed, the opportunities for the expression of free-flowing curiosity and for leisurely absorption of new information and knowledge have been markedly diminished. Critics of managed care decry the "bottom line" mentality which values economics over education and perhaps even over quality of care. Instead of encouraging a broader understanding of ways in which mental health and physical health intersect, managed care appears to give priority to indices like patient satisfaction and the rapidity with which physicians process their patients, whether in hospital or private office.

An attitude of "nothing extra" would appear to discourage efforts at learning how to attend to psychosocial factors in medical practice. However, there may be a saving grace in that primary care physicians (PCP), now assigned the role of "gatekeeper" for a patient's total care, may find that their own income will depend upon more cost-effective treatment and this may be a powerful incentive to learn more about the emotional aspects of medical care. Indeed, to encourage the primary care physician to incorporate awareness of mental health in medical practice, many agencies including the American Psychiatric and Medical Associations, Primary Care groups, and even pharmaceutical companies have devised screening measures and treatment guidelines that can easily be adapted to the current style of office practice.

A special set of guidelines and protocols for the primary care physician is based on the new classification DSM-IV[14], to make it more compatible with the kinds of patients seen in the general physician's office. And Upjohn[15] and Pfizer[16] have each designed a computer-assisted questionnaire which promises to help the primary care physician detect mental illness and to know when to treat and when to refer. Whether this "cookbook" approach to integrating psyche and soma in medical practice is more effective than previous efforts remains to be seen. It will be some time before relevant outcome studies will be available upon which assessment can be based.

1. DUALISTIC ROOTS

In the meantime, we might ask whether any of these approaches can result in a truly "integrated" biopsychosocial or psychosomatic medicine or is there some inherent rejection of this notion in organized medicine? Those who take the negative view repeatedly allude to the heritage of Descartes and attribute medicine's deficit to his dualistic philosophy of mind and body.[17] Others, however, believe that Descartes has taken a bad rap, that he was not only not this dogmatic but that this is mere scapegoating for some more pervasive and unrelenting problem in medical education.[18]

1.1. Separation of Psyche and Soma

Winnicott,[19] in a paper on the positive and negative aspects of psycho-somatic medicine, suggested that there was some deep-seated resistance embodied in most individuals--and this of course includes physicians--which set itself against a synthesis of psyche and soma. In certain instances, he suggested, cataclysmic events were apt to result from too urgent attempts to combine the two. Although he did not at the time know of the concept of alexithymia, we know of clinical situations in which what we have sometimes alluded to as lack of psychological-mindedness has appeared to manifest itself in a lack of language for emotion. And we have also seen that such individuals cannot be coerced into thinking of their physical distress as rooted in emotional conflict.

With other individuals who may not be designated alexithymic, we have noted a rigid defensiveness against acknowledgment of psychological causes of a variety of physical complaints. The process of working through these defenses toward some better integration in the individual is often a long, painstaking, psychotherapeutic course. In situations where too zealous pursuit of emotion in patients who resist it has resulted in psychotic reaction, Winnicott's reference to cataclysmic consequences appears to be supported.

1.1. Differences in Biomedical and Biopsychosocial Models

It is easy to see that physicians who have been trained in a medical model which reinforces their own preference for physical explanations will not likely be very receptive to educational efforts that emphasize the importance of psychosocial factors in illness. Several authors have pointed out the inherent conflicts and tensions between a medical and a psychiatric model. Brown and Zinberg[20] called attention to the way in which the biomedical model requires affective distance and isolation to counteract the tension of physical intimacy inherent in the physical examination. Others have suggested that the focus on objectivity of the medical model (as contrasted with the subjectivity or intersubjectivity of the psychosocial model) intensifies distancing from the patient with subsequent numbing, alienation and isolation. Furthermore, nonpsychiatrist physicians are not trained to tolerate complicated, ambivalent, or difficult emotional behavior. The biomedical approach tends to teach physicians to think of patients as reservoirs of specific diseases rather than as highly complex biopsychosocial persons.

1.1.1. Competition with Technology

Another barrier to psychosomatic or biopsychosocial education is what one may call the "technological imperative." We know well the seductive appeal of technology, whether it is in the manufacture of military weapons, space exploration, or the wonders of the computer age. In our lifetime we have witnessed remarkable technological achievements, which are dazzling, awe-inspiring, rapid and usually very effective. Furthermore, they are highly visible, in contrast to "psychosocial issues" which are essentially invisible. Psychiatry and psychology are regarded as "soft" sciences, referred to by medical students as "touchy-feely," or "fuzzy." Such areas of inquiry cannot easily compete with the spectacle of MRI's, laser surgery, the gamma knife, or the discoveries of neuroscience.

1.1.1. Attitudes Towards Psychosocial Factors

Except for those interested in the neuroanatomy or neuroendocrinology of the central nervous system, many physicians see the mind as mysterious, complex, and even threatening. Attempts to explain behavior or emotion are often experienced by the listener as "too close to home" and therefore personally rejected; it is, in a sense, more comfortable to assess illness in a non-personal, dehumanized, concrete way. There are very few studies that have examined attitudes toward psychosocial aspects of primary care, but they reveal some interesting findings. One study[21] demonstrated that physicians with positive attitudes towards psychosocial factors used more statements of emotion (like empathy and reassurance) in their communication with patients, and their patients more actively participated in their care by asking questions or expressing opinions.

In a medical world where "hard" science and technology are revered, it is difficult for students to express their interest in the "soft" areas of medicine. In spite of psychiatry clubs and other support groups for students interested in the social sciences, medical school does not foster curiosity about the "artful" side of medicine. Psychiatry is often ridiculed in sophomore plays and in general conversation so that there may be a tendency for interested students to disguise their curiosity. Furthermore, students selected for medical school admission often have majored in such subjects as biochemistry, genetics, and other so-called hard sciences. In addition, even those students who had majored in more humanistic studies are said, in four years of medical school, to become hardened, cold and cynical. Webster[22] has called attention to the ambivalent, compartmentalized thinking which characterizes many medical students and works against "integrating" psychosomatic concepts "into the deeper layers of (the) mind and into ... everyday clinical work." He believes that the essence of psychosomatic medicine could not be taught merely in courses or clinics but must be "woven into the overall design of the curriculum." While some medical schools have done much better along these lines by including courses on interviewing and communicating, as well as so-called humanistic topics, it would appear that turf wars of curriculum committees continue to deprive students of a more integrated experience in their medical school course.

1.1.1. Lack of Role Models

Another problem in medical school is the lack of sufficient role models for the kind of idealized medical practice that is espoused. Since most physicians are trained in the traditional medical model, this is the model which tends to be perpetuated. And especially in institutions which esteem scientific research above patient care there is likely to be a paucity of examples of the kind of physician who can enthusiastically teach a biopsychosocial perspective. Physicians who are action-oriented may not have an interest in the thought processes of patients; they may be more interested in what the patient **has** whereas the psychiatrist may be more interested in what the patient **says and does**. Furthermore, psychiatrists and internists respond differently to the chief presenting complaint, the psychiatrist using it to expand the patient's narrative and the internist using it to narrow down the options. When the physician is more wedded to his own agenda than to that of the patient, it is as though they speak entirely different languages.

The barriers to teaching a biopsychosocial model are not one-sided. It is not only nonpsychiatrist physicians who pose impediments. Psychiatrists themselves have contributed to this state of affairs by adopting a circumscribed mentalistic approach to all disease, by withdrawing from general medical settings, and perpetuating the "mystery" of their work by keeping themselves aloof from medical colleagues or by failing to communicate in comprehensible language the nature of their interventions. Some specialized pursuits by psychiatrists, such as psychoanalytic practice, have a tendency to isolate these physicians from the mainstream of medicine and thus to create wider gaps between the psyche and the soma. This is not to say that many psychoanalytically-trained psychiatrists are not heavily involved in medical school and hospital training programs.

1.1. Lack of Funding

Funding is another subtle factor in the way resources are assigned for the teaching of biopsychosocial medicine. Some department chairs, as finances become scarcer, are less inclined to assign time and personnel to other departments. And, of course, consultation-liaison psychiatry, as a matter of survival, has often had to curtail its teaching commitment because of a lack of reimbursement for services provided. These problems have intensified in the modern managed care context. Decreased hospital census, shorter lengths of stay, an emphasis upon cost-containment have all tended to diminish the use of psychiatric consultation and support. This means that house officers in training who already received very few hours of exposure to psychiatry in their entire training program, will now receive even less. There has been a noticeable shift, over the past several years, of requests for consultations from management and personality problems to questions of organic diagnosis, competency, and comorbidty. Furthermore, overburdened house officers, under pressure to discharge patients very quickly after initial workup, are disinclined to request additional interventions, lest they be reprimanded by their seniors for slowing down the process.

CONCLUSION: THE DILEMMA

It is difficult to know how these disparities between training in physical medicine and psychological medicine can be addressed. While undergraduate medical education has been greatly enhanced by the biopsychosocial teachings of educators like Leigh and Reiser[23,24] and others, it is not known to what extent these teachings influence the later attitudes and practice behavior of primary care physicians. Even in those who have been thus enlightened, it is likely that the new realities of medical practice strongly act against the application of the principles of comprehensive practice. Individual physicians, angry about changes in the health care system, are at risk to show less interest in their patients as people and this will severely affect how the patient-physician relationship influences the course of illness.

It can be hoped that economic incentives, if nothing else, will promote greater appreciation of how the biological and the psychosocial must interact in the best interests of the patient, as truly the most cost-effective and best quality of medical care which can be provided. If psychopharmacology and PET scans continue to displace interest in patients' feelings, behavior and emotional reactions, then the well-being of all patients will be in jeopardy. A powerful lesson has been learned from the astronaut physician recently returned from space travel saying that while much attention was paid to the science and physical effects of the mission, there appears to have been an unfortunate neglect of the importance of psychological factors in the expedition.

REFERENCES

1. Freedman DX: The search: Body, mind, and human purpose.
Am J Psychiatry 149: 858-866, 1992

2. Borus JF, Howes MJ, Devins NP, Rosenberg R, Livingston WW: Primary health care providers' recognition and diagnosis of mental disorders in their patients.
Gen Hosp Psychiatry 10: 317-321, 1988

3. Jencks SF: Recognition of mental distress and diagnosis of mental disorder in primary care.
JAMA 253: 1903-1907, 1985

4. Kessler LG, Amick BC, Thompson J: Factors influencing the diagnosis of mental disorder among primary care patients. Med Care 23: 50-62, 1985

5. Dunbar HF: *Emotions and Bodily Changes*. New York, Columbia Universities Press, 1935

6. Lipowski ZJ: Consultation-liaison psychiatry: the first half century.
Gen Hosp Psychiatry 8: 305-315, 1986

7. Witmer HL: *Teaching Psychotherapeutic Medicine*. New York, Commonwealth Fund, 1947

8. Kaufman MR: Role of the psychiatrist in the general hospital.
Psychiat Quart 27: 367-381, 1953

9. Cohen-Cole S, Bird J, Boker J et al. Psychiatric education for internists. A randomized controlled comparison of two teaching models. Psychosom Med 44: 122, 1982

10. Cohen-Cole S: Training outcome in liaison psychiatry: literature review and methodological proposals. Gen Hosp Psychiatry 2: 282-288, 1980

11. Lipsitt DR: Primary care: an "unrivaled opportunity for psychiatry"? (editorial)
Psychiatric Opinion 15:8, 1978

12. Engel GL: Resolving the conflict between medicine and psychiatry.
Res Staff Physician 26: 73-79, 1979

13. Luban-Plozza B: Empowerment techniques: from doctor-centered (Balint approach) to patient-centered discussion groups. Patient Educ and Counseling 26: 257-263, 1995

14. Broadhead WE, Leon AC, Weissman MM, et al. Development and validation of the SDDS-PC screen for multiple mental disorders in primary care. Arch Fam Med 4: 211-219, 1995

15. Spitzer RL, Williams JBW, Kroenke K, et al. Utility of a new procedure for diagnosing mental disorders in primary care; the PRIME-MD 1000 study. JAMA 272: 1749-1756, 1994

16. American Psychiatric Association: *Diagnostic and Statistical Manual of Mental Disorders, 4th ed., Primary Care (DSM-IV-PC)*. Washington, DC, American Psychiatric Press, Inc., 1995

17. Lipsitt DR: The influence of dualistic thinking on the role of psychiatry in medicine, in *General Hospital Psychiatry*. Edited by Lopez-Ibor Jr JJ, Saiz J, Lopez-Ibor JM. Amsterdam, Excerpta Medica, 1983, pp 18-24

18. Brown TM: Cartesian dualism and psychosomatics. Psychosomatics 30: 322-331, 1989

19. Winnicott DW: Psycho-somatic illness in its positive and negative aspects. Int J Psycho-Anal 47: 510-516, 1966

20. Brown HN, Zinberg NE: Difficulties in the integration of psychological and medical practices. Am J Psychiatry 139: 1576-1580, 1982

21. Levinson W, Roter D: Physicians' psychosocial beliefs correlate with their patient communication skills. J Gen Int Med 10: 375-379, 1995

22. Webster TG: Learning processes in physician education: integrating psyche and soma. Psychiat Med 2: 67-80, 1971

23. Leigh H, Reiser MF: Major trends in psychosomatic medicine. Ann Intern Med 87: 233-239, 1977

24. Leigh H, Reiser MF: *The Patient: Biological, Psychological, and Social Dimensions of Medical Practice*, 3rd ed. New York, Plenum, 1992

12

PSYCHOSOMATIC THINKING AS REFLECTED IN PRACTICE AND TEACHING OF PRIMARY HEALTH CARE - INTRODUCING THE SALUTOGENIC APPROACH[1]

In memoriam of Aaron Antonovsky

Benjamin Maoz, M.D., Ph.D.

Professor of Psychiatry
Ben-Gurion University of the Negev, Beer Sheva, and
Tel-Aviv University
Israel

Wolfram Schüffel, M.D.

Professor of Psychosomatic Medicine
Philipps University, Marburg
Germany

1. INTRODUCTION: Salutogenesis and Salutogenic Thinking as a Process

The symposium which was opened by an introductory paper by B. Maoz was dedicated to the late Aaron Antonovsky. Antonovsky was an outstanding sociologist of health in Israel with an international reputation. He developed the concept of salutogenesis, which means: Why do many people stay healthy? What are the inner and outer resources for this healthy coping? This question stands in contradiction to the question which is usually asked by physicians, namely why do people become sick?

One of the resources which enables human beings to remain healthy is a certain life style, a repertoire of states of mind, which Antonovsky (1987) called "sense of coherence" and which is composed of three components: comprehensibility, manageability and meaningfulness. This concept can fertilize our modern psychosomatic thinking in various ways: In the *practical* sphere of primary prevention it enables people to perceive tension-filled life situations either as neutral "noise" that can be ignored or neglected or as positive

[1]Proceedings of a Symposium at the 13th World Congress of Psychosomatic Medicine, held in Jerusalem, Israel, September, 1995. Correspondence to: Prof. Dr. W. Schüffel, Dept. Psychosom. Med., Centre of Internal Medicine, Philipps University of Marburg, D-35033 Marburg, Germany.

challenges for a new and creative development; and only if really necessary, as danger and stress. Even when there is a stress situation causing strain, many people will have the ability to perceive this situation with a strong and flexible sense of coherence and thereby mastering and controlling it. This concept can be broadened to secondary and tertiary prevention, which means early detection and treatment of disorders and the rehabilitation from diseases. Thus even when a person became already sick, one has to look for the still relatively healthy parts of the person and to encourage active coping. People who have developed a strong and flexible sense of coherence have the potential to be successful in this process.

A clinical example for the application of the salutogenic approach is coping with traumatic stress. It is known that after a massive disaster about 20% of the traumatized people will develop psychiatric symptoms that probably will need treatment. Antonovsky would have asked: Why do 80% of these traumatized people remain healthy, what gives them this strength? A salutogenic approach will tell us that certain interventions immediately after the disaster will increase the chances of more people coping actively and being able to master the traumatic experience and of not developing pathological symptoms. In the *theoretical* sphere Antonovsky's concept has enriched our psychosomatic thinking. In the 20th century the basic model of medicine became more and more one of bio-medical-technical reasoning, in a way, of *linear causality*: physical-chemical cause(s) produce pathological results and if one corrects or abolishes these causes one will cure the results. Psychosomatic medicine until World War II grew up in a paramedical area, using the (rather mechanistic) model of classical psychoanalysis and developed the hypothesis of specificity. This means that a certain specific subconscious and non-perceived conflict would cause a certain specific somatic disease.

During the last 30 years psychosomatic medicine has returned to the main stream of medicine by assimilating the bio-technical model with its *linear-reductional* causal thinking. By this it has contributed to the research of psychophysiology (especially psycho-biological stress research), brain research, research of eating disorders, sleep research, etc., and by gathering more accurate epidemiologic data especially in primary medicine. At the same time, concepts such as comorbidity were developed in which two or more independent circumscribed disorders, one somatic and one psychiatric, may be diagnosed at the same time in the same person. Slowly new models have emerged that could be integrated into psychosomatic medicine, like cybernetics, "fields", *open system hierarchies* with often complicated feedback mechanisms. Thus thinking in *circles and spirals and systems was accepted instead of linear lines*. Mutual relationships between two or more systems, e.g. between an organism and its internal and external environment, or in the inter-personal area particularly in the doctor patient relationship have become central issues. The individual is seen (again) in relation to his or her social-cultural background, as well in the present as in the past, in the light of one's personal biographical narrative. It became acceptable to perceive and understand medical problems in a multi-dimensional way, including psychosocial risk factors which are given equal validity as physical-chemical ones. Modern thermodynamic concepts were incorporated into medicine, conceptualizing, for example, chronic diseases as *unstable processes moving in one or more directions*, in which one can calculate at certain points only *probabilities and chances* for further developments. The salutogenic approach of Antonovsky should be seen in this frame of reference as another attempt to look at the facts and data from a new, until now neglected, angle which opens new possibilities.

Jochanan Benbassat elaborated on some of these points and discussed them in more depth in his paper entitled "Changes in Clinical Reasoning During the Past 40 Years". Benbassat described the dominant bio-medical paradigm of medicine which will be changed "only when it can no longer accommodate new facts or data". This bio-medical paradigm "reduced all diseases to a structural or biochemical dysfunction of the human body...causes were perceived as leading inevitably, rather than probabilistically, to their consequences, and chance and ambiguity had a very small role.... This attitude downplayed the importance of psychosocial factors in diseases and encouraged a deterministic reasoning...every disease has a *single* cause...." The main orientation was on outcomes.

In the frame of psychosomatic medicine this *bio-medical* model shifted gradually to the *bio-psycho-social* model; the orientation on outcomes shifted to an orientation on *processes*. Clinical judgment shifted from deductive, deterministic reasoning to inductive, probabilistic thinking. Disease is seen as "a result from a combination of etiological factors... there has been a growing acceptance of psycho-social factors of diseases and...there has been an increasing awareness of the confounding effect of false-positive and false-negative test results.... Terms such as risk indicators of disease, predictive values of tests and risk-benefit ratio are increasingly used."

Guidelines for medical diagnoses and treatments were developed in order to minimize medical errors, and not in order to reduce creative thinking, intuition and inspiration. The importance of these guidelines was also discussed by other speakers (see below). It is well recognized that many important medical inventions were the result of a single case report which could be generalized and reduplicated. As medicine becomes more probabilistic and less absolutistic, the patient's autonomy, his or her preferences and quality of life are slowly more and more being taken into account in clinical decision making. There is also more openness for modern and old-traditional concepts which have emphasized the need of harmony in human beings as a pre-requisite for health, as demonstrated in Chinese medicine and in Antonovsky`s concept of the sense of coherence to develop a better and more human kind of medicine.

2. Medicine Needs a New Language

Michael P. Weingarten addressed the topic of language in medicine. His paper was entitled "Old Ideas, New Words". Psychosomatics is a term which many psychiatrists do not use any more. It joins a long line of discarded words which were once at the forefront of modern jargon. However, when talking about modern family medicine, practicing a bio-psycho-social concept, etc., physicians and their patients are faced with the existence of the term "psychosomatics". Weingarten emphasized the need to *re-phrase* the term in present day words and to discover the old ideas seemingly forgotten. He observed that in China neither doctors nor patients think in terms of anxiety or depression, nor panic or phobic states. Instead different *organ* systems are related to different emotions like fear, happiness, anger etc. It's only when the Yin and Yang forces are out of balance one or more emotions start to domineer in a disturbing way. This *state* is treated by administering carefully selected herbs. They are known to act specifically on one or other organ systems which require support. According to Weingarten, Chinese doctors listen very carefully. They find, however, no need to talk to their patients: "...there is no place for (verbal psycho-; the authors) therapeutic transaction." Obviously the doctor himself is expected to apply exactly the right corrective drug. Seen with Western eyes the healing agent is the balance between two opposing forces within an "appropriately supportive emotional environment". Since this environment has become so complex the quantity and quality of interrelations between the individual and his environment have increased rapidly. Compared to old paternalistic days the question nowadays is how "more egalitarian, non directive" re-phrasing of the patient's problems can be introduced into today's Medicine.

"The main arena of both psychotherapy and biomedicine is the consultation." Weingarten quoted King Solomon: "The thing that hath been, it is that which shall be: and that which is done is that which shall be done: and there is no new thing under the sun (Eccl.. 1:9)". It is in this spirit of modesty that we may succeed in transmitting to our students old ideas in new words.

Comments

The consultation process deals with the individual on the one hand and with the inter-individual models or systems on the other hand. Thus we are constantly forced to rephrase the patient's problems in terms of models and systems and the latter ones have to be re-re-phrased describing the individual's situation. Adding to Weingarten's formulations one may say that modern medical convention provides DSM IV and ICD-10 as main dictionaries for the re-phrasing process. However, neither of them makes reference to the process of re-phrasing itself, neither of them explains how the dictionaries can be used in a sensible way.

Psychosomatic medicine on the other hand has always dealt with transactions and relationships, i.e., with translations. This is recognized and reflected by the very existence of the International College of Psychosomatic Medicine, being host to this symposium, of many other psychosomatic conferences, of psychosomatic journals around the world. They all prove that the term "Psychosomatics" has not been discarded at all. In Germany, Psychosomatic Medicine has been introduced as part of medical undergraduate training at all Medical Schools. There also exists a postgraduate training programme in Psychosomatics/Psychotherapy which comprises three streams:

1) Primary Psychosomatic Health Care (Psychosomatische Grundversorgung) see below (Schüffel, Brucks);
2) Integrated Psychotherapy (Zusatzbezeichnung Psychotherapie);
3) Psychotherapeutic Medicine as a speciality (Facharzt für Psychotherapeutische Medizin).

There are 9000 beds in Psychosomatic Clinics all over Germany. In Japan, there is a flourishing Psychosomatic Society (Japanese Society of Psychosomatic Medicine), a considerable number of Japanese medical schools have psychosomatic departments. The Chinese are increasingly asking themselves to what extent psychosomatic medicine is relevant to their health care (Japanese-Korean-Chinese Conference on Psychosomatic Medicine, Kyushu, 1994) which basically consists of traditional Chinese Medicine and modern Western Medicine. In the United States of America the content areas of Psychosomatic Medicine have been prominently discussed over the past sixty years. The psychosomatic pioneers of the world's most advanced medical culture are, among others, Franz Alexander, Flanders Dunbar, Stewart Wolf, James Henry, Morton Reiser, Herbert Weiner, Adam Krakowski, Bish Lipowsky, George L. Engel. It was G.L. Engel who righteously started re-phrasing when he coined the expression "Consultation-Liaison" (personal communication, 1972) and shortly afterwards the "bio-psycho-social model". When the term "Behavioral Medicine" was introduced the term "psychosomatic medicine" became unpopular, indeed. Nowadays an unfortunate split between Behavioral Medicine and Psychosomatic Medicine is seen, most prominently among researchers and less so among practitioners of health care.

Weingarten is one of the practitioners in the very best sense of the word. He is concerned with the basic elements of *process* oriented patient care which is based on an acknowledgment of the doctor-patient relationship. In so far as he is right to say that the ideas are old, now new words have to be connected with the old ideas. Systems theory will be of help in doing so as demonstrated by the following contribution:

C.A. Carel, a child and youth psychiatrist, presented also in the name of Y. Danziger, M. Mukamel, Y. Kaplan, M. Mimouni and S.Tyano a paper entitled: "The process of co-creation of a systemic treatment program: The particular case of a family based treatment program for eating disorders." The aim of this paper was the discussion of family based multi- disciplinary collaborations in health systems (services) in general, while eating disorders served as one of many possibilities. It demonstrates how family-system models influence the modern psychosomatic practice. The authors pointed to the possibilities of : (1) Joint collaboration on specific projects. (2) Multi-disciplinary health services.

A change in a multi-disciplinary direction may develop by chance and non-intentionally, or it may occur in an overtime-on-going-spiral. It may also develop as a result of mutual-interactive modifications of different parts of the health system. A multi-disciplinary program generates out of the confluence of a need for providing treatment for a certain patient population (in this case eating disorders of adolescent patients) and longitudinal psychiatric consultation-liaison services, in this particular case of child and adolescence psychiatry to pediatric services. There are several stages in the process of a co-creation of a systemic treatment program.

First stage: This is to provide an answer to the increasing need for treatment due to a deviance in the incidence and prevalence of the disorder; to further respond to the need to provide multi-model, long term treatment and follow-up because psychotherapy or physical rehabilitation, alone, seem to be insufficient. In this way therapists became more aware that a multi-disciplinary approach is really needed. The first order change that usually occurs is the acceptance of a collaborative program, which in the first stage is carried out by each discipline in parallel way; individual cases may be treated already jointly.

Second stage: The staff of the general medical system (in this case of pediatrics) becomes aware of the need to amplify interactional skills, e.g. in order to deal with low compliance. Thus an additional role of the psychiatrist develops, as he/she becomes a consultant of the staff in addition of being a therapist.

Third stage: The establishment of a multi-disciplinary team (this is a second-order change). A formal multi-disciplinary treatment program, a new treatment system, is thus created. This becomes possible because of the high motivation of all participants for change and collaboration; because of the support of the institutional hierarchy and the recognition of context and milieu as a part of the treatment program.

Fourth stage: Adding *families* (in our particular case parents) to the program (this is a second order change); understanding that the therapeutic system is composed of several sub-systems and functions each with its own professional identity, training and experience. As a result of the process of consolidation of the multi-disciplinary team, a common base of knowledge and information is developed, including cognitive elements as information and values, interactional skills and a clear description of accepted boundaries.

In conclusion, the process of co-creation of a systemic treatment program is a very complex process of change over time. This process is initiated and maintained for numerous factors. Prior analysis of these factors may facilitate the process of setting up such a program. Maintenance of such a program requires continuous awareness of the existence of contextual factors that will cause change in the system. The process presented may serve as a model for the creation of similar types of multi-disciplinary inter-system projects for treating different populations in health systems.

3. Experiencing the Team

Wolfram Schüffel and Ursula Brucks elaborated on the concept of a program on further education in Primary Psychosomatic Health Care. Their contribution was titled: "Can Further Education be Replaced by Consultation?". The program has been implemented at the Academy of the Hesse Medical College of Further Education at Bad Nauheim, Germany. Its schedule consists of ten Saturdays, each comprising eight teaching/learning hours totaling eighty hours over a period of one and a half years. The program started in 1989 and four consecutive courses have been conducted or are being conducted presently. Each course was attended by approximately 100 physicians, 40% of them being hospital-based and 40% practicing doctors, 20% being engaged at other places (e.g. occupational health, health authority, counseling etc.). The courses have been deviced[2] as a kind of an ongoing training program in peer consultation on health problems in Psychosomatic Primary Health Care. The salutogenic approach was emphasized throughout the programme. Basically each participant was told that he/she is regarded to be an expert of Primary Health Care who is *now* to be supported to exchange his/her experience with fellow experts. This is done in a problem oriented and resource oriented way using an interactive learning style.

Half of the program is dedicated to cognitive learning (see Table 1), the other half being reserved for attitudinal and psychomotoric learning objectives. As can be seen from the table there are dotted lines drawn both horizontally and vertically. Here the authors want to indicate that:

1) each of the ten *meetings* is understood to be an ongoing *process* and that there is always an overlapping of cognitive and affective/psychomotoric learning;
2) the *whole program* with its ten meetings is seen as a continuing learning and training *process* of eighteen months' duration. It also has no definite end, i.e.- it is a program of continuing education since the participants are encouraged to meet in peer groups on quality assurance after the ten meetings.

The ten meetings are composed of forty individual sessions which are held on a Saturday (see Table 2). The program starts by an introduction to the concept of *salutogenesis*. It is pointed out that 80% of the persons who have been exposed to the most traumatic stressors of disaster don't develop a Post Traumatic Stress Disorder (PTSD). This is partly due to a strong sense of coherence and Antonovsky (1987, p. 138) is quoted: "What a person with a strong sense of coherence (SOC) does is to select the particular coping strategy that seems most appropriate to deal with the stressor being confronted." And furthermore (p. 147): "...the person with a strong SOC is at an advantage in preventing tension from being transformed into stress." In particular the dimension of meaningfulness is introduced (p. 165): "...once the generalized view of the world as meaningful and comprehensible is focussed on the specific situation - one is ready to act."

This is underscored by providing four guidelines for coping with traumatic stressors:

1. Give good and clear information by demonstrating control;
2. Give a legitimization for experiencing anxiety and fatigue;
3. Care for the most basic needs of the victims;
4. Give a chance for ventilating and for telling the "story" (or narrative, see below).

---

[2]W.Shüffel G. Maass, both Internists and Psychotherapists/Psychoanalysts. U. Brucks evaluated the program.

Table 1. Curriculum on Basic Psychosomatic Health Care

Meeting	Objectives Session 1	Session 2	Session 3	Session 4
I	**Tension and Stress: Traumatic Stress Salutogenesis:SOC**	**Somatization and Health Care**	**The Office**	**The Psychosomatic Approach**
II	Psychlogical Development from birth to puberty	Traumatic Events	The Hospital	The AIDS/HIV positive person
III	Psychological Development from Ado-lescence to Senesence	Bodily expressed Depression	Counseling	Motivatng for a psychosomatic approach
IV	Neurosis and Deviant Behaviour	The PATIENT with Chronic Pain	Balint and Interven-tion Techniques	The Initial Talk
V	Symptom Formation	The PATIENT with breathing disorders	Balint and Interven-tion Techniques	Organ Language
VI	Psychosomatic Intervention	The PATIENT with heart/circulatory disorders	Balint and Interven-tion Techniques	Occupational Health
VII	Cooperation versus (?) Referral	The PATIENT with gastrointestinal disorders	Balint and Interven-tion Techniques	Family Health
VIII	Ethical Considerations	The PATIENT with disorders of the reproductive system	Balint and Interven-tion Techniques	Death and Dying
IX ill	Resources and Quality awareness	The PATIENT with skin disorders	Balint and Interven-tion Techniques	The chronically and the working alliance
X	Resources and Self Governing bodies	Coping with addiction	Balint and Interven-tion Techniques	Continuity and the **professional SOC:** teamwork

The program of further education on Basic Psychosomatic Health Care at the Hesse Medical College of Further Education, Bad Nauheim/Frankfurt (Germany) Each of the meetings consists of four sessions totalling 10 x 8 = 80 hours over a period of 1.5 years

Table 2. Curriculum on Basic Psychosomatic Health Care

The Functional Physician-Patient Relationships

1) The health progress is unsatisfying. The physician is worried by his/her lack of finding the adequate approach.

2) By reviewing the treatment course the physician identifies an adherence to a symptom oriented therapy. This has been done in the presence of (partly) missed causative illness factors.

3) Commitment to Misunderstanding: Both physician and patient feel unable to find a problem oriented solution and that's why they avoid referring to psychosocial issues.

4) Both physician and patient try to make up for (alleged) deficits in Health Care.

5) The patient plays down his/her own complaints assisted by the physician's unwillingly consenting to him/her.

6) By mutually agreeing the patient acts according to the physician's understanding.

7) The patient performs in a *coherent* and cooperative way being understood by the physician.

An interactive style is used, i.e., the participants are constantly asked to *consult* their peers who are present. Starting at the second meeting the patient and his key figures are introduced in vivo, i.e., the patient, the partner, the child, etc. are present personally. From then on the living patient is an integrated part of the program. In the second session of the first meeting the term somatization is introduced and reference is made to various pathological forms of dealing with stress.

The participants again consult each other on the topic of somatization which reflects a deficiency of salutogenic factors. In the third session of the first meeting particular emphasis is laid on the doctor's office and its specific problems. The session itself is seen as the precursor of regular Balint group work which is introduced in the fourth meeting. From then on the plenary is subdivided into four groups each consisting of 25 persons. They meet in two out of the four sessions of the meetings IV to X. The meetings take place every six to eight weeks. Gradually the group cohesion grows both in the plenary as well as in the four subgroups. Starting at the sixth (seventh) meeting the participants wonder how they may consult the colleagues outside the programme on an individual basis. The ninth and tenth meetings are used to form peer review groups on quality assurance and on contacting self governing bodies of the medical profession.

Schüffel and Brucks delineated aspects of systems theory. They superimposed Table 2 onto Table 1. It can be seen that the SOC of the professional team (topic of the tenth and last meeting) on one hand and tension, stress, traumatic stress (topics of the first session of the first meeting) on the other hand are connected within upwards and downwards movements within the whole program. On Table 2 this connection is symbolized by the vertical loop. They are part of a hierarchical system. - The (horizontal) loop as indicated in the middle of table 1 represents one of the ten particular meetings with its four sessions.

There are ten loops altogether. These loops are seen as circular feedback systems. Thus the SOC is part of the learning objectives of each of the ten meetings.

The functional physician-patient relationship was particularly emphasized by the authors. Table 3 was superposed on Table 1. Table 3 contains a hierarchy of seven particular functional physician-patient relationships (Brucks, 1995). They are called "functional" since each of them refers to a function of the particular relationship. According to Brucks (1995) numbers one to five represent a so called "potential for chronification" which is identical with the urge for somatizing. It refers to the "collusive element" as described by Ormel (see below). Relationships six and seven represent the most mature ways of transacting within the ongoing relationship and hence within the consultation process. By imposing table 3 onto table 1 the authors visualized that there are systemic upwards/downwards movements within the hierarchy of relationships. It is obvious that the seventh relationship, i.e. the stage of a *coherent* performance is the ultimate goal within an ongoing patient-physician relationship

Comment

Over a period of six years the educational program of Basic Psychosomatic Health Care has turned into an interactive process. The focus of this process is the doctor's problem as identified within the doctor-patient-relationship - whether in vivo or in Balint groups, etc. Consequently the participants regard each other as consultants and consultees and the process of consulting becomes the center of interest. Schüffel and Brucks even wondered whether future further education in the field of (psychosomatic) education may be replaced by refined methods of guided peer consultation. Future attempts to develop this program should consider the application of guidelines (see op't Root) and the intimate relationship between detection and management of mental disturbances (see Ormel).

4. Provision of Guidelines

J.M.H. op't Root's presentation was titled "Modelling the Consultation in General Practice; from a Conceptual, Psychosomatic Approach to an Open, Structured Approach". Improving the quality of primary health care has high priority in The Netherlands. This is achieved by laying emphasis on a) teaching the process of consultation to general practitioners and b) developing guidelines. Op't Root focussed on the consultation model. In order to understand its origins it is helpful to know that in developing the concept of primary health care, concepts of psychological, psychosocial, psychosomatic medicine and family medicine played an important role. The concept of primary health care was introduced in The Netherlands when the three year compulsory vocational training was started in 1974. This was preceded by a "flourishing period" of Balint group work, psychoanalytic and psychosocial interpretation of health problems by applying the social model in medicine, the comprehensive approach and by practicing cooperation between GPs and social workers. At present, in The Netherlands, the debate on the concepts and theories of psychosocial and psychosomatic medicine, the comprehensive approach and family medicine is coming to an end.

Now the focus lies more on clinical competence, guidelines, and more recently, on shared care between GPs and specialists. This development was made possible by the position of the Dutch practitioners whose professional organization is well established by the following four rules:

1. Everyone has a doctor and he/she is listed on the GP's list.
   There is freedom to choose one's own doctor.
2. Primary care is directly accessible.

Table 3

1	Introduction: Process Orientation	MAOZ BENBASSAT	Traumatic Stress and SOC
2	Medicine needs a new language	WEINGARTEN: There is no new thing under the sun CAREL: systems theory	„Complementary"
3	Experiencing the Team	Schüffel, BRUCKS	Relating to fellow man
4	Provision of Guide-lines	op't ROOT	Transgenerational exchange
5	The Intimate Rela-tionship between Detection and Manage-ment	ORMEL	Intimate Relationship between the Generations (see Germany/Nether-lands); between the Nations (see above)
6	Exploring the Rela-tionship between De-tection and Manage-ment	DAVINE	Thematic Poster Sessions
7	An Example of Detec-tion and Management	FRAENKEL	Limburg as a European Region
8	Detection and Man-agement as Rooted in Coherence - Illustra-ted by the Narrative Approach	RABINOWITZ et al.	Erzählgemeinschaften and the spirit of Lim-burg
9	Coherence as Con-strued within the Process of Consulta-tion - Consultation and Narrative Commu-nities seen as Com-plementary Terms	Schüffel	Erzählgemeinschaften Limburger Stils: eine europäische Konsulta-tion (coherence, conti-nuity, conflict resol-ving, understanding)

3. GP's are the gatekeepers for all kinds of health problems.
   More than 80% of patient complaints are solved by him/her.
4. It is the GP who makes the decision for a referral (including mental health referrals).

In primary care GP's have the opportunity to give personal, comprehensive, and continuing care to the individual and to the family. The Dutch GP clearly distances himself/herself from the position of a psychotherapist or family therapist. It is not his/her task to take up the content of psychosocial problems but "to trace and legitimate them in connection with the patient's complaints and health problems." *This is done within the consultation model for GP's "which is a systematic, although simplified representation of the actual doctor-patient communication.... The model does not describe the contents of somatic and psychosocial issues to be handled but it describes the process. It just indicates where things belong to in the process of consultation."* Stimulated by Weed's (1969) problem oriented (clinical) recording the Dutch GP's devised an *"enlarged and modified SOAP-scheme"*. SOAP stands for S-Subjective (patient/doctor; history taking), O-Objective (physical examination; laboratory), A-Assessment (interpretation of complaints and problems, differential diagnosis), P-Plan (treatment and therapy; management). The full scheme contains three parts.

The FIRST PART of the consultation model; this is identical with S = Subjective:

1. Past/Interval

2. Entry

1. Greeting and clarification of function, if needed
2. First impressions

3. General/overall orientation

1. General information on the reason(s) for encounter
2. Overall orientation

4. Exploration of questions

1. Exploration and clarification of the reasons for encounter
   What questions or messages, fears and expectations does the patient have?
   - open, accepting attitude and own (the doctor's)
   feelings and ideas
2. What event prompted the patient to come?

5. Consultation plan

1. Provisional diagnosis with attention to somatic and psychosocial aspects (a multiple track approach)
2. Planning the next step together

ad 1 Past/Interval: It can be important to know what happened to the patient before the consultation or in the time between this and the preceding consultation.

ad 2-4: During the first part of the consultation the patient is the expert. The doctor's role is an encouraging one. It is the patient who is working and telling. The doctor's first task is to sift out why and for what reason the patient comes to the office now. This part is the *narrative* part of the consultation.

ad 5: This is the *turning* point in the second part of the consultation process. The provisional diagnosis is made (with attention to bio-psycho-social aspects („multiple track approach")). The patient is informed. Doctor and patient agree how to progress. This is the explorational part of the consultation process.

The SECOND PART of the Consultation Model; this is identical with O = Objective and A = Assessment:

6. Diagnostic phase (O = Objective)

1. *History taking*
   (Is a new working-diagnosis needed?)
2. *Physical examination*
3. Additional laboratory, ECG etc.
   (Is a new working-diagnosis needed?)

7. Evaluation/Information (A = Assessment)
1. Evaluation of findings/problem definition/ working diagnosis(-es)/differential *diagnosis*
2. Informing the patient and checking for understanding

ad 6: The phase of history taking starts. Is a new working diagnosis needed? - The physical examination and laboratory tests follow. - Is another working diagnosis needed?

ad 7: The problem is defined and the (differential) diagnosis is made. The doctor makes sure that the patient understands him.

ad 6 and 7: The doctor is the *expert*. It is the doctor who is working and thinking. It is the *interpretation* part of the consultation process.

The THIRD PART of the Consultation Model; this is identical with P = Plan
8. Plan of action
1. Discussing possible further diagnostic measures, information, advice, treatment, *therapy*
2. Management, follow up

9. Evaluation of the consultation
1. Evaluation of the contents and form of the consultation
2. Ending this dialogue

ad 8: The doctor talks about his plans and asks for the patient's opinion.

ad 9: The doctor should make sure whether "this was what the patient came for, and checks if the patient is satisfied."

ad 8 and 9: Doctor and patient achieve mutual consent and work together.

J. op't Root finally emphasized that this model supports the structuring of the consultation process by inducing cooperation and openness. The GP will derive greater satisfaction from his work. At the same time the patient realizes that he/she has the opportunity for taking responsibility for health and life. The author finishes, "Patient centeredness and structuring the consultation are widely accepted in The Netherlands. Research shows that the Dutch GP works less disease centered than Belgian and British colleagues (Grol et al, 1990)".

Comments

The Dutch Consultation Model is invaluable for two reasons:

- It provides structure and encourages individual creativity at the same time.
- It is a model of intra- and interprofessional consultation.

Considering the first reason: The model is comprehensible and self evident because it is basic although its effectiveness tends to be underestimated by participants of further education programs. Their first reaction to a presentation of the scheme tends to be:

"Nothing new, that's what I have done all the time." Only by carefully applying it in a problem oriented way it proves to be a powerful tool in the hand of the physician. Every clinician knows how difficult it is to tune in into a dialogue *and* to distance oneself at the same time. In the first situation one may over identify with the patient and miss important data. In the second situation one may get the necessary data at the expense of missing basic feelings, however. Thus the consultation model serves as a constant reminder of particular basic elements in the process of consultation, i.e.- the clinician is helped to keep the balance. The procedure resembles George Engel's (1969) approach as devised for the clinical interview and further developed for this purpose in the German speaking countries by R. Adler (1994). By devising the patient evaluation grid (PEG) this approach had been formalized in a most practical and elegant way (Leigh, Reiser, 1980).

Considering the second reason: It has been said (Weingarten, see above) that the main arena of both psychotherapy and biomedicine is the mutual and deliberate consultation of members of the health professions. Unfortunately they have no common language since they are used to a language which is based on outcome as opposed to process and each discipline has its own outcome. A process oriented language as used here is much closer to both the patient's and the doctor's problems which are dealt with in a cooperative manner.

5. The Intimate Relationship between Detection and Management

Johan Ormel's and B. Tiemen's contribution was entitled, "Recognition and Treatment of Mental Illness in Primary care: Towards a Better Understanding of a Multifaceted Problem". Their starting point was the fact that "non-recognition of mental illness in primary care settings is a prevalent and complicated problem...a collusive phenomena as it serves the interest of both patient and physician...and an easy way out.... Rates of non-recognition based on a single day index may incorrectly classify cases as non detected." Detection in primary medicine is often a process that takes time (several visits). "Physicians do not always make a deliberate note of the presence of emotional distress.... This could explain that in a recent study 27% of the 'non-detected' cases received nevertheless some sort of mental health care from their Primary Care Physician (PCP)." Although there are cultural differences, usually the mild cases (and not the severe ones) are not detected.

Early and proper recognition and early adequate treatment of mental disorders in primary medicine is important also from the *socio-economic* point of view. "In the Netherlands with an active work force of 6,5 million, more than 30% of the one million receiving disability-benefits, do so because of mental health problems!" Detection often speeds up recovery if it is followed by adequate treatment. Detection without treatment has no prognostic value. "There is an intrinsic relationship between recognition and management skills." Even when mental disorders are treated in primary care, treatment is often "sub threshold": medication is not given in proper therapeutic doses and for not long enough. This, according to *the guidelines written by specialists in psychiatric hospitals*, who may see other patients and other, more severe diseases, but usually in a later phase and in an other setting.

It has also been concluded that the effectiveness of psychotherapeutic treatment modalities such as cognitive-behavioral and interpersonal therapy, is not much different from that of antidepressants, although drug treatment is more effective in severe depression." "Clinical costs were at least twice as much as routine GP care... research on prognostic factors and response prediction would yield specific indications for the most important treatment modalities, allowing better targeting in the next generation of randomized trials in primary care settings. Such studies should also take in consideration *long term outcome* because of residual symptoms, relapse and recurrence.

The multiple causes of non-detection are partly patient related, e.g., patients who present physical symptoms such as fatigue or multiple pains, or have a "co-morbid" physical disease. The tendency to somatize emotional distress is more frequently found in ethnic minorities, older people and patients of the lower social strata. But somatizing may be less persistent. Most patients are willing to consider seriously a non-medical explanation of their physical symptoms when the PCP sensitively and carefully probe for psychosocial cues. Other causes of non-detection are doctor and setting related. E.g., the communication style of the PCP, fear of the PCP of discussing psychosocial issues, lack of time, no proper payment and reward, etc.

How to improve recognition and treatment of mental disorders in primary care? First and foremost, it is essential to acknowledge the intimate relationship between recognition and management. Without sufficient skills for treatment, recognition will remain an illusion. The attitudes of the PCPs must be changed and relevant skills must be taught. Mental health consultation-liaison by itself, without *additional education and training*, seems to have no strong effect on the recognition and treatment. Educational efforts are needed. Good examples of such efforts are the US "Depression Awareness Recognition and Treatment" program; the British "Defeat Depression programme" and the special chapter on psychiatric disorders in primary medicine (which includes guidelines of management) published by the WHO (Ustün, Sartorius, in press). Training in interview and management skills can be provided in small groups with role playing and video feedback techniques.

Comments

It should be emphasized that Johan Ormel paid attention to the problem of cost-effectiveness. He did this by pointing out that early recognition of psychosomatic and mental health problems, followed by professional interventions and treatment given by a primary physician and consultation provided by skillful mental health professionals, may most probably save financial resources. It may be as efficient and satisfactory for patients as the more expensive treatment schemes offered by specialists.

6. Exploring the Intimate Relationship Between Detection and Management

John Davine`s contribution was titled, "Teaching about Somatizing to Family Practice Residents". Davine is a teacher of Behavioral Sciences and Psychiatry in the Residency Program of Family Medicine at the McMaster University, Hamilton, Ontario (Canada) and he acts as a permanent psychiatric consultant at non-academic Primary Care Clinics in Hamilton. He works in the framework of an Ontario State project, in which the effects of a psychiatric consultation-liaison program in Primary Medicine is tested and evaluated, concerning cost-effectiveness, improvements of services, patient satisfaction, quality of care, etc.

His teaching to family medicine residents is based mainly on group supervision of videotapes made by residents during their regular work with patients. Every resident has to present encounters with patients. The tape is supervised by his/her peers, by a senior family physician (who is seen by the residents as a role model), a social worker who belongs to the primary-medical team and by Dr. Davine. The presentation is often stopped and details of communication and content are discussed. In another session the residents watch Davine, via a closed circle television, interviewing a patient with a possible psychiatric problem. Besides that formal teaching also takes place.

Somatizing and Somatoform Disorders are an important part of the family physician's caseload. Some studies have shown that 10% to 30% of patients with somatic complaints who presented them to he doctor have no adequate physical cause to account for them. These patients are often referred to many specialists including psychiatrists and sent to many tests, X rays, and to other investigations. But they usually return to the family practitioner. Thus the "bulk of patients with somatoform disorders end up in the hands of the family physician". This kind of illness behavior is difficult to understand and to deal with; it seems to be a universal "natural" behavior. There are always great difficulties concerning the doctor-patient relationship, starting with the question of how to convey to the patient that his or her symptoms and complaints are neither a phantasy, nor a psychiatric illness (the patient is neither a liar nor crazy). These patients represent a behavioral spectrum reaching from those who manifest somatic symptoms which have unconscious motives to those who consciously play the sick-role. In the middle we find the "half conscious" factitious disorders. Co-morbidity with other psychiatric disorders may exist. Thus somatization can develop on the basis of depression, anxiety, delusional disorders etc.

Somatic symptoms often express interpersonal, including sexual, problems, low self esteem, perception abnormalities (of the body), low tolerance (e.g., for pain), increased attention of bodily functions, cognitive abnormalities, alexithymia and others. The treatment that can be given to those patients in the frame of primary medicine should usually be pragmatic, practical, and simple. First of all iatrogenic medical procedures and medication should be avoided as a preventive measure. Psychotherapeutic interventions should include operant models, supportive approaches, relaxation, bio-feedback, and sometimes anti-depressant medication. An assessment of the intervention should always follow. It is certainly the task of the teacher and of the liaison-consultant to support the family physician in this difficult relationship and to enable him/her to care for these often chronic and sometimes not curable patients and to share with them their frustration, so that the treatment of somatizers can be perceived by the doctor as a challenge.

Davine's activities as a liaison-consultant was described also briefly: There is a permanent (part time) counselor, usually a social worker, in every primary clinic. The psychiatrist, as Davine himself, visits the primary clinic every two weeks for at least 4 hours and is constantly in contact with the family physicians, who can always phone him and consult him. During the bi-weekly consultations the psychiatrist examines a number of patients who are referred to him by the family physician during the short personal contact they have before seeing the patients. After examining the patients, findings and recommendations are reported orally to the family physician and notes are written in the general chart of the patient. Some patients are treated further by the psychiatrist, others are referred to the counselor, who works closely with the psychiatrist. This liaison-consultation model is also accompanied by some formal educational activities.

7. An Example of Detection and Management

Y.M. Fraenkel, M. Leibovits-Zezak, and R. Aronzon presented their paper under the topic "Consultation-Liaison for Family Practitioners: A Preliminary Report - The Jerusalem Report". Y.M. Fraenkel reported on the therapeutic results achieved within a community based consultation-liaison service just established in Jerusalem. The service was offered to family practitioners whose patients were suffering either under psychological factors affecting medical conditions (PFAMC) or anxiety disorders.

When offering their service Fraenkel and his coworkers had in mind:

1) most patients with PFAMC are not referred for a mental health consultation by their family practitioners.
2) Even when referred patients refrain from seeking consultation since they are afraid of stigmatization.

3) Patients will benefit most when they are treated by both the family practitioner and the member of the liaison group on a short term basis.

Painstaking efforts were undertaken to establish a good working relationship between the referring family practitioner and the members of the liaison group. This was accomplished by regular and personal contacts and by sending out questionnaires to the referring practitioners. Therapy was limited to the above described group of patients (no somatization syndromes) and to ten sessions. Thereafter the patient was expected to see the GP as his sole therapeutic partner.

So far, forty-four patients were referred to the consultation liaison group. 37 patients were accepted for treatment. They had an average of 7.1 sessions; the therapeutic modalities being pharmacotherapy (32%), relaxation (23%), consultation (16%), all three (26%).

The majority of patients benefitted and the practitioners felt satisfied in most cases. The reutilization of medical resources (unexpected office calls, specialist consultations, laboratory check ups) was greatly reduced. The practitioners acknowledged the liaison's strength in providing useful information via a reliable consultation process.

Comments

The paper may be seen to be a kind of case study dealing with the relationship between consultant and consultee being the most crucial part of the study. It seems that the referring doctors knew that detection of disorder was followed by adequate management. Thus a strikingly good managerial result was achieved despite a very low number of treatment sessions. Hopefully the authors will be able to continue with this type of field experiment.

8. Detection and Management as Rooted in Coherence - Illustrated by the Narrative Approach

Stanley Rabinowitz, Benyamin Maoz and Reva Kassan reported on "The Narrative Approach, Medicine, and Psychotherapy". They pointed out that the narrative or story telling approach has received increasing interest in recent years. An old medical tradition is thus taken up since story telling has always been part of clinical medicine. It was only in this century that "the third person passive has become the voice of the medical writer and conference presenter; objectivity has become the tool, and IMRD (Introduction, Methods, Results, Discussion) the sacred model."

The practice of medicine is largely based on interpretation of data. The vast amount of information presented by the patient needs structuring by the physician, i.e. "narrative organization of the medical case". Not different from the Chinese doctor quoted above the doctor listens to the patient's narrative and tries to adjust it to his understanding of disease.

This is done in a empathic way and reflects the rhythm of passivity and activity of the consultation model as described by J. op't Root. But tension and even pain can be caused by telling the patient a poorly constructed physician's narrative. One is reminded of Antonovsky's referring to tension as the point of departure for well-being or for falling ill: According to Antonovsky it is in the state of tension when the person with a strong sense of coherence (SOC) may perceive the situation as a challenge. Such a person is able to prevent tension from being transformed into a state of stress.

A severe or unbearable state of stress, i.e., a state of distress may be transformed into somatization. Somatization can be seen as the communication of personal and interpersonal stories in physical idioms of distress and patterns of behaviour that emphasize the seeking of help. The stories center around unresolved conflicts between opposing motives. The act of revealing and exposing motives may be in itself therapeutic or it could contribute directly to improved outcome through the support and care implicit in attentive and nonjudgmental listening.

The narrative approach seeks "narrative truth", not objective nor historical truth. The narrative truth is "in the service of coherence, continuity, conflict resolving, and understanding."

This kind of truth can be told by the patient or by the physician.Two case vignettes were presented for illustration,the first related by the patient,the second by the physician:

Mike, a 36-year-old engineer, was referred to the clinician because of a sudden, increasingly irrational fear of being attacked by a terrorist. The fear had become so great that he insisted on spending the nights with his wife and children locked in the security room of their home. In therapy, he disclosed several traumatic incidents relating to his army experiences which resulted in mild PTSD. However, there was another traumatic story in the family concerning Mike's father who had spent his early life in the concentration camp of Buchenwald, but had never spoken about it to anyone. The father had recently begun to talk about his experience. Mike quickly understood that his father was not only referring to the material aspects of his state but also to his life experiences including his holocaust experiences. As Mike's father had always been withdrawn and reticent about his past and Mike had been conveniently unwilling to listen, the two had never had the opportunity to develop a close and open relationship. This point was raised in the patient's interactional story with the therapist. Mike understood that he would have to decide whether to listen to his father's story. If so, he would have to create the right atmosphere for his father to tell his story and would need the therapist's assistance in choosing a suitable scenario.

And now the circumstances which led to the second story.

A young widow presented for treatment a ten-year-old daughter who did not sleep for several weeks some time after the death of her father. She spent the nights roaming the house and her schoolwork and social life suffered as a consequence of being exhausted all day. It transpired that the daughter was totally obsessed with and opposed to the idea of her mother remarrying although at this stage the possibility was remote. The clinician simply told her the Grimm's fairy tale of the dancing princesses. Without having to say another word, the clinician had made it clear to the girl that he understood what she was up to and almost overnight her sleeping patterns returned to normal.

As in the stories outlined above the clinician's role is passive-active rather than conventionally active. The clinicians are even *expected* to conceal the extent of their influence and discretely guide the patients, thus leaving it up to them to use their imagination and initiative to create an alternative version to their lives to take *control* (emphasized by the authors) and behave independently. This does not mean that the clinicians are opinion less and are being driven by the patients. Clinicians are guided by their attempts to identify *progressive* elements, *stable* elements, and *regressive* elements in the patient's life. At the same time symptom formation and symptom shift are the ongoing red line which is woven as a narrative truth, namely serving *coherence*, *continuity*, *conflict resolving*, and *understanding*. In two final statements Rabinowitz and coworkers stated that more systematic research into the narrative process itself and its application is needed. Secondly it is unknown to which extent the clinician's own personal story will trespass professional boundaries and to which extent we as professionals want to be discussed or remembered as storytellers.

Comments

The narrative may turn out to be the via regia to salutogenesis. Although this concept was not used by the authors explicitly their contribution is clearly rooted in salutogenic soil. This becomes even more obvious when their statement on narrative truth is slightly reformulated. "Narrative truth is in the service of coherence which itself results from the interaction of continuity, conflict resolving, and comprehending."

Continuity stands for meaningfulness, conflict resolving for manageability, comprehending for comprehensibility. On the other hand these terms are not identical. This is particularly true in the case of manageability and conflict resolving. Antonovsky (1987, p.17) defines manageability: The extent to which one perceives that resources are at one's disposal which are adequate to meet the demands posed by the stimuli that bombarded one, and he adds that "at one's disposal" in his understanding will refer to resources under one's own control or to resources controlled by legitimate others - one's spouse, friends, colleagues, God, history, the party leader, a physician - whom one feels one can count on, whom one trusts.

Conflict resolving on the other hand refers to actively clarifying, confronting, and *interpreting* seemingly contradicting forces. Also it leaves space for subconscious motives and defense mechanisms such as denial and projective identification. Narrative truth, however, is not identical with coherence and its interacting components but it is in its service. It is the result of a transaction as can be demonstrated in the two case vignettes quoted above. Mike and the little girl are both in need of a safe and trusting relationship with the therapist. The therapist will enable them to control, to legitimize, being nurtured vis à vis the therapist, the helper, to probe (Schüffel, Brucks, see above) feelings and reactions connected with the traumatic situation which is reenacted in therapy. It is up to the patient to re-form his/her life story by consulting the therapist how to solve particular problems.

The therapist's task is to make use of his/her professional consulting tools. In the case of an interactionally/psychoanalytically oriented therapy transference will be used. Mike will reenact the impaired relationship with his father in the presence of his therapist. The little girl has to reexperience a supportive fatherly figure to whom mother will be able to confide her sorrows. Mother's confiding in the physician was followed by the daughter's relaxation and recovery.

9. Coherence as Construed within the Process of Consultation and Narrative Communities - Conclusions

A principal motive running through the whole symposium was the motto of consultation. The term "consultation" points to a joined action provided by two or more persons or by a system. One speaks about cooperation, mutual activities, multi-disciplinary interventions, integration, liaison, shared care and responsibility etc. This phenomenon starts by referring to models of theoretical thinking and medical reasoning. It continues in reflecting medical practice. It can be observed during the encounter between an individual and his/her environment, between physicians and patients and their families. A patient consults his/her doctor and they agree within open communication and based on a more "egalitarian", i.e.- non-authoritarian and coherent attitude: This is the problem and this will be the treatment (op't Root).

On another level, the general (or even the specialized) physician will often consult colleagues, specialists or paramedical health workers. In order to be able to make a working contract they have to establish a common language and better mutual understanding (Ormel) of their expectancies or to construe a multi-disciplinary system (Carel). Thus the process of consultation moves into the center of modern psychosomatic thinking as reflected in the practice and teaching of primary health care. It is even suggested to transform traditional further education into "refined methods of guided peer consultation" (Schüffel, Brucks). Modern psychosomatic thinking is more process oriented and less outcome oriented than it used to be. It is based on general systems theory and yet it is firmly rooted in the emotional part of the doctor patient relationship.

Guidelines are accepted as a powerful tool to structure this relationship in a dynamic and open way. Wisely used guidelines do not hinder but foster creativity within the doctor patient relationship. The diagnostics of mental disorders is more complicated than believed so far: Physicians do observe signs of mental disturbances, however these are often not diagnosed as such as adequate management is lacking. One may even summarize: No management - no detection; the better the management the better the detection. Management will improve if physicians discover the professional sense of coherence. This is achieved within peer groups exhibiting a trusting atmosphere and where members respect each other. Both patient and physician have to negotiate in how far the patient can solve a problem by himself/herself. Basically the physician's main role is in letting the patient know that she/he can trust the *other* person and *how*.

Conclusions

J. op't Root who described the Dutch developments and trends said, "Now the focus lies more in clinical competence, guidelines, and more recently, on *shared care* (emphasis by the authors) between GPs and specialists." Shared care is based on trust - no trust, no share. The physician's most important clinical competence lies in structuring the consultation process empathically and problem orientedly. It allows the patient to probe actively himself/herself in a coherent way and thus experiencing his/her own sense of coherence. If future health care is going to depend on shared care between GPs and specialists - which is very likely - the future of health care will depend on the physician's consulting capabilities.

Summary

Delegates of different health systems agree that modern psychosomatic thinking is based on both circular reasoning and on a non-authoritarian and person centered attitude. This is reflected by the process of consultation in primary health care. There is the consultation between patient and physician and between two (or more) physicians. The process of consultation is to be structured as described by guidelines. Disturbances will be detected depending on the physician's capability of managing them. Management of disturbances will improve if physicians discover a professional sense of coherence (SOC) enabling patients to rely on the ongoing functional physician-patient relationship. Seven different functions may be discriminated. This will allow the patient to probe himself/herself actively in a coherent way thus experiencing the own sense of coherence as the central element of salutogenesis (Antonovsky, 1987).

Key words

Psychosomatics, Teaching, Consultation, Sense of Coherence, Salutogenesis

REFERENCES

Adler, R., Hemmeler, W. (1992): Anamnese und Körperuntersuchung. 3rd Ed., Fischer, Stuttgart, Jena, New York

Antonovsky, A. (1987): Unraveling the Mystery of Health - How People Manage Stress and Stay Well. Jossey-Bass, San Francisco, London

Engel, G.L., in: Morgan, W.L., Engel, G.L. (1969): The Clinical Approach to the Patient. Saunders, Philadelphia, London, Toronto

Engel, G.L. (1972): personal communication with the author W. Sch.

Grol, R., Maesseneer, J., Whitfield, M., Mokking, I.I. (1990): Disease-centered versus patient-centered attitudes: comparison of general practitioners in Belgium, Britain, and the Netherlands; Family Pracitioner 7, 100-103.

Japanese Society of Psychosomatic Medicine (1994): Guidelines on Diagnosis and Treatment in Psychosomatic Medicine, Fukuoka.

Japanese Society of Psychosomatic Medicine (1995): Shinshin - Igaku. Japanese Journal of Psychosomatic Medicine, Tokyo.

Leigh, H., Reiser, M.F. (1980): The Patient - Biological, Psychological, and Social Dimensions of Medical Practice. Plenum, New York, London

Ustün, T.B., Sartorius, N. (eds.): Mental Illness in Primary Care: an international study. WHO, Wiley&Sons (in press)

Weed, L.L. (1969): Medical records, medical education, and patient care; Year Book, Medical Publishers Inc., Chicago

13

REDUCTIONISM REVISITED: RETURN OF THE BIOMEDICAL MODEL

A. A. Howsepian, M. D.[1]

Department of Psychiatry
University of California, San Francisco
Fresno Medical Education Program

INTRODUCTION

It has become quite fashionable over the course of the past two decades, in many clinical circles, to repudiate the biomedical model (BMM) and, in its stead, to embrace the biopsychosocial model (BPSM) in medicine. The impetus for this significant shift in conceptual allegiance amongst medical practitioners is commonly traced most directly to the work of George L. Engel, M.D. (1977) who is widely believed to have successfully undermined the BMM in a seminal essay which appeared in the prestigious journal *Science*. As medical sociologist David Armstrong (1987) conceptualizes it, the biopsychosocial ideology as developed by Engel "was intended to save psychiatrists, who were then (and largely still are) torn between pursuing a biological reductionist model of mental illness...and [pursuing] a more psychosocial approach." (p 1213). Although the seeds for such a conceptual shift predated Engel's published work,[1] it was Engel's influence which most forcefully propelled biopsychosocial ideology into the psychiatric and general medical arenas.

The BPSM was meant to replace what is alleged to have been the old guard's conceptual scheme which had, according to Engel, long dominated how clinicians had come to think about medicine. Currently, in some medical circles - particularly those that are well represented by psychiatrists and primary care physicians - one's rejection of biopsychosocial medicine is tantamount to a betrayal of one's profession. Such a rejection has, in those circles, come to be viewed as constituting a retrograde movement in the otherwise inexorable march of humanistic progress that has been made in the psychiatric and general medical fields during the past fifty years. Much of this recent progress has been credited directly to Engel.

I shall shortly argue that there is in fact nothing conceptually novel about Engel's biopsychosocial proposal and, in light of this, that Engel's primary contribution to this

[1]Correspondence: Department of Psychiatry, UCSF-Fresno, 2615 E. Clinton Ave, Fresno, CA 93703

discussion has been merely rhetorical in nature. In addition, I shall demonstrate that many professing disciples of Engel appear to have fundamentally misunderstood his central claims and that this misunderstanding can, at least in part, be traced to those conceptual infelicities found in Engel's own work. Finally, I shall attempt to show that, ironically, certain key misunderstandings of Engel's *anti*-reductionist thesis have served as catalysts for the revival - and more virulent transformation - of biomedical *reductionism*.

I shall be assisted in the above tasks by posing and attempting to answer a series of questions concerning the biopsychosocial ideology: (1) Is there only *one* BPSM available or are there *several*? (2) What is it that a BPSM is most properly a model *of*? (3) How precisely does a BPSM differ from a BMM? (4) Are BPSMs superior to rival models? (What, for instance, are BPSM's actual or potential (dis)advantages over BMMs?)

As best as I understand them, there is, according to Engel and many (although not all) of his disciples, a *single* BPSM, it is most properly a model of *disease*, it radically differs in several specific ways from what preceded it, namely, the BMM, and it is clearly *superior* to its rival(s). I intend in this essay to argue that Engel and many of his most ardent followers are mistaken on all four counts. I shall, that is, (i) argue that there is a multi-membered *family* of mutually incompatible BPSMs, (ii) argue that these models are most properly models of how best to understand the functioning of *human persons* in health *and* disease, (iii) argue that some of what are categorized as being full-bodied biopsychosocial schemes are actually disguised biomedical variants, and (iv) suggest that the BPSM advanced by Engel and variations on it advanced by others should be replaced by rival, more comprehensive, and more historically entrenched, anti-reductionistic models.

1. Is There Only One BPSM Available or Are There Several?

Engel repeatedly refers to <u>the</u> BPSM, apparently implying that there is available only one such model. This single BPSM is meant to replace its alleged single competitor and lone conceptual predecessor in the medical domain, viz. *the* BMM. In Engel's view, the primary distinction between the BPSM and the BMM is that the latter embraces and the former rejects what he calls *reductionism*. The conceptual vehicle by which Engel rejects reductionism is powered by his reliance on General Systems Theory (GST), a world-view the construction of which he credits to Weiss (1969, 1977) and von Bertalanffy (1952,1968).

According to GST, the natural world is ordered on an hierarchically structured continuum with each level in the hierarchy representing an organized dynamic system arranged in such a way that the larger, more complex units in the hierarchy are superordinate to the smaller, less complex units. In addition, each system (except the highest-ordered system) is itself a component of at least one higher-ordered system. By no means, though, do complexity and size exhaust the features which demarcate one system unit from another. Thus, if one were wondering about where to place a small (ten piece) jigsaw puzzle in this hierarchy in relation to a large (million piece) jigsaw puzzle, one would be making a mistake if one were to place the larger puzzle in a position that is superordinate to the smaller puzzle. For, what is critical in differentiating one level from another involves not merely features involving size and complexity but, in addition, features which are *emergent* in nature, i.e., special features that are not shared by systems on subordinate levels in the hierarchy. Engel (1980) explains this critical notion as follows: "Each system implies qualities and relationships distinctive for that level of organization, and each requires criteria for study and explanation unique for that level. In no way can the methods and rules appropriate for the study and understanding of the cell as cell be applied to the study of the person as person or the family as family." (p 535) The aforementioned puzzles therefore would share the same level in the hierarchy for, its size and complexity notwithstanding, the larger, more complex puzzle possesses no emergent features relative to the smaller, more simple puzzle.[2]

General systems theorists, including Engel, are therefore explicitly committed to some variety of *emergentism*. This commitment warrants careful examination, for emergentist theories have a very long and honorable history and current work in emergentism has become quite subtle and sophisticated, yet almost none of this rich history and very little of this conceptual sophistication is reflected in the work of contemporary purveyors of the biopsychosocial ideology.

Intuitively stated, as for example, philosopher C.D. Broad (1925) has stated it, one can properly infer the existence of emergent properties wherever "the characteristic behavior of a whole could not, even in theory, be deduced from the most complete knowledge of the behavior of its components, taken separately or in combinations, and of their proportions and arrangements in this whole." (p 59) It does not appear that current discussions of emergence found in the biopsychosocial literature have advanced to a theoretical level which surpasses Broad's informal, relatively rough, intuitive characterization of property emergence. Fortunately, there has been a significant amount of conceptual work done on emergentism in the comtemporary philosophical literature to which we may appeal. One especially noteworthy essay in this domain has recently been written by philosopher Timothy O'Conner (1994).

According to O'Conner, any satisfactory account of property emergence must incorporate the following three features: supervenience, non-structurality, and novel causal influence. Yet, claims O'Conner, previous thinkers have attempted to explicate the notion of property emergence drawing upon only one or another of these conceptual features. O'Conner's (1994, p 98) proposal may be stated more formally as follows: A property P is an *emergent* property of a (mereologically complex) object O if and only if (1) P supervenes on properties of the parts of O, (2) P is not had by any of O's parts, (3) P is distinct from any structural property of O, and (4) P has a direct 'downward' determinative influence on the pattern of behavior involving O's parts. Each part of this characterization will require further elaboration.

First, O'Conner appeals to a strong form of *supervenience* in his account. In doing so he is following a suggestion made by philosopher James van Cleve (1990) who has proposed that we consider property emergence to be a subtype of what philosopher Jaegwon Kim (1984) calls 'strong supervenience.' In an attempt to be sensitive to the mereological (i.e., whole-part) features of emergent systems, O'Conner modifies Kim's notion of strong supervenience in the following manner (O'Conner, 1994, p 96): A-properties of objects supervene on B-properties of their parts = df Necessarily, for any object O and A-property a, if O has a, then there are B-properties b, c, d,...(which include relational properties) such that (i) some proper parts of O have (variously) b, c, d,...and (ii) necessarily, for any things collectively having all of b, c, d,...there is an object of which they are parts that has a. (A-properties and B-properties are intended to be certain *families* of properties. In discussions concerning emergentism, A-properties constitute the set of *emergent* properties, and B-properties constitute the set of non-emergent, or *base*, properties.)

Imagine that you have a glass of water in front of you. Water, we all know, is composed of molecules of various isotopes of two hydrogen atoms and one oxygen atom. We also know that, at room temperature, water is liquid. In this example, the water in the glass is the object in question, O. Liquidity is an A-property a had by O. The B-properties in question are constituted by a set of properties (b, c, d,...) exemplified by those molecules of which water is composed. In accord with O'Conner's definition, then, the liquidity of water supervenes on the molecular properties of water's parts if and only if, necessarily, if water at room temperature has the property of being liquid, then there are molecular properties such that some proper parts of this water (namely the molecules themselves) have all these properties and, necessarily, for any other thing that has all of these particular molecular properties, there is an object that is liquid of which these molecules are parts.[3]

Notice how O'Conner's definition of supervenience successfully captures two central ideas, designated by clauses (i) and (ii). The former clause spells out the condition that no object can have A-properties unless it (in whole or in part) has B-properties. A-properties (i.e., the emergent properties in question) *depend upon* the B-properties (i.e., the non-emergent, or base, properties). Call this the *dependence* condition. The latter clause spells out the condition that no object can be exactly similar to another object with respect to its (or its parts') B-properties without also being exactly similar to that object with respect to its A-properties. The B-properties, thereby, *determine* the A-properties. Call this the *determination* condition.

O'Conner cogently argues that although the determination condition and the dependence condition capture elegantly one form of strong supervenience, they are not, by themselves, sufficient for adequately characterizing the notion of emergence. What more is needed is, first, some manner in which one may screen out *structural* properties which may also fulfill the determination and dependence conditions where, "A property, S, is structural if and only if proper parts of particulars having S have some property or properties not identical with S, and this state of affairs is, in part at least, constitutive of the state of affairs of the particular's having S." (O'Conner, 1994, p 93) The mass M and shape H of a table are in this regard structural properties of the table, for the table's proper parts (e.g., the molecules which compose it) do not themselves possess the mass and shape exemplified by the table, and these parts' micro-properties *constitute* the table's exemplifying its macro-properties, in this instance, having mass M or shape H. Structural properties, therefore, are certain macro-properties exemplified by composite objects which are nothing over and above the summation of micro-property causal potentialities exemplified by those objects' micro-constituents. Because this is so, emergent properties must be *non*-structural in nature.

Finally, O'Conner requires emergent properties to possess what he calls *novel causal influence*. This requirement is meant to insure that the causal influence of the emergent property is *irreducible* "to that of the micro-properties on which it supervenes: it bears its influence in a direct, 'downward' fashion, in contrast to the operation of a simple structural macro-property, whose causal influence occurs via the activity of the micro-properties that constitute it." (O'Conner, 1994, pp 97-8) Human consciousness, for example, is thought by some to be an emergent property of the brain (or part of the brain) which provides conscious organisms with novel 'downward' causal powers in the sense outlined.

To philosopher John R. Searle (1992), for example, it appears "obvious from everything we know about the brain that macro mental phenomena are all caused by lower-level micro phenomena. There is nothing mysterious about such bottom-up causation; it is quite common in the physical world. Furthermore, he adds, "the fact that the mental features are supervenient on neuronal features in no way diminishes their causal efficacy. The solidity of the piston is causally supervenient on its molecular structure, but this does not make solidity epiphenomenal [and, therefore, causally inefficacious]; and, similarly, the causal supervenience of my present back pain on micro events in my brain does not make the pain epiphenomenal." (Searle, 1992, pp 125-6)[4]

The above theory of property emergentism, thereby, entails a commitment to *anti-reductionism*. In fact, *any* theory of emergentism *must* entail a commitment to some variety or other of anti-reductionism in virtue of the fact that emergentist theories are, by definition, theories about features of the world which are *not*, in *some* sense of the term 'reducible', reducible to certain of the world's other features. Engel appears to recognize this. He is clearly committed to a GST model of the world; he clearly claims to be rejecting the BMM's commitment to reductionism; and he appears to make the appropriate conceptual connection between GST and anti-reductionism. What he fails to do, though, is to make explicit what kind of reductionism he is rejecting. Although I might be mistaken about this, it at least appears that this failure is a function of his being unaware of the fact that the term 'reductionism' as it is employed in metatheoretical discourse is multiply ambiguous.

J.R. Searle (1992), for example, has chronicled five varieties of reductionism.[5] (1) *Ontological Reduction*: Objects of type T consist in nothing but objects of type T*. For example, it is fairly uncontroversial to claim that amoebae are composed of nothing but collections of elementary particles configured amoebae-wise. It is even less controversial to claim that chairs are mere collections of molecules arranged chair-wise. According to Searle, it is ontological reduction which is the ultimate aim of the remaining four types of reduction. (2) *Property Ontological Reduction*: Properties of type P consist in nothing but properties of type P*. For example, we are told by physicists that a gas's property of being hot consists in nothing but the mean kinetic energy of those molecules which make up that gas. (3) *Theoretical Reduction*: Laws of a reduced theory RT can (more or less) be deduced from the laws of the reducing theory RT*. An often repeated example of theoretical reduction in the scientific literature is the reduction of classical gas laws to the laws which govern statistical thermodynamics. (4) *Logical* (or *Definitional*) *Reduction*: "a relation between words and sentences, where words and sentences referring to one type of entity can be translated without any residue into those referring to another type of entity. For example, sentences about the average plumber in Berkeley are reducible to sentences about specific individual plumbers in Berkeley." (Searle, 1992, p 114) (5) *Causal Reduction*: Causal powers of the reduced entity are entirely explainable in terms of the causal powers of the reducing phenomena. The causal powers of solid objects (e.g., their powers to resist pressure, to be relatively impenetrable to other solid object, etc.) can be reductively explained by appealing to the causal powers of the vibratory properties of their molecular lattice structures.

Now we are in a position to ask: To precisely which of these forms of reductionism is the biomedical model (BMM) wed? And precisely which of these forms of reductionism are incompatible with Engel's biopsychosocial model? After all, not all of these forms of reductionism rise and fall together. Some philosophers, for example, believe that numbers have successfully been *logically* reduced to sets, but they deny that because this is the case that an ontological reduction has occurred; that is, they both claim that all sentences about numbers can be translated without any residue to statements about sets and they claim that this does not imply that numbers do not exist. Logical reduction, they claim, does not entail ontological reduction.

Similarly, very few people would disagree with the claim that thrips are wholly physical objects, i.e., that all of their parts and all of their properties are wholly composed of and realized in collections of elementary particles arranged thrip-wise. It is relatively uncontroversial, therefore, to claim that thrips are ontologically reducible to certain collections of elementary particles. Yet quite a significant number of philosophers who endorse this ontological reduction also *deny* that thrips' behavioral properties, for example, are *property* ontologically reducible to collections of elementary particles arranged thrip-wise or that the (perhaps yet to be discovered) laws that govern thrip behavior can be *explained* by, and hence are *theoretically* reducible to, the laws that govern the behavior of elementary particles.

Engel's troubles with reductionist discourse begin with his apparent ignorance of the fact that 'reductionism' is multiply ambiguous. Were Engel to have appreciated this fact, it would have been obvious to him that one can go about either accepting or rejecting 'reductionism' in several different ways. It is easy merely to repeat the claim that the BMM is reductionistic without specifying the kind(s) of reductionism it embraces. Likewise, it is easy simply to claim that 'the BPSM' is not reductionistic without further specifying the kind(s) of reductionism it denies.

Suppose that Engel, or someone on his behalf, were to counter with the following riposte: Engel meant that 'the BMM' embraces *all* contemporary varieties of reductionism and 'the BPSM' rejects *all* such varieties. But, surely, this response would be *ad hoc* and implausible, for first not all contemporary varieties of reductionism were being considered when the contemporary biopsychosocial ideology was being forged by Engel and disseminated by his disciples; and, second, at this level of conceptual discourse one would certainly expect to find a prominent diversity of medical opinion (once the issues were presented, grasped, and reflected upon), not the simple pre-BPSM (i.e., BMM) consensus and the present growing BPSM consensus (at least in some noteworthy domains of medicine) alleged by several authors in the biopsychosocial literature. Rather, one would expect to find, for example, that some adherents of BMM models will endorse some versions of reductionism and reject others, while other adherents will embrace all present (and projected future) reductionistic schemes.

There is reason to believe that Engel's troubles with reductionism are even more basic than those which I have thus far outlined. According to Engel (1977), "the biomedical model embraces both reductionism...and mind-body dualism, the doctrine that separates the mental from the somatic." (p 130) He adds that reductionism is "the philosophic view that complex phenomena are ultimately derived from a single primary principle" (p 130) and that "[h]ere the reductionistic primary principle is physicalistic; that is, it assumes that the language of chemistry and physics will ultimately suffice to explain biological phenomena. From the reductionist viewpoint, the only conceptual tools available to characterize and experimental tools to study biological systems are physical in nature." (p 130)

What is most striking about Engel's above claim that the BMM embraces both reductionism and mind-body dualism is that it is conceptually incoherent. There are, to be sure, several varieties of mind-body dualism, but every such dualistic view is *essentially anti-reductionistic*. It is, therefore, impossible consistently to be both a reductionist with respect to a given phenomenon and to attribute to that phenomenon (mind-body) dualistic characteristics.

One reason one might give for being a mind-body dualist is that one can see no possible way in which mental phenomena could be composed wholly of physical simples; or no possible way in which mental phenomena could wholly be explained by appealing only to explanatory schemes available to physicists or chemists; or no possible way in which all sentences about mental phenomena can be satisfactorily translated, without residue, to sentences about neurons; etc. This is, in fact, how many dualists do argue. (See, for example, Jackson [1982] and Swinburne [1986].)

So, either Engel is attributing to adherents of 'the BMM' a position that is conceptually incoherent or he is using the terms 'reductionism' or 'mind-body dualism' in strangely idiosyncratic ways. I find it hard to believe that Engel is charging adherents of 'the BMM' with incoherence in this context, if only because he never comes right out and *charges* them with conceptual incoherence as one would expect if he, in fact, thought this. Rather than attempting to dispose of 'the BMM' quickly and easily in this manner (since, obviously, no conceptually incoherent model could possibly be adequate for modeling a given phenomenon) he instead opts to supplant 'the BMM' with 'the BPSM' by arguing for the superiority of 'the BPSM' on *empirical* grounds. Perhaps then Engel is using the terms 'reductionism' or 'mind-body dualism' in idiosyncratic ways. Is he?

We have already seen that Engel appears unaware of the multiply ambiguous nature of the term 'reductionism.' This impression is further reinforced by his conflation of several types of reductionism in his single characterization of reductionism. By stating that, according to reductionism, "complex phenomena are ultimately derived from a single primary [physicalistic] principle," (Engel, 1977, p 130) he appears to be equating reductionism with ontological reductionism. But later he at least appears *also* to claim that the reductionist principle he has in mind is either logical or theoretical or both.

Most curiously, Engel (1977) states that, "From the reductionist viewpoint, the only conceptual tools available to characterize...biological systems are *physical* in nature." (emphasis added, p. 130) How can this possibly be true if, as Engel claims, BMM adherents are also mind-body *dualists*? Perhaps it is Engel's understanding of mind-body dualism, then, which is at the root of this particular confusion.

Engel characterizes mind-body dualism as that view which *separates* the psychic from the somatic. 'Separation' is an odd choice of words in this context. As typically used, the term 'separation' (and its cognates) refer(s) to being *spaced apart* or *disunited*. At least neither of these senses, when taken literally, appear to be appropriate so far as traditional dualistic hypotheses are concerned.

There are, as has already been stated, several distinct versions of mind-body dualism. One such version is called substance dualism of which traditional (or classical) *Cartesian dualism* (or *Cartesianism*) is one variety. As its name implies, traditional Cartesian dualism is that version of dualism based upon the thought of the great 17th century French philosopher and mathematician, Rene Descartes.[6] According to traditional Cartesianism, minds are things in their own right; *things*, that is, which can exist independently of bodies and bear properties which the body *cannot* bear. In other words, on the traditional Cartesian view, minds are what some philosophers have called *immaterial substances*.[7]

According to Descartes, live physical bodies are substances which are essentially extended in space as opposed to minds which are essentially unextended substances. In other words, live physical bodies are physical objects which are spatially located while minds necessarily exemplify neither of these properties. Given these characteristics attributed to minds and bodies in the Cartesian tradition, it follows immediately that minds and bodies *cannot possibly* be separated in the sense of being literally 'spaced apart,' for according to traditional Cartesianism, necessarily, minds do not exist in space at all.

It is of significant importance to point out that Descartes' actual philosophy of mind appears to entail an even tighter link between mind and brain than does traditional Cartesianism. Conceiving of Cartesian minds as being separated from Cartesian bodies in the sense of being 'disunited' from them is, therefore, also seriously to misconstrue what is arguably Descartes' own (rather than the Cartesian tradition's) philosophy of mind, for Descartes (1975) himself has clearly stated that, "I am present to my body not merely in the way a seaman is present to this ship, but...I am tightly joined and, so to speak, mingled together with it, so much so that I make up one single thing with it." (p. 50)[8]

An additional important feature of classical Cartesian dualism is that the human mind - which is conceived as being both immaterial and the essence of the human person - may continue to exist after the body has died. From where did these immaterial minds originally derive their being? According to Descartes, directly from the creative hand of an omnipotent God. Furthermore, Descartes believed that, should God wish to continue sustaining them in existence, minds would continue to exist after the death of the body. Perhaps this is what Engel had in mind when he claimed that the doctrine of mind-body dualism 'separates' the mental from the physical. But, of course, not all *substance dualism* is *Cartesian dualism*.

One manner in which to be a non-Cartesian substance dualist is to be a certain kind of emergentist, namely, an emergentist which claims that brains which have attained a certain level of complexity *generate* minds conceived of as substances in their own right. Such minds are not directly created *ex nihilo* by God at the moment of 'enmindment' (whenever that moment happens to be), but rather *arise from* the physical substrate of brains which have reached the requisite level of complexity. A 'sustance-emergentist' could posit that this emergent substance is, like the living body, intrinsically corruptible, but at a rate which does not exactly coincide with the corruption of the body. In such a case, perhaps the body would die, the mind would then 'live on' for a specified period of time and then it too would cease to exist. I know of no one who holds such a view. Rather, those individuals of whom I am aware who seriously entertain substance-emergentism, claim that the dependence relation between mind and brain is not restricted to its genesis, but also to its sustenance. On this view, when the brain dies, the mind ceases to be.

Most mind-body emergentists, though, are not *substance-emergentists*. Rather, most mind-body emergentists are *property-emergentists*. The claim is not that a thing called 'the mind' comes into existence once the brain attains a certain level of complexity, but that certain *non*-physical mental properties come into existence at this point. It follows from this view that non-physical mental properties are not properties of minds, since minds are not, on this view, substances in which properties can inhere. Rather, mental properties are thought to be properties of those neurobiological processes which govern the workings of the brain itself. The term 'the mind' is misleading on this view, for the definite article is not meant to pick out a *thing*, but only a set of properties (namely, non-physical mental properties) exemplified (at least in humans) by a set of neurons.

It is of great importance to point out that although the countenancing of *some* emergent properties have lead *some* philosophers toward *some* version or other of dualism, there is no necessary link between a property's being emergent from a physical medium and that property's being *non*-physical in nature. The extended discussions of emergentism and reductionism above were, in part, meant to make this point diaphanous. This, in review, is the critical point: One may consistently be both an emergentist with respect to a given phenomenon P and be a *non*-dualist with respect to P. In fact one can be both an emergentist with respect to P and a monist of the physicalist variety. It follows from this that one can consistently be both an emergentist with respect to P and an (in principle) *ontological* reductionist with respect to P. It is in this manner that, *contra* Engel, reductionism and emergentism with respect to one and the same phenomenon (but, again *contra* Engel, *not* reductionism and mind-body dualism) can happily coexist.

Some examples of this confluence of emergentism and reductionism have already been provided: The solidity of the piston, we are told, is an emergent property of the vibratory motions in its molecular lattice structure; the liquidity of water is believed to be an emergent property of its underlying molecular structure, etc. But, one might ask, can the same be said about at least some *living* systems? Again, the answer appears to be yes.

Living organisms were, of course, studied and taxonomized long before the advent of modern (Baconian) biological science. The most prominent of these pre-modern biologists (then called 'natural philosophers' or 'philosophers of nature') was Aristotle. Aristotelian biology was vigorous in its rejection of several schemes of reductionism (e.g., what we would now call logical, causal, and theoretical reductionisms). Yet it was equally vigorous in its insistence that the vast majority of biological systems were nothing more than very complex physical objects.

Aristotle would, for example, claim that living thrips are nothing more than unified collections of elements arranged thrip-wise and yet, he would insist, the behavior of living thrips could not, even in principle, be explained simply by invoking the explanatory schemes employed in order adequately to explain the behavior of its parts.[9] Instead, Aristotle thought it essential for one's attaining a thorough understanding of living systems that one's explanation of the behavior of whole unified systems utilize concepts foreign to those disciplines which would otherwise be quite appropriate for explaining the behavior of those systems' parts. On Aristotle's view, then, the whole could not be thoroughly understood simply in virtue of having a thorough understanding of that whole's parts. This is Aristotle's doctrine of 'holism.' It is also a deep posit of GST and, thereby, it is a doctrine embraced by Engel.

What Engel (and others[10]) has (have) apparently failed to recognize, though, is that this doctrine did not die when Aristotle died, and it was not resurrected with the work of Weiss and von Bertalanffy. It has survived, in fact *flourished*, in the work of a multitude of Aristotelians and Thomists (i.e., adherents of the philosophy of the remarkable 13th century philosopher and theologian, Thomas Aquinas, also called 'the Thomistic philosophy' or simply 'Thomism') over the past two millennia. Aquinas was heavily influenced by Aristotelianism and, to a lesser extent, by Platonism. In addition he was a Christian. Some of what Aquinas had to say was Aristotelian or Platonic philosophy Christianized. Some of what he had to say, though, was strikingly original. All of what he had to say deserves our intellectual respect. His influence on Western thought has been enormous, in large part because his influence on Roman Catholic thought has been enormous. The Thomistic philosophy, and with it the biology of Aristotle, has been and continues to be an important part of Roman Catholic intellectual life.[11] These Roman Catholic intellectuals have kept alive this intellectual tradition in the face of stiff opposition from prevailing currents in biological thought which had banished teleology and holism (distinctive Aristotelian-Thomistic doctrines) from serious consideration in scientific circles.

It has always struck me as curious that the conceptual core of what many (Engel included) have taken to be a kind of twentieth century paradigm shift - some have even referred to it as a 'revolution' - in the psychiatric and general medical arenas - a GST-mediated shift toward 'the BPSM' and away from 'the BMM' - had been conceived and intricately developed in ancient Greece and further deepened and extended over several centuries in the context of that institution (viz., the Christian Church) which the scientific community has often vilified as being the enemy of scientific progress. I say that it's about time to set the record straight. (I plan, more fully, to do just this in Part 3.)

What I find equally curious is that several recent writers on the biopsychosocial ideology appear to have failed to appreciate one important entailment of that ideology intended by Engel, namely a commitment to some variety of emergentism.[12] I say that this is one important entailment of that ideology that was intended by Engel rather than saying that this entailment is *essential* to biopsychosocial ideology *simpliciter* in virtue of the fact that it is wholly unclear in Engel's writings and those who follow him precisely which particular elements of what are properly called 'biopsychosocial models' are meant to be essential to them. Thus, when Peter Vitaliano et al. (1988) speak of "complex combinations of biological and psychosocial factors" (p 311) and when they claim to have found that "a comprehensive model explained distress better than any variable used alone" (p 325) it is wholly unclear whether they, like Engel, are committed to a form of emergentism or simply to a complex confluence of, in principle, reducible causes. One would think that if they were, in fact, committed to some form of emergentism, they would have made this clear. But they did not. Rather, they speak in a manner which is annoyingly *ambiguous* between a commitment to emergentism, a commitment to thorough-going reductionism, and commitments to *other* incompatible metaphysical views. Because emergentism is such a deep philosophical posit, one would have predicted that were Vitaliano et al. committed to it, they would have made this explicit. Given that they did not, I am left to infer either that they do not realize that any such metaphysical commitment was ever intended in this domain, or that they do realize this but reject it.

Vitaliano et al. are not alone in this regard. According to J.W. Dwyer et al. (1988), "The biopsychosocial model interrelates the social and psychological conditions experienced by the patient to a diagnosis derived from the standard biomedical model." (emphasis added, p. 20) Len Sperry et al. (1991) believe that "changing from a biomedical to a biopsychosocial perspective involves a major paradigm shift in health care," (p. 99) in part because "the biopsychosocial perspective has been advocated as being *more comprehensive and humane* than a strict biomedical approach." (emphasis added, p 99) Cairns Aitken (1987) assures us that by taking a biopsychosocial approach to diagnosis and treatment, "factors in *all three dimensions* are taken into account." (emphasis added, p. 130) Gregory J. O'Shanick et al. (1986) identify 'the biopsychosocial model' with a model that emphasizes "*multifactorial causation of disease* and patients' reactions and adaptations to physical illness." (emphasis added, p 366) Zeev Ben-Sira (1990) states that "The concept of bio-psychosocial approach, developed by Engel in the seventies, refers to the *integrated* application of biological, psychological and social factors in the understanding and treatment of health problems." (p 565) Thomas N. Wise (1993) claims that "Psychosomatic medicine is best conceptualized as understanding health and illness from a *multifactorial perspective* that includes biological, psychological and social factors. This approach is the biopsychosocial model of Engel and Reading." (emphasis added, p. 100) J.Z. Sadler and Y.F. Hulgus (1990) call Engel's BPSM "one of the most influential developments in psychiatry and medicine in the latter part of this century." (p. 185) They go on to state that "the BPS model can briefly be described as a medical model where clinical data in the biological, psychological, and social spheres are given equal weight in clinical formulations. In addition, these *spheres function* interdependently." (emphasis added, p 185) Finally, Alan Beigel (1995) avers that "the biopsychosocial model...underscores the role of *complex interactions* between the biological and the psychosocial." (emphasis added, p. 32)

What I find most striking about the aforementioned characterizations of BPSMs is that these appeals to interrelatedness, comprehensiveness, multifactorial causation, integration, spheres that function interdependently, and complex integration are, as stated, all conspicuously *ambiguous* between reductionist and holistic ways of understanding these phenomena. Compare the aforementioned ambiguous characterizations with the more nearly univocal, substantive claim made by Z.J. Lipowski (1986) who writes that, according to the biopsychosocial ideology, "a person should be viewed as an integrated *whole*, a psychobiological unit, which could not be reduced to one of its aspects only[.]" (p 348) But although Lipowski appears explicitly to embrace an emergentist alternative to reductionism in medicine, neither he nor Engel make at all clear how *this* particular emergentist ontology is *superior* to a thorough-going form of reductionism which *also* takes into account biopsychosocial variables albeit under different (viz. reductionistic) descriptions.

One might, at this point, raise the following query: Is it not the case that anyone who uses biopsychosocial language, i.e., anyone who speaks of psychological and social as well as biological determinants of human behavior is, by definition, an anti-reductionist? The answer to this query is clearly no. The reason for this is that reductionists of many stripes *commonly* resort to the use of theoretical and practical vocabularies which merely *appear* to convey anti-reductionist sentiments. In such cases, the apparently anti-reductionist vocabularies in question serve merely as place-holders. Although they freely employ a psychosocial vocabulary, such reductionists are explicitly committed to the thesis that such a vocabulary is, in principle, temporary, dispensable, ultimately replaceable by a more sophisticated (bio)physical vocabulary.

The reductionists' claim here is that, eventually, if we were able to master the enormous complexity of human (bio)physics, we would also be able to carry out all of the proper reductions. Thus, an appeal to 'social factors' is not meant, in this context, to be an appeal to some emergent 'social' property of human beings; rather, it is an appeal to some set of yet uncharacterized properties of elementary particles which, at least for the time being, are conveniently referred to as 'social factors.' Once these elemental properties are elucidated, the reductionist meaning of the term 'social factors' will become manifest; social causes will be shown to consist in, and be explainable in terms of, nothing but complex systems of reduced (microphysical) causes. In this sense, the use of an apparent anti-reductionistic vocabulary serves a critical pragmatic function, namely, it allows one the convenience of speaking about reductionistic processes prior to one's having elucidated the (inferred) reduced structure of the determinants in question.

But, one might ask, is this kind of reductionistic model a 'BPSM'? It certainly appears to be, simply in virtue of its making appeals to superordinate determinants which the prior biomedical ideology allegedly failed to appreciate. Such biopsychosocial models are not, to be sure, biopsychosocial models which are identical to Engel's. But then, it is unclear - given Engel's own obvious unclarity on this matter - what Engel's requirements for a model's being *biopsychosocial* in character *are*.

It is in this manner, then, that reductionistic biomedical thinking has been reintroduced into the medical medium disguised as anti-reductionistic biopsychosocial thinking. (A second manner in which such a reintroduction has been effected may be found in what Z.J. Lipowski [1985] calls 'methodological reductionism' in which he argues that psychiatrists ought both to adopt an integrative approach in clinical practice and theory, and to practice reductionism in research.) And it is in this sense that the biomedical ideology has returned; returned in a form that is more subtle and pernicious than the biomedical ideology which it had previously supplanted.[13] One might say that this apparently prominent reductionistic strand in biopsychosocial ideology is the 'Trojan Horse'[14] of psychiatry and medicine. It is, in this manner, an ideology which had been formally expelled under one guise and, under a different guise, has been invited back onto medicine's theoretical stage.

2. What is it that a BPSM is most properly a model *of?*

According to Engel (1977), 'the BPSM' is most properly a model of *disease*. If it is meant to model all human diseases, this characterization is inaccurate. It is, first of all, not the case that *all* disease states have a biological, psychological and social component to them. Anencephalic infants, for instance, suffer from a disease if any one does and yet such infants, we are told, instantiate no *psychology* at all.

On the other hand, there is good reason to believe that mature, well-functioning, flourishing human beings enjoy states of optimal health only if they are properly ordered along (at least) biological, psychological, and social axes. Deficits in any of these three areas constitute a movement away from healthy human functioning. The *absence* of a psychology, social contacts, or an intact biology could prove to be disastrous. I would like to suggest, therefore, that BPSMs (at least in the domain of *human* medicine) be viewed as being models, not of disease itself, but of *how* human persons function in health *and* disease.[15]

3. How, Precisely, Does a BPSM Differ From a BMM?

We have already noted (in Part 1) that not all models which appear to have a justifiable claim to being called a 'BPSM' are incompatible with models which are thought to be biomedical in nature. (One could, of course, simply *stipulate* that every BPSM is incompatible with every BMM, but this move would have the strange consequence of disqualifying a significant number of what appear to pass for BPSMs in the literature - and in hospital halls - as being genuine instances of BPSMs. The principal difficulty with this exclusionary maneuver is that it rides, for the most part, on a deep metaphysical point about emergence which, as I see it, almost no one in the biopsychosocial corpus appears to understand.) The reason for this, I said, is that there is a bewildering array of BPSMs, some of which, *contra* Engel, appear unselfconsciously to countenance various forms of thoroughgoing reductionism.

The picture becomes significantly more complicated when one notices that neither do BMMs come in only a single variety. Engel's characterization of 'the BMM' as possessing a strict 'factor-analytic' structure is a caricature. In fact, Engel (1977) himself admits that, "The contrasting posture of strict adherence to the medical model is *caricatured* in Ludwig's view of psychiatrist as physician[,]" (emphasis added, p 129) and then goes on to explicate this caricature as one of his main targets in this domain. Of course, it would not be a caricature, if this is simply what Engel was *stipulating* as being what the structure of a BMM is. If this is what Engel were doing, then he has every right to designate whatever model he would like and call it 'the BMM.' But this is not what Engel took himself to be doing. Rather, he imagines that he has discovered the kind of model that *dominated* the pre-BPSM era; the kind of model employed by mainstream American medicine; the kind of model that served as the structural dogma upon which modern medical ideology had been poised. Is he right about any of this?

Engel is neither a sociologist nor a historian. The reasons he adduces for believing that a *single* medical model dominated Western psychiatry and medicine and, furthermore, that the single model in question is what he calls 'the BMM' are reasons that are neither sociological nor historical in nature; rather Engel's reasons appear to derive from his selective reading of some of his medical and psychiatric contemporaries. Engel (1980) allegedly deduces from this fragmentary evidence that 'the BMM' which, he surmises, at that time provided the dominant conceptual framework in Western psychiatry and medicine "does not include the patient and his attributes as a person...[and that it] can make provision neither for the person as a whole nor for data of a psychological or social nature." (p 536)

Of course, many reductionists would vigorously resist Engel's suggestion that 'the patient as a person' has been left out of their conceptual systems. The counter-claim would go something like this: "What are you talking about? Our reductionist models are models of patients as persons in health and disease. We simply happen to believe that human persons are nothing more than the sum of their (elementary) parts and that the psychology of persons as well as their social nature is (in some sense of the term 'reducible') *reducible* to the behavior of elementary particles." Now Engel may *disagree* with the reductionist on this score; that is, he may be convinced that there *can be* no successful reduction (in any significant sense of that term) of human persons to any collection of their parts. This would indeed be a substantive metaphysical claim. But nowhere does Engel defend *this* particular claim against its reductionistic detractors.

What Engel does do (for example, in his 1980 paper, "The Clinical Application of the Biopsychosocial Model") is to argue that it makes for better medical care when physicians consider psychological and social variables as well as biological variables in the context of health care. What he does not do though - and what he *must* do if he is properly to highlight his position's theoretical and practical advantages over the position of the reductionists - is to show how it is that one's construing psychological and social properties as properties which are (in some sense) *irreducible* provides the clinician with theoretical and practical advantages over one who construes such properties as, in principle, *reducible* to other (non-psychological and non-social, respectively) properties.

What Engel has also failed to do is to have shown in any convincing way that there has been anything like a consensus in the Western medical community concerning how best to model the functioning of human persons in health and disease. There is not, nor has there ever been, to my knowledge, a medical pontificate whose authority extends over the members of the medical profession and who, thereby, could have properly elevated what Engel calls 'the BMM' to the status of a dogma. Neither have there been, to my knowledge, any polls of physicians which questioned their allegiance to one metaphysical view concerning the nature of human beings over another. But I am confident that if such polls had been taken, one would have found a wide variety of positions on this issue. I would not be surprised if many practicing physicians polled held *no* view at all on this relatively rarefied metaphysical issue. Of those who *did* hold a view, one would expect that some would be reductionists but not know what kind. Other would be reductionists of one kind or other. And, given the significant number of Catholic hospitals and Catholic-educated physicians in the West, it would not be surprising (to me, at least) if a significant number of physicians polled were anti-reductionists of some variety or other.

I imagine that the discovery of a significant number of anti-reductionist physicians prior to the biopsychosocial era would be quite surprising to Engel, especially if such physicians were found amongst those who were practicing medicine a century or more ago, for according to Engel (1980), 'the BPSM' "is based on a systems approach, a development in biology hardly more than 50 years old." (p 535) Now it may in fact be the case that Engel's incarnation of biopsychosocial medicine was constructed from the building blocks supplied by GST as developed by Weiss and von Bertalanffy during the early parts of this century. But anti-reductionist BPSMs are not *essentially* tied to a *general theory* of emergent systems.

As mentioned in Part 1, Aristotle was an anti-reductionist who would have rejected a general systems approach to understanding the world. Rather, he restricted his anti-reductionist commitments largely (and according to some Aristotle scholars, solely) to the proper understanding of living organisms. According to Aristotle, iguanas, thrips, and plankton would be considered emergent systems, while social networks of human beings would not; neither, according to Aristotle, would subatomic particles, atoms, molecules, organelles, families, cultures or almost any other 'system' found in Engel (1980).

Aristotle presented some deep reasons for thinking these things, reasons that have to do with what is sometimes called his *hylomorphism,* or his *matter-form ontology.* The details of this metaphysical system cannot be adequately developed here; neither can the hylomorphism of Aquinas which borrowed heavily from Aristotle.[16] Fortunately, the relevant points can be stated without appeals to the subtle and difficult philosophies of nature elaborated by Aristotle and Aquinas. The points to which I am referring are, first, the fact that well-developed and well-entrenched anti-reductionist models of human beings had been developed long before the advent of GST and, second, the fact that a significant number of practicing physicians who were well-versed in Aristotelianism (principally in virtue of being Thomists, i.e., principally in virtue of being living members of the Catholic philosophical tradition) were anti-reductionists with respect to human organisms long before the promulgation of Engel's biopsychosocial ideology.

One need not, of course, countenance hylomorphism in order to be an anti-reductionist with respect to human beings. Engel, for example, appears to be ignorant of both Aristotelian and Thomistic metaphysics and yet his BPSM is anti-reductionist in character. In a like manner, Peter van Inwagen (1990) is a contemporary metaphysician who has developed a metaphysical system (without explicitly relying upon the Aristotelian-Thomistic tradition) that entails a form of anti-reductionism but which does not entail hylomorphism.

What is it, precisely, that has driven Engel to embrace an *emergentist* version of the biopsychosocial ideology (again, assuming for the time being that there are possible *non*-emergent versions of this ideology). Engel does not appear to be driven to this emergentist ideology by prior, more basic metaphysical commitments. (If he is being driven by such commitments, he has not yet made these known to us.) It also does not appear that he is driven to his specifically emergentist version of the biopsychosocial ideology by practical considerations either, since one would think that *non*-emergentist versions of BPSMs would have sufficed in this regard: All one would need to have done is to point out that there are pathogenic variables, none of which are emergent in nature, which have been neglected by many (although not all) Western physicians and which, if properly reflected upon in the context of medical practice, could greatly improve patient care.

4. Are Biopsychosocial Models (BSPM's) Superior to Rival Models?

The answer to this question depends (at least in part) on (i) what there *is* and on the *nature* of what there is, (ii) whether or not the term 'BPSM' is meant to be understood *literally*, and (iii) what the intended *purpose* of BPSMs is meant to be. We will consider (iii) first.

It might appear that one's primary motivation for constructing a model of anything x is in order to achieve a *comprehensive understanding* of x. This is, in fact, not always the case. Sometimes models *obscure* one's understanding of several key features of that x which is being modeled, yet adequately serve to illuminate one particular feature of x - perhaps a feature which serves some *pragmatic* purpose. So, for example, Ptolemaic astronomy modeled the solar system in a geocentric manner, a manner in which we now believe does not accurately reflect the proper relationship between the Earth, the Sun, and the other planets. Yet geocentric astronomy's *predictive* power was quite impressive. If one were to have asked a Ptolemaic astronomer where a certain planet could be found on a given night, his answer would certainly have been at least as accurate as the answer of an (early) astronomer of the Copernican persuasion. Copernicus's heliocentric astronomy was simply not, during its theoretical infancy, any more predictively accurate than its Ptolemaic counterpart.[17]

Geocentric astronomy significantly obscured the proper relationships between the Sun and its planets, yet in part because of the premium placed on the *predictive* power of astronomical theories in the 16th century, the much more complex, more *ad hoc*, and hence less plausible (from a structural-relational point of view), epicycle-ridden geocentric model was favored over the more simple, less *ad hoc*, heliocentric model.[18] Several physicists (including Einstein) have held out for an analogous Copernican revolution in the microphysical world, for the 'picture' of reality that has been painted by contemporary quantum mechanists has appeared to many to be inelegant, implausible, even fantastical. Yet the predictive power of quantum mechanics has been enormous, and in 20th century physics - just as in 16th century astronomy - the value placed on the predictive power of a physical theory is immense.

In this context, consider again emergentist BPSMs. *How* precisely are these models meant to deepen our understanding of human beings in health and disease? Are they meant accurately to portray the structure of healthy and diseased human beings? Or are they meant merely to serve some other, *pragmatic* purpose? Perhaps they were intended to accomplish both of the aforementioned tasks. According to Engel (1980), "How physicians approach patients and the problems they present is very much influenced by the conceptual models in relationship to which their knowledge and experience are organized. Commonly, however, physicians are largely unaware of the power such models exert on their thinking and behavior." (p 535)

It appears, then, that according to Engel, one very important feature of 'the BPSM' as he conceives it is its potential role in restructuring the manner in which health care professionals deliver patient care. And one manner in which to formulate this hypothesized relationship between BPSMs and patient care is to claim that psychiatrists, for example, who approach their patients with their medical knowledge and psychiatric experience organized by a BPSM will *ceteris paribus* be in a position to deliver patient care that is either quantitatively or qualitatively superior to the patient care delivered were their knowledge and experience organized by any other available model. But, of course, even if this pragmatic advantage of BPSMs were well established, this does not entail that human beings actually *are* structured in those specific manners implied by the pragmatically successful BPSMs in question.

It is at this point that a key question arises: What pragmatic advantage is there in one's endorsing an *emergentist* (e.g., Engelian) BPSM over a *non*-emergentist model in which the same variable categories are invoked? It is this question that Engel does not answer, but it is a question which he *must* answer if he is to persuade sophisticated reductionists who are convinced that, in principle, biological, psychological, and social variables are *all* reducible to microphysical variables. What Engel or his defenders first need to specify in order to demonstrate the superiority of emergentist BPSMs over rival non-emergentist models is the intended *purpose* of the emergentist BPSMs in question. Once this purpose is specified, then one can go about comparing emergentist BPSMs to their non-emergentist rivals along the specified axis.

The axis in question could, of course, be something other than a pragmatic purpose involving patient care. Suppose, instead, that the axis of interest were the fundamental structure of human beings. Engel (1980) has, for example, claimed that "The crippling flaw of the [biomedical] model is that it does not include the patient and his attributes as a person[.]" (p 536) An analogous situation in the field of astronomy might involve a model which approximated the fundamental structural relations among astronomical bodies but which did not include clear mathematical guidance for accurately tracking this structure's diachronic behavior. It may be the case, that is, that one model is well-suited for capturing one of these features but ill-suited for capturing the other.

So, too, for models of human patients in health and disease. A model which had been conceived in order to capture the nature of human beings in health and disease would be superior to its rivals insofar as it actually captured the nature of human beings more accurately than its competitors. And, of course, whether or not one model captures human nature better that another depends critically on what the nature of human beings is as well as what the natures of extra-human variables which shape human nature happen to be. In this case, emergentist BPSMs would be superior to their rivals insofar as human beings *actually* do exemplify emergent properties as these are specified by the theory or, in other - specifically GST - terms, actually do constitute emergent systems. *Mutatis mutandis* for other extra-human variables which, for example, according to GST, constitute systems of various sorts with just those emergent properties countenanced by GST.

Consider in this light the content of certain widespread religious beliefs. Suppose, for example, that certain religious beliefs concerning the nature and existence of God and angels are true. Then, although being a theist may, in fact, afford one certain psychological and social benefits, one's relationship with God could not itself be reduced to mere psychological or social variables. If *strict* BPSMs were, therefore, to be taken as *excluding* one's relationships with supernatural beings, such BPSMs would be inferior to more comprehensive models which included at least the possibility of such natural-supernatural interactions.

Whether or not biopsychosocial models are or are not sensitive to variables that are neither biological, psychological, or social in nature depends on whether or not the term 'biopsychosocial' is meant to be taken literally.[19] Some thinkers, for example, appear to believe that, by definition, 'BPSMs' strictly understood exclude spiritual or environmental or cultural variables. (See, for example, Hiatt [1986] and Burkett [1991].) This, to me, is not so obvious, for the term, biopsychosocial, may properly be viewed to be a kind of *shorthand* that denotes models which include supernatural, environmental, cultural, and numerous other variables.

The main point of the preceding discussion can be summarized as follows: Whether or not a certain model is superior to its rivals depends upon the axes along which these models are compared; and the axes in question depend, in part, upon the intended purpose for which the models were constructed. Thus, if two models are being compared along purely structural axes, the criteria for whether or not one model is superior to another will depend upon *what there is* and on the *structure* of what there is. This is not the case when comparing models along more pragmatic axes (e.g., along axes having more to do with prediction, or, alternatively, with clinical utility[20]). In this latter domain, what there is and the structure of what there is may, in fact, be wholly irrelevant to the comparison in question.

I have, in this essay, attempted to draw attention to a number of complexities in biopsychosocial theorizing which all writers on this topic (of whom I am aware) have, either in whole or in part, managed to elide. My principal point has been that there are a large number of mutually incompatible models which appear to deserve the 'biopsychosocial' title, some of which are, in some relevant sense, reductionistic in nature. I have further argued that no one in this discussion has, to my mind, yet made explicit how precisely the deep metaphysical commitment to emergentism required by GST provides physicians with any clinical advantage when it comes to issues relating to patient care over those who are committed to a thorough-going reductionism.

Rather than being driven by any such anti-reductionistic metaphysical commitments, the engine that drives contemporary biopsychosocial ideology appears to be powered merely by the desires of clinicians to explore the etiological roles - under *no particular* metaphysical description - of a wider range of variables than had previously been explored, in their attempts to best meet the clinical needs of their patients in health and disease. But even this, we have seen, is not entirely accurate, for there have always been amongst us significant numbers of physicians who have explored not only those variables specified by Engel, but other variables as well. Some of these physicians have been Catholic, others have not. Some have been emergentists, others have been anti-reductionists of other stripes, and yet others have been thorough-going reductionists.

It appears then that Engel's explicit attempt to extricate the general medical and psychiatric professions from the mire of biomedical reductionism has, unexpectedly, failed on at least the following two fronts. First, it is clear that anti-reductionism in the context of medicine has, for centuries, been alive and well, having been well-represented in communities of physicians throughout the West long before the development of GST. In fact the principal variety of anti-reductionism there represented, viz. Aristotelian-Thomistic anti-reductionism, had been developed and refined into a conceptual tapestry the power and elegance of which can only be adequately appreciated after years of careful study. Engel's model is, in comparison, an attempt at re-inventing the anti-reductionist wheel, but an attempt which, as I see it, is a mere shadow of the historical pattern which it unwittingly has aspired to resemble. Second, in virtue of the apparent fact that the anti-reductionism inherent in Engel's work has not been shown (at least in the biopsychosocial literature) to be any more relevant to patient care than a parallel BPSM which is reductionistic - and thereby *biomedical* - in nature, and in virtue of the practical difficulties inherent in conveying to others the critical entailments of emergentist - or other anti-reductionist - metaphysical schemes, what appears to have flourished in the contemporary biopsychosocial literature is a many-membered family of *reductionist* BPSMs. But, as we have seen, *reductionist* BPSMs are nothing more than disguised *BMM* variants. It is therefore the strangest irony of all that Engel, in an effort to rid psychiatry and the general medical arenas of biomedical reductionism, appears actually to have been instrumental in reductionism's return and re-entrenchment in a much more subtle, pervasive, and virulent form.[21]

ENDNOTES

1. I am grateful to Hoyle Leigh, M.D. for having brought to my attention Karl Menninger's (1963) *The Vital Balance* as an example of careful and cogent biopsychosocial theorizing in psychiatry prior to Engel. One might, in this context, also refer to James E. Sabin's (1990) account of eminent New England internist Joseph Hersey Pratt's biopsychosocial approach to medicine. I shall shortly argue that such theorizing can further be traced back to an ancient Greek philosophical tradition which originated with Aristotle and which has been further deepened and extended in the writings of St. Thomas Aquinas.

2. Never mind that jigsaw puzzles are arguably not *systems* in the sense intended by systems theorists. Nevertheless, this example provides an elegant illustration of the insufficiency of size and complexity criteria alone for making distinctions between system units. According to Engel (1980), the "designation 'system' bespeaks the existence of a stable configuration in time and space, a configuration that is maintained not only by the coordination of component parts in some kind of internal dynamic network but also by the characteristics of the larger system of which it is a component part." (p 537) Note that given this understanding of 'system,' the universe as a whole (understood as all that there is) could not form a system, for the universe as a whole could not be a component of any larger system.

3. Although water *supervenes* on its molecular parts, this does not, on O'Conner's view, entail that water's liquidity is an *emergent* property of its molecular parts. In fact, O'Conner explicitly denies that liquidity is an emergent property of water molecules. (Personal Communication) Other philosophers disagree with O'Conner on this point.

Note that some philosophers do not believe that there *are* any such *objects* constituted only by a collection of water molecules. Nevertheless, I ask that we all suspend our native metaphysical reservations concerning this point, assume that a collection of water molecules is a genuine object, and acknowledge the manner in which reflection on a glass of water can help elucidate the mysteries of supervenience.

4. Searle (1992) would insist that O'Conner's 'novel causal influence' requirement is not a proper requirement for that variety of emergence which Searle finds to be ubiquitous. Thus, Searle's preferred view of emergentism is significantly weaker than O'Conner's. For a second contemporary explication and defense of an emergentist theory of consciousness, see R.W. Sperry (1980, 1991).

5. Searle (1992) readily admits that consciousness' being an irreducible property of the brain is merely an artifact of how reductions are presently being carried out. He confidently predicts that, in principle, once the conceptual machinery used to carry out reductions is appropriately refined, a thorough-going reductionism will be possible, for he is convinced that all human mental properties are wholly caused by and realized in those entities called 'human brains.' See Searle (1992), pp. 188-124.

6. I mean to imply that there are other, non-Cartesian, varieties of substance dualism, a taxonomy of such varieties being beyond the scope of this essay. I mean also sharply to distinguish traditional Cartesianism from Descartes' actual philosophy of mind.

7. The term 'substance' is also multiply ambiguous. The history of its use is long and complex. Suffice it to say that I shall be using the term in the following, rough sense:

x is a substance if and only if x bears properties and x can exist (in some important sense of 'on its own') on its own. In this sense, thrips, human beings and Cartesian minds are substances, while being a better wrestler than Plato, being colored green, and Socrates' being snub-nosed are not.

8. This strong claim to mind-body unity appears to be inconsistent with substance dualism and, hence, it also appears to be inconsistent with traditional Cartesian dualism. The strongest claim to mind-body unity amongst those who embrace a species of mind-body dualism (broadly construed) is found not in Descartes, but in those Aristotelian-Thomistic 'hylomorphic' schemes the complexities of which preclude detailed discussion in an essay of this nature.

9. See Aristotle's *Physics*. What more is needed, according to Aristotle, is an appeal to the *natures* of living things, i.e., an appeal to what might be called *nature explanations*. A discussion of what nature explanations are and why they were thought by Aristotle to be essential for understanding biological phenomena would require a substantial amount of conceptual background which space constraints prohibit my attempting to impart here.

10. Z.J. Lipowski (1986), for example, claims that the 'holistic' or 'biopsychosocial' approach to issues of etiology and treatment of mental disorders was "developed by Adolf Meyer early in this century[.]" (p 347) And according to Aviel Goodman (1991), 'the BPSM' is "[l]ess than 20 years old" and "is now the most coherent, comprehensive, and empirically valuable conceptual framework within which to understand the human being in health and in illness." (p 554) Goodman, like Lipowski, appears to be unaware of the rich tradition of holism in early Greek and latter Medieval thought.

11. Pope Pius V pronounced Aquinas the *Angelic Doctor* in 1567. In 1880 Pope Leo XIII named Aquinas Patron of Catholic Schools.

12. Note that although GST entails a commitment to some form of emergentism, it is not the case that the entailment holds in the opposite direction. Some emergentists would not countenance any composite *things* (in the strict, philosophical sense of the term 'things') in which properties could inhere *except* living organisms. The systems theories in these cases would not be *general* systems theories. See, for example, Peter van Inwagen (1990).

13. David Armstrong (1987) endorses the provocative thesis that Engels specific BPSM is, at its root, a disguised biomedical variant: "Engel clearly is firmly fixed into biomedicine and its root biological context. His 'new model' is therefore nothing of the kind. It is simply the old one with a gloss." (p 1217) He finds Engel's original model to be "grossly medicocentric and sociologically naive." (p 1213) He goes on to state that, "far from systems theory creating a 'new model' based on an integrated hierarchy, it would seem to offer... a strengthening of traditional biological, reductionist medicine." (p. 1213) Armstrong argues that Engel's BPSM was motivated by potential threats to biomedicine from the psychosocial quarter and that his model merely incorporates psychosocial concepts in order to 'neutralize' them "all in the name of a progressive model of disease." (p 1213)

Although I have sympathies with some of Armstrong's central concerns, my primary thesis in this essay differs from Armstrong's principally with respect to his implausible claim that *GST* itself strengthens medical reductionism. On the contrary, general systems theory is conceptually inimical to biological reductionism; rather, it is how this theory has been *misunderstood* and *misapplied* that has strengthened the grip of reductionist biomedical models on the theoretical commitments of psychiatrists and primary care physicians.

14. This illuminating metaphor of the 'Trojan Horse' was related to me by Lev Gertsik, M.D. in conversation.

15. Jasnoski and Warner (1991) advance a similar suggestion concerning what it is that BPSMs model in the context of developing an alternative ('synchronous systems') model. Note that Jasnoski and Warner also claim to have detected the return of reductionism into psychiatric and general medical theorizing but for reasons that differ from my own: "The old phrase 'biopsychosocial model' is still reminiscent of the old biomedical model, both of which emphasize parts rather than wholes." (p 254)

16. See St. Thomas Aquinas, *Summa Theologica*, I, qq 75-87. For an intriguing, vigorous, and spirited contemporary explication and defense of hylomorphism as it applies to human beings, see David Braine (1992).

17. *This*, (along with the fact that it certainly does not *seem* that the Earth is in rapid motion) and *not* the alleged fact that a geocentric astronomy was a religiously-driven dogmatic demand of the ecclesiastical authorities of Copernicus' day was one of the primary reasons for Copernican astronomy's initially being forcefully resisted by Catholic Church authorities. See Kuhn (1970, 1977).

18. The noted 'simplicity' of the heliocentric model needs to be appropriately qualified. Copernican astronomy was more simple in *some* respects, but not in others. See Kuhn (1970, 1977).

19. What the term 'biopsychosocial' is supposed to mean is a live issue. Paul J. Fink (1988), for example, points to what he considers to be "the gradual loss of meaning that has followed the original power of the term 'biopsychosocial'" (p 1061), further claiming that this term "has become an intellectualized, overused shibboleth (password) in psychiatry and [that it] is destined to follow the fate of such other hollow terms as 'eclectic' and 'mental health' which have lost their power as metaphors." (p 1061)

20. Worries about the clinical action-guiding utility of BPSMs are forcefully raised in Michael Alan Schwartz and Osborne P. Wiggins (1985). The provocative suggestion advanced by Schwartz and Wiggins is that BPSMs result in a gain of theoretical comprehension at the expense of clinical utility.

21. I am grateful to Timothy O'Conner for helpful comments on an earlier version of this essay.

REFERENCES

Aitken C: Psychosomatics for all - Past, present and future. Psychother Psychosom 47:128-138, 1987.

Armstrong D: Theoretical tensions in biopsychosocial medicine. Social Science and Medicine 25:1213-1218, 1987.

Beigel A: A proposed vision for psychiatry at the turn of the century.
Comprehensive Psychiatry 36:31-39, 1995.

Ben-Sira Z: Primary care practitioners' likelihood to engage in a bio-psychosocial approach: An additional perspective on the doctor-patient relationship.
Social Science and Medicine 31:565-576, 1990.

Braine D: *The Human Person: Animal and Spirit.*
Notre Dame, University of Notre Dame Press, 1992.

Broad CD: *The Mind and its Place in Nature.*
London, Routledge and Kegan Paul, 1925.

Burkett GL: Culture, illness, and the biopsychosocial model.
Family Medicine 23:287-291, 1991.

Descartes R: *Meditations on First Philosophy.*
Cress DA (trans.), Indianapolis, Hackett Pub. Co. ,1979.

Dwyer JW, Detweiler NL, Kosch SG: Medical students and comprehensive patient care: Attitudes, perceived competence and demonstrated ability.
Medical Education 22:19-26, 1988.

Engel GL: The need for a new medical model: A challenge for biomedicine.
Science 196:129-136, 1977.

Engel GL: The clinical application of the biopsychosocial model.
American Journal of Psychiatry 137:535-544, 1980.

Fink PJ: Response to the presidential address: Is 'biopsychosocial' the psychiatric shibboleth? American Journal of Psychiatry 145:1061-1067, 1988.

Goodman A: Organic unity theory: The mind-body problem revisited. American Journal of Psychiatry 148:553-563, 1991.

Hiatt JF: Spirituality, medicine, and healing.
Southern Medical Journal 79:736-743, 1986.

Jackson F: Epiphenomenal qualia.
Philosophical Quarterly 32:127-136, 1982.

Jasnoski MB, Warner RM: Graduate and post-graduate medical education with the synchronous systems model.
Behavioral Science 36:253-273, 1991.

Kim J: Concepts of supervenience.
Philosophy and Phenomenological Research 45:153-173, 1984.

Kuhn T: *The Structure of Scientific Revolutions. 2nd ed.*
Chicago, University of Illinois Press, 1970.

Kuhn T: Objectivity, value judgment, and theory choice, in Kuhn T: *The Essential Tension: Selected Studies in Scientific Tradition and Change.* Chicago, University of Chicago Press, 1977.

Lipowski ZJ: To reduce or to integrate: Psychiatry's dilemma. Canadian Journal of Psychiatry 31:347-351, 1986.

Menninger K: *The Vital Balance.* New York, Viking, 1963.

O'Conner T: Emergent properties. American Philosophical Quarterly 31:91-104, 1994.

O'Shanick GJ, Levenson JL, Wise TN: The general hospital as a center of biopsychosocial training. General Hospital Psychiatry 8:365-371, 1986.

Sabin JE: Joseph Hersey Pratt's cost-effective class method and its contemporary application: Some problems in biopsychosocial innovation. Psychiatry 53:169-184, 1990.

Sadler JZ, Hulgus YF: Knowing, valuing, acting: Clues to revising the biopsychosocial model. Comprehensive Psychiatry 31:185-195, 1990.

Schwartz MA, Wiggens OP: Science, humanism, and the nature of medical practice: A phenomenological view. Perspect Biol Med 28:331-361, 1985.

Searle JR: *Rediscovery of the Mind.* Cambridge, Mass., MIT Press, 1992.

Sperry L: Teaching the biopsychosocial perspective: A comparison of two approaches. Psychological Reports 68:99-102, 1991.

Sperry RW: Mind-brain interaction: Mentalism, yes; Dualism no. Neuroscience 5:195-206, 1980.

Sperry RW: In defense of mentalism and emergent interaction. Journal of Mind and Behavior 12:221-245, 1991.

Swinburne R: *The Evolution of the Soul.* Oxford, Clarendon Press, 1986.

Van Cleve J: Mind-dust or magic? Panpsychism versus emergence. Philosophical Perspectives. Action Theory and Philosophy of Mind, 4: 216-226, 1990.

Van Inwagen P: *Material Beings.* Ithaca, Cornell University Press, 1990.

Vitaliano PP, Maiuro RD, Russo J, Mitchell ES, Carr JE, Van Citters RL: A biopsychosocial model of medical student distress. Journal of Behavioral Medicine 11:311-331, 1988.

Von Bertalanffy L: *Problems of Life.* New York, John Wiley and Sons, 1952.

Von Bertalanffy L: *General Systems Theory.* New York, Braziller, 1968.

Weiss P: The living system: Determinism stratified, in Koestler A, Smythies JR (eds): *Beyond Reductionism*. New York, Macmillan Pub. Co., 1969.

Weiss P: The system of nature and the nature of systems: Empirical holism and practical reductionism harmonized, in Schaefer KE, Hensel H, and Brody R (eds): *Toward a Man-Centered Medical Science*. Kisco, New York, Futura Pub. Co., 1977.

Wise TN: Teaching psychosomatic medicine: Utilizing concurrent perspectives. Psychother Psychosom 59:99-106, 1993.

14

RELIGION AND SPIRITUALITY IN THE PRIMARY CARE SETTING: TOWARD THE 21ST CENTURY[1]

Shimon Waldfogel, M.D.

Assistant Professor
Department of Psychiatry and Human Behavior
Behavioral Medicine Consultant
Department of Family Medicine
Jefferson Medical College

INTRODUCTION

Religion and medicine have a common tradition of alleviating suffering, yet, throughout much of the twentieth century the religious /spiritual dimension of the person has rarely been addressed in the medical literature and more rarely incorporated in clinical training. Thus, an important therapeutic tool that can enhance the patient's coping with illness and improve their well-being has not been part of the clinician's medical treatment repertoire. Recently, there is a growing recognition that the biopsychosocial model of health could be expanded to include the spiritual dimension (1,2). The primary care setting is the logical locus for this expanded paradigm to sprout as we enter the twenty-first century.

The United States is a highly religious nation with 94% of Americans professing a belief in God, 57% report praying daily, 42% attending religious services regularly. Nearly three-quarters of Americans say that their approach to life is grounded in their religious beliefs.(3) 82% of adults surveyed recently believe in the healing power of personal prayer and 77% believe that God sometimes intervenes to cure people who have a serious illness. Twenty-eight percent of the sample of 1,004 adults believed in the ability of faith healers to make people well through their faith or personal touch. (4)

It is assumed that religion has a unique influence on individuals during times of personal crisis and suffering. It therefore seems likely to have an impact on the person's health and response to disease. This association has been demonstrated in numerous studies that have been reported in the medical, nursing, medical sociology and epidemiology

[1]Correspondence: 1651 Thompson Building, 1020 Sansom St, Philadelphia, PA. 19107
Tel: (215) 955-8115.

literature. The inclusion of religious and spiritual problems in DSM IV further supports the importance of addressing this aspect of the person in the clinical setting. In this chapter the author will explore the role that religion and spirituality play in the medical setting in general and the primary care setting in particular.

RESEARCH

General reviews of the literature

There is a growing body of scientific literature supporting the observations of many clinicians and patients that religious resources contribute to coping with medical disease.(5-7) The relationship between religion and spirituality and medicine is complex. Religion and spirituality are multi-dimensional variables and very few studies have controlled for potential confounding or mediating variables. Additionally, there is a lack of a theoretical framework with which to conceptualize the relationship. Generally there are a number of problems related to research of the role that religion plays in well being: 1. Selection of the variables used for religion (belonging, participation, rituals) 2. Outcomes used to assess benefit.

A review of 1,036 articles that were published in the Journal of Family Practice over a ten year period by Craigie, Larson and Liu (5) found that fifty two, or approximately 5% of the articles contained references to religion. These studies contained 64 references to religion, religious denomination, or religious commitment. 25 of the 64 religious items were associated with clinical benefit: 9 were found to have a negative clinical impact: the remaining 30 items were found to be neutral with no statistical clinical relationship.

Levin, in a review of two hundred and fifty studies that have appeared in the medical literature since the 19th century concludes that there is an association between religion and health, that the association is probably valid, and it maybe causal (6). Levin offers the following alternative hypotheses for these findings:

1. Behavior- Religiously sanctioned health related behaviors.
2. Heredity- Health related to genetic characteristics of a particular religious group.
3. Psychosocial effects- Due to religions promoting of social support, sense of belonging.
4. Psychodynamics of belief systems- Religious beliefs may engender peacefulness, self confidence, and a sense of purpose: alternatively they may produce guilt, self doubt shame and low self esteem.
5. Psychodynamics of religious rites: Rituals of religious worship and spiritual practice may serve to ease anxiety and dread, defeat loneliness, and establish a sense of being loved and appreciated.
6. Psychodynamics of faith: The mere belief that religion or God is health-enhancing may be enough to produce salutary effects akin to the placebo effect.
7. Multifactorial explanation: A combination of the above explanations.
8. Superempirical force: Levin suggests that while the previous explanations engage social, psychological and biological phenomena which can be measured scientifically, super-empirical phenomena cannot be subjected to scientific examination. This dimension involves a mystery force or power that goes by various names such as life force, orgone, prana, ruuach, chi (6).

A recent National Institute of Health Conference to explore the research on the relationship of health and religion led to a review by Mathews et. al (7). This review of over four hundred published empirical studies in the medical, epidemiological, sociological and nursing literature dating back to the 19th century explore the effects of religion on various constructs of medical outcome and utilization. The authors point out that "although most of these studies are correlational, use inadequate measures of religious commitment such as religious denomination or other single-item measures, and seldom assess the intensity of religious commitment, they generally have suggested a beneficial, or salutary, effect for religious or spiritual involvement on physical and mental health status."

I will present a selective review of the literature focusing of the following areas:
1. Prevention of disease
2. Response to disease
3. Coping with illness

Prevention of disease

Religion may have specific influence on dietary habits, exposure to cigarette, sexual behavior, drugs, alcohol. Oleckno and Blacconiere studied 1077 college students and found that religiosity was positively correlated with wellness and inversely with health compromising behaviors (8). Watson studied the mortality rates from heart disease in 24 industrial countries (9). He found the mortality rate to be inversely related to the proportion of Catholics to Protestants. He speculates that the mortality is related to the culture's attitude to time, i.e. "waste of time is... The first and in principle the deadliest of sins." Comstock and Partridge (10) studied health related variables of 91,000 people in Washington County, Maryland. They found a decreased risk for Ischemic Heart Disease (IHD) death, cirrhosis of liver, emphysema, and suicide in the religious individuals who regularly attended church. Others have noted the benefit of religion in the prevention of depression and as a coping strategy among the elderly (7).

Coping with illness

Multiple studies in various clinical populations have demonstrated the frequency with which patients use religious and spiritually-based coping mechanisms in responding to their illnesses. The role of the health care team's recognition of, and promotion of these resources, can lead to a beneficial outcome by enhancing well-being. Oxman et al. (11) studied 232 patients 55 years old or older who were preparing to undergo elective heart surgery. Those that described themselves as being more religious had a better outcome. Pressman (12) found that religion improved the patient's emotional response to illness and at times led to quicker recovery from hip surgery. Coward (13), studying 107 women with Stage IIIb and Stage IV breast cancer, found that a sense of self-transcendence decreased the distress associated with illness, enhancing emotional well-being. Others have shown that patients with increased religious faith viewed their health as better then that of others. They reported less anxiety, less depression, greater self esteem, and greater physical and emotional well-being (7).

Mental Health

Williams examined the effects of religious attendance and affiliation on psychological distress in a longitudinal study of 720 adults (14). Religious affiliation was found to be unrelated to mental health status. Religious attendance does not directly reduce psychological distress, it buffers the deleterious effects of stress on mental health. Williams concluded that in the face of stressful events and physical health problems, religious attendance reduces the adverse consequences of the stressors on psychological well-being.

Addiction

There are numerous studies that show the benefit of various dimensions of religion in the prevention of substance abuse (15-16). There are however no double blind statistically significant studies showing the benefit of a religiously/spiritually based program in the treatment of addiction problems. From clinical experience, the role of religious and spiritually based interventions, especially twelve step programs, are often reported by patients to be positive.

Response to disease

- **Prayer:**

There have been a number of studies that suggest the positive relationship between intercessory prayer and outcome of medical illness. The role of prayer as a clinical intervention has been gaining publicity as evidenced by the best selling books by Larry Dossey and Herbert Benson (17-18). The most often quoted research was conducted by Byrd in San-Francisco (19). In his study, patients who were prayed for had a lower rate of complications after a myocardial infarct. The study suffers from methodological problems and has not been replicated. Other studies assessing the role of intercessory prayer in various medical conditions have not shown a clear-cut association between prayer and healing.

- **Spiritual healing**

The efficacy of faith healing and spiritually based clinical intervention as the therapeutic modality for medical illness has not been scientifically researched (20). Yet faith healing has a fair following. Faith healing is carried out by a religious leader who prays for a person's healing, privately or at a public meeting. It is often accompanied by touching the person while the leader prays. The research in this area is focused on the perception of physicians and patients about faith healing. King et. al. state that faith healers may be one of the most potent and dangerous types of alternative medicine used by patients today (21). People consult faith healers in addition to physicians. In a rural family practice population, 21% of patients had attended a faith healing service. Twenty-nine percent believed that faith healers can help some people whom physicians cannot help. In a study of inner city patients in Kentucky 10% of patients stated that they had attended faith healing services, and 80% of them stated they had been cured. Of the physicians surveyed, 23% agreed that faith healers can divinely heal some people (21).

Future research

1. Prevention- What is the role of the religious dimensions on prevention of illness/ disease? How can religious factors be used to enhance early detection and prevention of physical and mental disease?
2. Intervention- Does religious intervention affect outcome of disease? The impact of religiously informed intervention on the outcome of addiction treatment.
3. Coping- How do religious and spiritual resources affect well being and function in response to medical disease?

Although there is indication from the research that religion and spiritual factors may have an impact on well being, Levin rightly concludes that without a discussion of the therapeutic relevance of these findings, religion will remain, as it should, a marginal issue for epidemiology and medicine (6). The next section will focus on clinical aspects of the role of religion in the medical setting.

CLINICAL APPLICATIONS

Patients often incorporate religious beliefs and practices in coping with the stress of physical illness (22,23). Religion can be used adaptively or maladaptively, and can have a positive or a negative impact on health (24). Adaptive religious beliefs and practices can enhance well-being (25), improve quality of life, and speed recovery from illness (12). Maladaptive religious responses may lead to refusal of necessary treatment, and may even be the cause of self-injury (26). Failure to explore a patient's religious beliefs and practices in the clinical evaluation can lead to an incomplete diagnostic assessment that overlooks important intervention options (2).

Religious life may consist solely of ritual acts at designated times, or a religious sensibility may pervade a person's life, informing every decision and providing a filter through which they interpret experience and information -- including medical information. Without an understanding of the role of religion in psychological life, the physician's own biases can also lead to conflicts with religious patients in the clinical setting (27).

Attitudes toward religious and spiritual matters influence patients' attitudes about their medical problems. But questions about the impact of these attitudes on medical outcome remain unanswered. What, for example, is the impact on quality of life of the attribution of illness and healing to a divine being? How does belief in an afterlife influence the anxiety that accompanies illness? More generally, what role does belief in God play in a patient's perception of being valued, and how does this influence the outcome? In order to explore the clinical role of religion in the medical setting we have to define what we mean by these terms.

The concepts of religion and spirituality have varied definitions and conceptualization. Ultimately, the meaning that religion and spirituality have for a particular individual is idiosyncratic, reflecting multiple variables including cultural, developmental, and even biological factors. This section will focus on a concrete way to define religion and spirituality, and use this definition to explore ways that religion and spirituality can be incorporated into the medical setting.

There is no consensus about the boundaries between religiousness and spirituality. Religiousness usually refers to "adherence to the beliefs and practices of an organized church or religious institution" (28). Spirituality is used to describe the transcendental relationship between the person and a higher being, a quality that goes beyond a specific religious affiliation(29). More specifically, religion has been defined as any specific system of beliefs, worship, and conduct involving a code of ethics, a philosophy of life and a way of understanding the world. Religion is best understood as a multidimensional and complex aspect of human life.

Based on Glock's (30) typology of religion along five dimensions, Waldfogel and Wolpe (2) suggest six dimensions of religion that can help the practitioner categorize and conceptualize religious behavior in a way that can be helpful in the clinical setting.

The six dimensions of religion are:

1. Ideological (religious beliefs)
2. Intellectual (religious knowledge)
3. Ritualistic (participation in religious rituals)
4. Experiential (having a religious experience)
5. Consequential (the influence of religiosity on non-religious activities)
6. Supportive (affiliation with a religious community that provides social and spiritual support).

Each of these aspects of religion can emerge in the medical setting, though they are clearly integrated to some degree or another in the lives of most religious people (31). I would like to discuss these six dimensions in turn, using case examples (where possible) to illustrate how each might appear in the clinical setting. Examples of interventions are offered that incorporate the patient's religious beliefs and practices.

1. THE IDEOLOGICAL DIMENSION: RELIGIOUS BELIEFS

A central responsibility of the clinician is to understand what the illness means to the patient and what the patient's attitude is toward it (32). However, the significance of an illness for a patient is determined in part by how he frames his understanding of the illness in his larger belief system. Religious themes are often employed to infuse the illness episode with a larger meaning.

Ellison recently described how religious symbols and beliefs provide an interpretive framework through which some individuals make sense of everyday reality and which modulate the harmful effects of stress on psychological well being (31). Religious symbols and values can help the individual interpret potentially stressful events as less threatening, and make traumatic events easier to bear. Religious faith often redefines potentially negative life events as opportunities for spiritual growth or as part of a broader divine plan.

Religious beliefs such as those related to the divine force, human relationships, death and the afterlife, offer a framework for many people to make sense of their experiences, including illness and health care experiences. For example, belief in God, depending on how it is understood by the person, may lead to feelings of being loved and cared for or to feelings of being rejected or punished. Thus a belief in God may lead to enhanced self-esteem in some, while for others it may be the basis for severe distress in times of adversity.

Case A: The Maladaptive and Adaptive Role of Religious Beliefs

Ms. A. was a 53 year-old female who had been suffering from abdominal pain that was later found to be due to Diverticular Disease. The patient initially turned to her pastor for help. The pastor attributed her pain to being punished by God and noted that she was possessed by demons. The pastor initiated rituals to exorcise the demons. She felt better for a few days. However the symptoms recurred. As she was not improving she become increasingly anxious and concerned and finally sought medical attention.

Due to her significant anxiety, she was referred for psychiatric evaluation. Over time the patient was able to process her frustration with her pastor and chose to join a different church. As she became more involved in her new church, she started seeing her illness as a challenge from God rather then punishment.

In seeking healthcare and choosing specific modalities the patient brings with them their beliefs and values. These values and beliefs are of prime importance in the clinical encounter. Working within the patient's beliefs can enhance clinical outcome of the treatment provided. Ms. A. used religion as a template by which integrated her illness experience. Lipowski suggests that illness can be interpreted in eight ways: as a challenge, an enemy, a punishment, a personal weakness, a relief, a strategy, an irreparable loss or damage, and\or as a value (32). Ms. A.'s religious beliefs led her to frame her symptoms in a religious manner and thus she was willing to allow her pastor to treat her.

It has been shown that belief in God or the divine other may have a significant impact on the decision-making process of the individual in the clinical arena. In a study of heart transplant patients, 66% claimed to have prayed and have consulted God when they had to make decisions and 69% felt that God guided them in making decisions (33). For certain religious groups such as the Jehovah's Witnesses, refusal to accept blood products is well-known and respected. For many Jehovah's Witnesses, it is more important to comply with the religious tenets and be at peace for eternity than to have a potentially life-saving procedure that violates their religious beliefs. Pargament (23) has suggested three styles of problem-solving in individuals who incorporate God in decision making:

1. Self-Directing (God grants me freedom to solve my own problems by myself)
2. Collaborative (God and I actively work together to solve my problem)
3. Deferring (I turn my problems over to God and wait for his solutions to emerge)

Recognizing the style of problem solving of a particular individual may help the physician better understand the patients response in stressful medical situations. Occasionally the patient's religious beliefs will appear to be in conflict with the recommended treatment for the patient. The following case highlights the impact of the patient's beliefs on their decision making regarding the treatment of a psychiatric problem.

Case B. Refusal of Psychiatric Treatment due to Religious Beliefs
Ms. B. is a 46 year old female who was seen by the primary care physician on a regular visit. During that visit the patient noted her fear of leaving the house alone. (She came to the visit accompanied by her son). She noted increasing anxiety manifested by dizziness when she is alone outside. The symptoms have been going on for four years and have increased in intensity. The patient was referred to the psychiatrist for a diagnostic evaluation.. The patient noted the onset of symptoms, including ideas of reference after sustaining a head injury in a motor vehicle accident. The patient attributed the accident to punishment by God, and declined the recommended pharmacological intervention claiming that God will cure her.
In this case the patient framed her problems in a religious framework and the recommended treatment was not acceptable to her as it didn't fit in her frame of reference. The physician may attempt to enlist the assistance of a "cultural broker", to have her consider the medical recommendation.

2. THE INTELLECTUAL DIMENSION: RELIGIOUS KNOWLEDGE

Religious knowledge includes scriptural or other information, symbols, and stories, usually integrated into an organized theology. The world-view of a patient educated in a particular theology or with reference to a particular set of scriptures will influence a patient's outlook on health and disease. In addition, scripture or a particular theology will have a specific attitude towards medical illness, or even to a certain medical problem. The Jehovah Witness's refusal of blood products is a familiar manifestation of this aspect of religion. Patients who belong to the Jehovah Witness community will often review with their physicians, advance directives related to their refusal of blood products under any circumstances. For these patients as Barnard points out, the biological survival may not be as significant as the loss of their soul (34). For these patients their transgression on earth will lead to living in sin for eternity.

In the primary care setting religious knowledge can be used to assess the extent to which the patient uses religious stories as metaphors, identifies with religious figures, and casts their responses to questions in an appropriate religious context. The knowledgeable clinician can incorporate these religious stories and themes into the treatment plan of a particular patient. For example, appropriate religious imagery can be used in visualization techniques and hypnosis when indicated.

Case C: The Use of Religious Imagery in Psychiatric Treatment

Ms. C., a 43 year-old female hospitalized on the surgical service for severe abdominal pain, received a psychiatric consultation for pain management. Ms. C. developed severe abdominal pain at the age of 16 after her mother died of pancreatic cancer. She underwent numerous abdominal surgeries to look for the cause of the pain, until finally diagnosed with Chronic Pancreatitis. Ms. C. was initially reluctant to have a psychiatric consultation as she believed that it might challenge her strong Christian religious beliefs. She relented when her concerns were addressed by the psychiatric consultant, who reassured her that her religious beliefs would not be challenged. The psychiatric consultant also suggested she discuss his intervention with a trusted pastor. Upon further assessment, it became clear that religious issues were a central component of her coping ability and had been of great support in the past. While dynamic issues appeared to be of great importance in the origin and maintenance of Ms. C.'s abdominal symptoms, the psychiatrist chose to explore her religious beliefs and to offer therapeutic interventions that capitalized on her strong religious identity, especially the comfort she received from her acceptance of the Holy Ghost. To aid in pain management, the psychiatrist suggested hypnotherapy that incorporated religious imagery. The patient was a good hypnotic subject and was able to focus on the Holy Ghost while in trance. Although she came to feel more comfortable with the psychiatrist, she refused to consider secular psychotherapeutic interventions fearing that her religious beliefs would be challenged. Upon discharge, she chose to see a spiritual counselor for psychotherapy. At that time her complaints of pain had significantly diminished, and she was being tapered off of her analgesic medications.

This case highlights a number of important issues. First, it demonstrates the importance of acknowledging the patient's religious orientation and treating it with respect. Second, it reminds us of the mistrust often felt by religious patients for psychiatry, and the potential for resistance if the fear is not addressed. Third, it illustrates the potential benefits of using familiar religious imagery in treatment when indicated. Finally, the case illustrates the potential benefit from collaboration with a "culture-broker," an intermediary who is acceptable to the patient and who may assist in translating the religious aspects of a patient's decision-making process (35).

3. THE RITUALISTIC DIMENSION: PARTICIPATION IN RELIGIOUS RITUAL

Religious rituals often play a central role in the daily life of the religious individual. Illness may disrupt or prevent daily prayer, participation in ceremonies, exposure to religious music, and church attendance. At just the time when there is the greatest need for the sense of comfort afforded by religious ritual, an important mechanism for religious coping may not be available. Rituals are central in many religious traditions. One purpose they serve is to reinforce the religious beliefs held by the group and the individual. As such, they may be sources of great comfort for religious persons. Prayer, meditation, and reading of scriptures, as well as community religious activities, often increase the individual's ability to cope with medical problems.

Case D: Religious Ritual in Coping

Ms. D. was a 39 year-old female with C4-C5 fracture which she sustained in a motor vehicle accident while on a church-sponsored outing five months prior to the current psychiatric consultation. Psychiatric consultation was requested to assess her for depression. Ms. D.'s religious identity was strong, she was an active participant in her church, and she reported that prayer and faith were an important component of her ability to cope with her injury. She also noted that she missed the religious and spiritual practices she had performed prior to hospitalization. Ms. D. displayed symptoms consistent with a depressive disorder. The recommended treatment plan included antidepressant medication, and psychotherapy with an exploration of her religious beliefs in light of her accident. It was also recommended that she obtain a Walkman to listen to her favorite spiritual music. Efforts were also made to involve local clergy of her faith, in addition to her own minister, in her care. Ms. D. commented on the benefit of the religious-spiritual intervention.

This case illustrates how using familiar rituals and bringing associated religious objects (such as music) into the hospital setting can calm patients and enhance their sense of continuity and connection to their religious community. Assessing the patient's daily religious routines may suggest other rituals appropriate to the hospital setting. The recent APA guidelines (36) note that religious interventions are not substitutes for appropriate therapeutic interventions; however, "religious prescriptions" may constitute an ethically sound treatment to complement other medical and psychiatric interventions.

4. THE EXPERIENTIAL DIMENSION: INTENSE RELIGIOUS EXPERIENCE

Religious experiences can range from feeling a general sense of connection with a Supreme Being to a specific event by which one perceives oneself to be in a personal relationship with a Supreme Being. Such experiences often profoundly influence or alter a person's attitudes toward life and death. Religious experience as defined by Glock and Stark (30) consists of "occasions defined by those undergoing them as an encounter -- some sense of contact between themselves and a supernatural consciousness". They describe four levels of religious experiences, ranging from feeling a sense of connection with a Supreme Being who does not specifically acknowledge the person in return to perceiving oneself to be the confidant or fellow participant in action with a Supreme Being. Such an experience may have a profound effect on the patient, often leading to a significant alteration of their attitudes toward life and death. Patients who have undergone traumatic medical events such as cardiac arrest or required resuscitation for other reasons may have near death experiences that can be of great significance to them. Without an understanding of that event the patient may be unable to integrate that experience into their life.

Case E: Religious Experience and Coping

Ms.E. a 44-year-old woman with chronic steroid-dependent asthma, was hospitalized for respiratory distress and septicemia. During the hospitalization she developed painful deep vein thrombosis of her lower extremities. She requested a do-not-resuscitate order; because of her despondency, psychiatric consultation was sought to assess her capacity to request the order. During her evaluation, Ms. E. was very anxious and appeared in significant distress. She expressed a deeply felt desire for relief from the pain she was experiencing. She related that during a seizure ten years prior to her current hospitalization, she experienced a the presence of a "beautiful man" who wiped her hair to the side and told her that everything will be alright. She believed that the man was the Lord and felt that the experience profoundly effected her ability to cope with her illness. She expressed a desire to be in the arms of God, who would protect her from the consequences of her worsening condition. Although she had little contact with religious organizations, she drew on her religious experience for emotional support.

Ms. E. drew on her religious experience to construct a view of a benevolent God who would protect her from the fears of her medical condition. The experience had a profound effect on her ability to cope with serious illness; during an exacerbation, she could anchor her feelings in the memory of her religious experience. Pollner has found a correlation between "relationships with Divine Others" and several measures of well-being -- even when controlling for such things as church attendance (37). Psychotherapeutic exploration of her fears, supportive attention to her religious experience, and improvement in her medical condition led to a decrease in her anxiety. Transcendence has been identified as a powerful spiritual experience that may help the patient cope with severe physical pain, or terminal illness. The person can either resist, submit to or transcend suffering. Transcendence involves facing the pain in clear perspective. Self-transcendence consists of the experience of extending self-boundaries inwardly, outwardly, and temporally to take on broader life perspectives, activities and purposes (38).

4. THE CONSEQUENTIAL DIMENSION: THE INFLUENCE OF RELIGION IN NON-RELIGIOUS ACTIVITIES

Religious beliefs can influence behavior in areas of life that have little to do with formal religion. For example, research has shown a positive correlation between religiosity and health-enhancing behaviors (7). Particularly strong is the relationship between certain religious beliefs and the avoidance of alcohol, illicit drugs, cigarette smoking and promiscuous sexual behavior. Spiritually-based interventions such as the twelve-step programs, which rely heavily on acceptance of God, have become standard treatment for addictive disorders. The twelve-step programs encourage the individual to surrender control to an "external" Supreme Force, however the individual conceives of that force. Patients with Psychoactive Drug Use Disorder (PSUD) often report high levels of religiousness, though their participation in organized religion tends to be low, either because they feel unwelcome in their church or because they consider themselves to be sinners. The twelve-step programs are often responsible for bringing PSUD patients back to organized religion by restoring a sense of self-esteem and self-worth.

5. THE SUPPORTIVE DIMENSION: AFFILIATION WITH A RELIGIOUS COMMUNITY

Religion and spirituality provide support systems for the individual within the group as well as in relationship with a divine being. Findings suggest that functional, need-based social supports is uniquely beneficial for individuals under high levels of recent life event stress. This is based on a perception that one is cared about and loved, esteemed and valued and that support is readily available when needed. Religious institutions are able to provide this kind of support.

However religion and spirituality may also offer the patient a system of support beyond that of the religious community. Alongside the individual's "real" social networks there exists a network of others which partly overlaps the network of actual acquaintances but includes unmet, or unmeetable, others as well. The divine support that is available to the religious individual may also be of great comfort in times of stress (37). The support of a religious community can be very helpful to patients who are isolated from their normal support structures or who lack any support structure whatsoever.

Religious institutions usually have impressive volunteer pools and often have committees whose sole purpose is to visit the sick. It should become standard practice to inquire into the desirability of religiously based visits for patients who are socially isolated. Contact with a religious community can initiate the development of a new set of social supports for the socially isolated. These supports should be considered in treatment planning.

It can also happen that an existing religious support system is suddenly made unavailable to the patient, as when a patient opts for a treatment option that is contrary to the religious beliefs of his community. In these situations, choosing such an option may lead to a conflict with the patient's family and result in additional stress if they withdraw their support. In cases where the family or the religious community withdraws support, a culture-broker might be called in to see if a compromise might be reached or if an exception might be made to religious strictures. In some cases, an alternative religious community of the same faith might be located who are less strict about their interpretation of the scripture. Psychotherapeutic support may help the patient see his or her options and facilitate a positive, adaptive response to feelings of abandonment or rejection.

Social science research on stress buffering role of social support has demonstrated the importance of religious organizations in providing instrumental and emotional support to the sick. The infrastructure of the religious communities is particularly suited for providing the services needed by individuals and groups (39). The culture and values of the religious group can be helpful in promoting health enhancing behaviors. The religious group can encourage a positive approach to health maintenance and preventive care. Moderation in alcohol consumption and eating behavior may be encouraged. The religious group may even explicitly promote screening activities.

Conversely, religious organizations and beliefs may lead to the refusal of recommended medical treatment. Some organized religious groups have proscriptions against seeking health care or against certain kinds of treatment. Many individuals seek medical help from religious figures or religiously acceptable healers instead of seeking conventional medical care. Some seek religious-based treatment exclusively and stay out of the medical arena. However, most religious and spiritually based treatment is used as an adjunct to traditional medical care.

TREATMENT IN THE MEDICAL SETTING

Attending to the religious dimensions of the patient can provide the physician with a variety of therapeutic tools and can greatly facilitate the patient's coping ability, thus enhancing their well being. This section will focus on the treatment application of the role of religion in the medical setting.

General Approach

In 1990, the American Psychiatric Association's Committee on Religion and Psychiatry issued the following guidelines regarding the possible conflict between psychiatrist's religious commitment and psychiatric practice (36):

1. Physicians should maintain respect for their patients' beliefs. It is useful for the physician to obtain information on the religious and ideological orientation of their patients so that the may properly attend to them in the course of treatment.
2. Physicians should not impose their own religious, anti-religious, or ideological systems of beliefs on their patients, nor should they substitute such beliefs or rituals for accepted diagnostic concepts or therapeutic practice.

These general guidelines are applicable to any medical encounter.

The physician should familiarize themselves with religious and spiritual resources within their community. This may include information on outreach by religious institution to medically ill individuals, sponsorship of 12 step meetings, religious based counseling, prevention and early detection activities through the religious organization. Additionally, the physician may identify clergy in the community that the can serve as a cultural broker if needed. In general, it is important for the physician to accept the patient's religious beliefs in a non-judgmental manner, even if these beliefs are contrary to the physician's beliefs. In some circumstances, if consistent with the physicians' beliefs, they may find it useful to pray with or for patients, read scripture with them as a therapeutic modality, or encourage them to get in touch with their spirituality in order to transcend their physical illness.

Addressing Religious and Spiritual Issues in the Clinical Encounter

With whom and when to discuss religious and spiritual issues:

Maugans(40) writes that spirituality can be effectively discussed with patients of most age groups including children and young adults. He points out the importance of addressing these issues not only with children but also with their families. The depth and focus of the spiritual conversation will vary based on the cognitive and developmental ability of the patient as well as the comfort level of the physician.

The nature and depth of the religious and spiritual issues discussed in the patient interview will depend on multiple variables. These may include the circumstances of the clinical encounter, the time available, the role of the physician in the care of the patient, patient's response and physician comfort. Discussion of religion and spirituality in the face of life threatening illness including a discussion of advance directives lends itself to a more in depth exploration then a visit for a minor medical problem.

Health maintenance visits provide an opportunity to explore the patient's religious and spiritual identification and practice in context of an overall assessment of the patients lifestyle, risks, and coping resources. Additionally, by addressing these issues in a non judgmental way the physician "legitimizes" the importance of religion and spirituality to the patient and its relevance in the medical setting. When appropriate, the physician can make suggestion regarding the utilization of religiously/spiritually based supports such as meditation and prayer for coping.

Religiously Informed History

A religious/spiritual history can be included in questions assessing the various dimensions of religion. Additionally, the exploration of changes in the patient's religious commitment and practice is often revealing, as they may suggest conflicts the patient has experienced in this area.

A comprehensive religious/ spiritual history is time consuming and rarely indicated, usually a number of questions exploring the six dimensions of religion discussed earlier will provide an insight into health-related religious and spiritual issues. Asking the questions in the context of exploration of the patient's coping allows for a non-judgmental exploration of the religious dimension.

Sample questions:

- Tell me of your belief in God or a higher power?
- What does your belief in God mean to you? Has it changed during your illness?
- How important is your religious and spiritual identification?
- Tell me about your religious and spiritual practices such as prayer, meditation?

- Do you belong to a religious or spiritual community?
- What aspects of your religion or spirituality would you like me to be aware of as your physician?

A more targeted history can be undertaken if the patient has a life threatening illness. This may include specific questions about the patient's beliefs as they relate to end of life decision making, about their previous experience with religion in periods of stress. Has the patient sought treatment from a faith healer, or other religiously based provider? Additionally, questions to identify religiously based community support system can be useful to better address the patients' needs. For patients with substance abuse disorders, a targeted history about their religious/spiritual experience as well as changes in their religious and spiritual practice often can identify areas of strength that can be incorporated into treatment planning.

Of course the physician will develop his/her own approach to religious and spiritual issues in the clinical setting. The comfort in addressing this delicate topic will increase with their experience gained by incorporating these questions into their patient interview.

RELIGION AND SPIRITUALITY OF THE PHYSICIAN

For many physicians religion and spirituality are central in their lives and contribute to their choice of medicine as a career. The physician's religious faith can provide tools for coping with the rigors of medical training and practice. Very little is known of the impact of physicians' (or other health providers') religious and spiritual beliefs on their decision making processes in medical situations. Physicians are rarely educated as to the importance of the patient's and their own religiosity and spirituality in the clinical arena. Physicians may experience tension when the patient's decision about medical care is religiously unacceptable to them. Lack of awareness of the conflict can lead to ethical dilemmas. Maugans (40) recommends that the physician reflect on their own spirituality and how it impacts on their concept of self, their relationships, and their practice. Physicians may benefit by their awareness of this aspect of their lives as they confront the challenges of medical practice.

CONCLUSIONS

Religious beliefs and rituals add meaning to life and are often relied upon to adapt to major life events such as birth, illness and death. Religion is a central component of the personal identity for most Americans and, as such, for many of the medical patients that are encountered by the clinician in the primary care setting. The patients' religious beliefs may affect their understanding of, their emotional response to, and their ability to cope with, their physical illness. The clinician should not judge these religious claims, but seek to understand their clinical impact. By attending to the religious concerns of the medical patient, the clinician can greatly enhance the patient's ability to cope with his illness.

A patient should be understood as a bio/psycho/social/spiritual whole. In this conceptualization, the person can be located in a larger landscape and be brought "closer to a transpersonal source of meaning and to the human community that shares those meanings" (41). Such support can be of particular value when a patient faces a physical illness that challenges their religious belief system.

Physicians need not be knowledgeable in a patient's particular religious system. When needed, a *culture broker* can be used to assist in the dialogue with the patient. A culture broker may also be helpful when the clinician encounters resistance in the religious patient who perceives the physicians recommendation as anti-religious. When psychiatric evaluation is indicated, incorporation of clergy, when indicated, may enhance the acceptance of the psychiatric evaluation and the treatment plan.

Occasionally, a patient may ask about the religious beliefs of the physician. The physicians may choose to reveal their religious beliefs or may politely explain why they will not do so. If they prefer not to reveal their personal beliefs, it is often helpful to acknowledge the importance of the search for meaning and the awareness that not everything about our universe can be scientifically explained. Such an acknowledgment may be enough to open the dialogue with patients who fear their religious beliefs will be challenged or minimized.

Physicians should be better trained about the role that religion plays in psychological life. It is also important for the physician to explore and recognize his or her own religious-spiritual needs and beliefs to minimize the potential bias that these beliefs may have in the clinical encounter. Scientifically-based research exploring the impact of the dimensions of religiosity on physical and quality of life outcome to medical illness will be helpful in further defining the role of religion in the response to medical illness.

Note: Part of this chapter was adapted from Waldfogel S, Wolpe P. Using Awareness of Religious Factors to Enhance Interventions in Consultation-Liaison Psychiatry. Hosp Comm Psychiatry 1993:44:473-477

REFERENCES

1. Hiatt JF. Spirituality, Medicine, and healing. South Med J 1986; 79:736-43

2. Waldfogel S, Wolpe P. Using Awareness of Religious Factors to Enhance Interventions in Consultation-Liaison Psychiatry. Hosp Comm Psychiatry 1993;44:473-477

3. Gallup G, Castelli J: *The People's Religion: American Faith in the 90's.* New York, Macmillan, 1989.

4. Time. June 24, 1996. p.62

5. Craigie FC, Larson DB, Liu IY. References to religion in the Journal of Family Practice: Dimensions and valence of spirituality. The Journal of Family Practice 1990; 30 (4):477-480

6. Levin JS. Religion and Health: Is there an association, is it valid, and is it casual? Soc Sci Med 1994; 38: 1475-1482

7. Matthews DA, Larson DB, Koenig HB, Swyers JB. The Relationship Between Religious and Spiritual Factors and Health Status: A Review of the Research. Unpublished manuscript

8. Oleckno WA, Blacconiere MJ: Relationship of religiosity to wellness and other health-related behaviors and outcomes. Psychological Reports 1991; 68:819-826.

9. Watson JR. Religion as a cultural phenomenon, and national mortality rates from heart disease. Psych Reports 1991; 69: 439-42

10. Comstock Gw, Partridge KB: Church attendance and health.
J Chronic Dis 1972;25:665-672

11. Oxman TE, Freeman DH, Manheimer ED. Lack of social participation or religious strength or comfort as risk factor for death after cardiac surgery in elderly.
Psychosom Med 1995; 57:5-15.

12. Pressman P, Lyons JS, Larson DB, et al.: Religious belief, depression, and ambulation status in elderly women with broken hips.
Am J of Psychiatry 1990;147:758-760.

13. Coward DD. Self-transcendence and emotional well being in woman with advanced breast cancer. Oncology Nursing forum 1991;18: 857-863.

14. Williams DR, Larson DB, Buckler RE, et al. Religion and psychological stress in a community sample. Soc Sci Med 1991;32:1257-1262.

15. Larson DB, Wilson WP: Religious life of alcoholics.
Southern Medical Journal 1980;73:723-727.

16. Zucker DK, Austin F, Fair A, et al.: Associations between patient religiosity and alcohol attitudes and knowledge in a alcohol treatment program.
International Journal of the Addictions 1987;22:47-53.

17. Dossey L: *Healing Words: The power of prayer and the practice of medicine.*
Harper San Francisco, San Francisco Ca, 1993

18. Benson H. *Timeless Healing*. Scribner NY, NY, 1996.

19. Byrd R, Positive therapeutic effects of intercessory prayer in a coronary unit population.
South Med J 1988; 81: 826-9.

20. Hodges RD, Scofield AM. Is Spiritual healing a valid and effective therapy?
J Royal Society Med 1995; 88: 203-7.

21. King DE, Bushwick B. Beliefs and attitudes of hospital patients about faith healing and prayer. J Fam Practice 1994; 39 (4) 349-352.

22. Whitehead PL, Stout RJ: Religion as ego support, in A Task Force Report of the APA: *Treatment of Psychiatric Disorders, Vol.3*. Washington DC, APA Press, 1989.

23. Pargament KI: God help me: Towards a theoretical framework of coping for the psychology of religion. American Psychological Association Division 1988; 36. 13:2

24. Jarvis GK, Northcott HC: Religion and differences in morbidity and mortality.
Social Science and Medicine 1987;25:813-24.

25. Koening HG, Smiley M, Gonzales JAP: *Religion, Health and Aging: A Review and Theoretical Integration.* New York, Greenwood Press, 1988.

26. Favazza AR: Why patients mutilate themselves. Hosp Comm Psych 1989; 40:137-145.

27. Galanter M, Larson D, Rubenstone E. Christian psychiatry: the impact of evangelical belief on clinical practice. Am J Psych 1991;148:90-95.

28. Shafranske E, Maloney HN. Clinical psychologists' religious and spiritual orientations and their practice of psychotherapy. Psychotherapy 1990;27: 72-78.

29. Peterson EA, Nelson K. How to meet your client's spiritual needs. J Psychosoc Nurs. 1987;25: 34-39.

30. Glock CY, Stark R: *Religion and Society in Tension.* Chicago, Rand McNally, 1965.

31. Ellison CG: Religious involvement and subjective well- being. Journal of Health and Social Behavior 1991; 32:80-99.

32. Lipowski ZJ: Physical illness, the individual, and the coping process. International Journal of Psychiatry and Medicine 1970;1:91-102.

33. Harris RC, Dew MA The association of religious beliefs and behaviors with the well-being of heart transplant recipients. Unpublished abstract.

34. Barnard D: Psychosomatic medicine and the problem of meaning. Bulletin of the Menninger Clinic 1985;49:10-28.

35. Greenberg D, Witzum E: Problems in the treatment of religious patients. American Journal of Psychotherapy 1991;XLV:554- 565.

36. American Psychiatric Association: Guidelines regarding possible conflicts between psychiatrists' religious commitments and psychiatric practice. American Journal of Psychiatry 1990;147:542.

37. Pollner M: Divine relations, social relations, and well-being. Journal of Health and Social Behavior 1989;30:92-104.

38. Reed P. Spirituality and well being in terminally Ill hospitalized adults. Research in Nursing & Health 1987;10: 335-44.

39. Shelp EE, DuBose ER, Sunderland RH . The infrastructure of religious communities: a neglected resource for care of people with AIDS. Am J Public Health 1990; 80: 970-972.

40. Maugans TA: The SPIRITual History. Arch Fam Med 1996;5: 11-16.

41. Cassel EJ: The nature of suffering and the goals of medicine. New England Journal of Medicine 1982;306:639-645.

15

A BIOPSYCHOSOCIAL CRITIQUE OF MANAGED MENTAL HEALTH CARE AND ITS RELATION TO PRIMARY CARE

Seth Wigdor Robbins[1], M.D., M.P.H.

Clinical Instructor, Department of Psychiatry
University of California, San Francisco

> Planning for systems of medical care and their financing is excessively influenced by the availability and promise of technology, the application and effectiveness of which are often used as the criteria by which decisions are made as to what constitutes illness and who qualifies for medical care. -George Engel, 1977

INTRODUCTION

The quality of health care for any given problem is influenced by many factors other than the presence or absence of objective knowledge about the problem and the availability of effective treatments for it. George Engel recognized this more than 20 years ago when he proposed the incorporation of social and psychological factors into the reductionistic biomedical model of his day (1). Engel worried that the healing power of medicine was being diminished by an exclusionary devotion to science, fortified by the professionalism of physician-scientists. His work has provided the philosophical basis for today's renewed emphasis on the role of the generalist in clinical care. However, his cynicism about economic forces and about superficial enthrallment with technology remains relevant as the health care industry organizes itself around business principles and management technologies.

Systems factors and economic motives are prominent determinates of health care process, content, and outcome, with particularly strong impact on the treatment of mental health problems and the clinical relationships between primary care and specialty mental health care providers. This chapter will critique the influence of managed mental health system structures and clinical practices on outpatient mental health care and its relation to

[1]Correspondence: 2475 Washington Street, San Francisco, California 94115, Telephone: 415-292-6044

primary care. This will be done in the light of the biopsychosocial model, which comprises many core intellectual and humanistic values from the tradition of medicine and psychiatry.

MENTAL DISORDERS IN PRIMARY CARE

In the United States, about 20% of the population experience symptoms of a mental disorder in a given year (2). Prevalence rates in primary care populations are even higher, with up to 30% of patients having an active diagnosis (3-5). Rates of psychiatric disorder are especially elevated among persons with medical illnesses (6), and up to one third of patients with chronic illness have depressive symptoms (7).

About half of persons treated for psychiatric or substance use disorders are treated in primary care only (8), and a great deal of attention has been given to assessing and improving the quality of care delivered in that setting (9). It is commonly acknowledged, however, that treatments of psychiatric disorders in primary care are frequently sub-optimal (10), with many missed diagnoses and failed treatments (11-13). The basis for these problems is complex, but is likely due to the interactive effects of inadequate training of primary care providers in the diagnosis and treatment of psychiatric problems, ever-increasing time constraints in the primary care setting, and an all-too-common bias among medical practitioners to emphasize somatic problems over psychosocial concerns.

Although the multifaceted debate about which psychiatric problems can and should be treated in primary care versus specialty mental health settings will not be resolved for some time, there can be little doubt that we are still in great need of improving the clinical linkages between primary care and mental health practice. The current rise to power of managed systems of medical and mental health care brings with it the opportunity to thoughtfully shape the functional relationships that exist between these disciplines, rather than consolidating the interdisciplinary rifts and biases of the past. Because primary care is a pivotal sector of our "de facto" mental health system (14), and because primary care providers are being designated as coordinating figures in clinical care systems, it is essential that primary care providers understand managed mental health care, its benefits and limitations, and their relationship to it.

THE ARRIVAL OF MANAGED CARE

During the last decade, an increasing number of Americans have begun to receive their mental health care through insurance plans that use a variety of "managed care" methods to control costs and standardize treatments. Although managed care methods may include initiatives to assess and improve the quality of care, there is growing consensus that the emphasis in most plans has been on controlling service use and costs (15,16), and many experts say that managed care has "subordinated the quality of care to the drive for profits" (17). This trend has been met with significant dismay by patients and health care providers alike, as managed care practices have restricted many of the freedoms previously enjoyed in unfettered fee-for-service systems. Complaints have centered around the intrusion of third party management practices into two general areas: constraints in freedom of choice in the selection of particular providers and treatments, and pervasive interference in the patient-doctor relationship.

Nonetheless, health care administrators working in both the public and private sector have argued that managed care practices remain a necessary means of controlling spiraling health care costs (18). Indeed, many medical care practices occurring in traditional unmanaged systems have been seriously lacking in terms of cost-containment and self-evaluation. Supporters of managed care contend that managed care practices will allow individuals, employer groups, and government to continue to purchase health services that had, in an unrestricted third party payment system, become exorbitantly expensive, and will limit spending to treatments of proven efficacy. Indeed, many provider groups and hospital systems are responding to the financial pressures of managed care contracts by developing differentiated clinical services that allow for treatment of a spectrum of diagnostic and acuity needs at reduced cost. In the midst of these profound changes, a central question has arisen: does managed health care have the intention and capability to improve access and quality of care while reducing costs, or will it merely restrict access and redistribute clinical decision-making power and financial remuneration away from health professionals toward third party business interests? As we assess the merits and deficiencies of managed care in future years, this question will likely remain an ongoing source of tension.

Managed Care: Economic Constraints Limit Mental Health Service Allocation

For mental health practitioners, the rise of managed mental health care (also commonly called "managed behavioral healthcare", a name which may signify a new emphasis on behavior, rather than subjective emotional well-being, as the primary focus of attention) has been especially harrowing. Managed care practices have placed especially stringent restrictions on the allocation of mental health specialty services, relative to other medical specialties. These restrictions have the purpose, in the words of the industry leaders, of "limiting authorization of benefit expenditures to reimburse only necessary and appropriate care. . . " in order to control costs (19). This has occurred for two main reasons. The first issue is accountability for expenditures: to health professionals from outside the mental health field, treatment objectives in mental health appear relatively vague, and treatment endpoints, however carefully thought out, may appear subjective and rather arbitrary. Second, insurers fear that patients will consume mental health services (which the insurers may perceive to be of unproven utility) in an open-ended manner. Nonetheless, the debate about what criteria should be used to define "necessary" and "appropriate" care remains largely unresolved.

In determining the nature and quantity of mental health care to be made available to patients, both clinical and economic factors must be considered. Increasingly, however, managed care insurers and the provider groups that contract with them are defining authorization criteria and treatment plans based on what is deemed affordable by the corporate or public-sector purchasers of mental health benefits, rather than based on what is likely to provide for optimal long-term mental health among the beneficiaries in question. This "bottom line" emphasis has been particularly distressing to mental health providers, because it results in an economically driven redefinition for large segments of our population of what constitutes a mental health problem, what problems deserve to be treated, and how such problems should be treated.

Though it is known that expenditures for mental health care account for about ten percent of total health care dollars nationally, capitation rates for mental health care presently amount to only about three percent of the total health care premium (19). Considering that only about one fifth of patients with an active psychiatric problem receive any treatment for that problem in a given six month period (2), evidence of a great deal of untreated psychiatric morbidity, one may conclude that current capitation rates are too low to meaningfully address the real need for mental health services. In any event, very limited mental health benefits are becoming the accepted norm, despite convincing evidence that mental disorders cause functional disability as great or greater than many prevalent chronic medical conditions (20), and evidence that most common mental disorders can be effectively treated.

In private and public managed care systems economic factors exert significant influence on clinical priorities, mental health care is generally a low priority, and afflicted persons suffer as a result. Within the private sector, where most managed care methods have been developed, benefit structures are limited, but many employees have the ability, in the situation of mild to moderate psychopathology, to purchase substitute or supplemental mental health services outside of their insurance plan. More severely afflicted employees may find their benefits to be inadequate in addressing their mental illness, a situation that may ultimately allow for the development of impairment so severe that it causes long term disability or job loss. To whatever degree restricted mental health benefits fail to meet their needs, employed persons with mental health problems generally lack a voice in bringing attention to their need, since calling attention to their need brings the risk of stigmatization and rejection, if not dismissal, by their employer.

As the methods of private sector managed care programs are applied in public sector populations (i.e., Medicaid and other state and county health plans), there are additional problems. Private sector managed care practices and capitation rates require significant modification for use in public sector populations, where the prevalence and severity of psychopathology is much greater than in the private sector. In addition, because public sector patients by definition lack financial resources that would allow them to supplement their care with additional care paid for out-of-pocket, restrictions on service use inevitably result in increases in morbidity.

The Biopsychosocial Model: Central to the Traditions of Medicine and Mental Health Care

In recent years most physicians have embraced, at least in theory, the biopsychosocial model, put forth by George Engel about 20 years ago (1,21). Engel proposed his model as a comprehensive improvement on the biomedical model, as a way for medicine to provide ". . . room within its framework for the social, psychological, and behavioral dimensions of illness" (1). His model stemmed from a concern over the direction of medicine and psychiatry in the 1960's and 70's. Engel felt that the biomedical model was overly reductionistic, encouraged an artificial mind-body dualism, and failed to account for important clinical phenomena. He offered the biopsychosocial model to the medical and psychiatric communities as a rational basis for movement from a narrow scientific medicine to a more integrative model for research, teaching, and clinical action.

Since Engel expressed his concern about the emphasis on science and reductionistic thinking within psychiatry, there has been continued debate about whether a biomedical or biopsychosocial model is more useful in conceptualizing mental phenomena (22). Since Engel's time, mental health practitioners have become a differentiated and pluralistic group, spanning the spectrum of thought from strict reductionism to holism. Across this spectrum, there can be no doubt that psychiatry and the allied mental health professions have been profoundly impacted by concepts derived from social, cultural, philosophical, religious, and artistic thought and experience, in addition to obvious contributions from medicine, neuroscience, and psychology. While the practices of some non-psychiatric physicians may still emphasize biomedical over psychosocial phenomena, the practices of most psychiatrists and allied mental health practitioners are consistent with the biopsychosocial model.

Managed Mental Health Care Narrows the Practice Model

It is important for us to remain aware of the richness of what has been accomplished within the mental health field, consonant with the biopsychosocial model. Mental health practitioners have in the last 25 years greatly refined methods for treating psychological and psychiatric problems. These methods derive their strength from a broad range of theoretical perspectives used to explain mental phenomena (i.e., psychoanalytic, developmental, cognitive, and neuro-scientific perspectives), and from complex techniques that have great emotional depth and personal meaning for patients (i.e., individual and group psychotherapies). Central to the efficacy of most mental health treatment methods are two principles: first, that emotional and behavioral change is most likely to occur in the context of a trusting relationship with a clinician; and second, that lasting improvement requires considerable self-reflection, which is best developed through repeated contacts with a mental health provider. These principles hold true for brief or long-term psychotherapies and group psychotherapy, as well as most psychopharmacologic treatments. Even if we postulate that long-term psychotherapies are beyond the financial reach of most health plans, we should be clear that psychotherapeutic principles are essential to any effective therapeutic alliance, however brief the treatment. These principles are increasingly challenged by the economic scientism of many managed mental health care systems.

Managed mental health care systems are redefining basic elements of the *content* and *process* of mental health care, advocating treatment approaches that are quite discrepant with tradition. In terms of the *content* of care, years of experience have shown that insight about the origin and perpetuation of symptoms can alleviate emotional and behavioral dysfunction. Self-awareness allows patients to mobilize intra-psychic, inter-personal, cultural, and spiritual structures of meaning which can have lasting impact on symptomotology and direction in life. But under managed care, the core content of most mental health treatments is determined by more superficial and short term goals: crisis resolution, the amelioration of commonly observed and easily measured symptoms, and the restoration of minimum standards of personal safety and social and occupational role functioning. The de-emphasis on insight, with an increased focus on behavior and symptoms, reflects a devaluation of the psychological and social components of the biopsychosocial model.

In terms of the *process* of care, mental health treatments work best when there is the creation of a safe relationship between patient and provider, continuity over time, an individually tailored treatment plan, and flexibility in determining the particular topical focus and depth of examination of the patient's complaints. In contrast, managed care practices increasingly shorten and/or make uncertain the length of treatment, thereby reducing the patient's sense of safety in the therapeutic situation. Moreover, many managed care systems attempt to standardize treatment methods in ways that may artificially restrain the topical focus and depth of treatment, for example through treatment-manual-based therapies and highly structured psychoeducational groups. They may also require patients to work with multiple providers within an episode of care (separating psychotherapy from psychopharmacology) or in subsequent episodes of treatment.

These changes in the content and process of mental health care represent an under-estimation of people's capacity for psychological growth and change, and may deprive many people from the meaning derived from such growth. Moreover, as managed care policies increasingly determine the mental health care accessible to most Americans we must look beyond the impact on individuals, to consider the impact of such practices at the population level. Given a high population prevalence of mental health problems, the impact of superficial treatments on the collective American psyche is not likely to be positive.

The Necessity and Opportunity to Expand the Managed Mental Health Care Paradigm

Many of the management concepts currently emphasized in managed care are not specific to health care, they could be applied to the production or delivery of any good or service. The managed care paradigm considers clinical services and treatments to be commodities responsive to generic market forces (23). This paradigm fails to acknowledge that psychosocial needs are not neatly or easily manipulated or measured, as may be desirable from a business perspective. Attempts to define clinical services as particular commodities may dangerously gloss over the most human psychosocial needs.

Synthesis of business requirements with biopsychosocial clinical objectives could create movement toward a system that would honor the psychological needs and capacities of patients as well as the capabilities of providers. Although unmanaged systems have allowed for significant innovations in health care delivery, such systems have lacked the authority found in managed systems to define clinical relationships and priorities on a large scale. Management of large groups may make it possible to develop biopsychosocially oriented systems where clinicians in different disciplines could orchestrate their activities in order to facilitate mental health referral and provide comprehensive and integrated care (24). Movement in this direction may occur if those impacted by managed mental health care actively question the trends now occurring. When Engel proposed the biopsychosocial model, he noted the importance of efforts to "neutralize the dogmatism of biomedicine and all the undesirable social and scientific consequences that flow therefrom" (1). In this era we must be careful to avoid entrenchment in the dogmatism of an economically driven managed mental health paradigm, so that we may embrace a conceptualization of health that more fully respects psychological experience, needs, expression, and capacity for growth.

Assumptions of the Biopsychosocial Model Important to Clinical System Design and Evaluation

The biopsychosocial model has been referred to frequently as a standard for judging the qualities of our health care system (22,25,26). The model suggests several factors important to the quality of a system of clinical care. First, as Engel pointed out, clinical care must embrace more than narrowly defined biomedicine: illness can only be fully understood and addressed in the context of psychological and social factors (1). The biological, the psychological, and the social are each important domains in the etiology of illness, its expression, and in the assessment of health status and treatment planning. Acknowledgment of the importance of these three domains requires that an effective system of health care has accessible multi-disciplinary staff and resources to detect and address problems in each domain: biological, psychological, and social.

Second, the model suggests that these three domains are inter-related: changes in one of the domains may effect health status in the other domains. To illustrate this: marital discord (a social problem) may result in anxiety or depression (psychological symptoms) and a worsening of back pain or GI symptoms (biological phenomena). Alternatively, a flare of multiple sclerosis (a biological phenomenon) may impact on mood (through psychological or biological mechanisms), or on employment status (a social phenomenon). Moreover, changes in any one of these domains may alter the subjective experience in any of the other domains. As Engel put it, " These [domains] cannot be understood merely as an assemblage (or reassemblage) of constituent parts" (21). Thus, the model suggests that systems that integrate care in these domains will be most effective in improving health. There must be functional integration of staff, resources, and clinical activities in different departments and disciplines.

Third, Engel put forward his model because of his observation that the complex interaction between biological, psychological, and social factors in the etiology, course, and response to treatment of illness may not be immediately evident or easily understood by patients, or in many cases by health professionals. An important purpose of the model is to facilitate rational attention and integration of psychological and social phenomena, phenomena previously considered outside the realm of a strictly scientific medical model of disease (21). Based on this, we can predict that systems of care that educate patients about the inter-relatedness of bio-psycho-social phenomena will be most effective in improving patients' knowledge, health behavior, and health status.

Finally, Engel would probably have argued that implementation of the model would depend on structural support for the model in the composition of the clinical care system. It is not sufficient to present a theoretical approach to providers in an effort to garner voluntary support. Truly integrated care only occurs when multi-disciplinary staff have personal and financial incentives to collaborate.

Evaluating the Characteristics of Managed Mental Health Care Systems Based on Assumptions of the Biopsychosocial Model

The remainder of this chapter will consider in detail some of the common explicit policies, as well as some of the implicit attitudes of managed mental health programs, and their impact on our ability to work within the assumptions of the biopsychosocial model. We will review 1) large scale organizational structures, 2) common benefit restrictions, and 3) clinical practice behavior, to evaluate the degree to which managed care is adopting, ignoring, or rejecting the biopsychosocial model.

1. System Organizational Structure and the Biopsychosocial Model

Let us begin by examining managed care practices at the "macro" level of system organization, to elucidate structural improvements and impediments to biopsychosocial care. Historically, mental health services have been dualistically separated from medical services, in the form of free-standing mental hospitals, community mental health centers, and private practice mental health providers and groups. These groups usually have had only informal relationships with their counterparts in the medical community, and neither group has had much financial accountability to the other. Exceptions have existed, in the form of inpatient and outpatient consultation programs, behavioral medicine and health psychology programs (27), and multi-disciplinary pain clinics (28), but most people who have been treated for a mental health problem have been treated by a specialist in the private practice realm, or, more likely, by a primary care provider (14).

Under managed care, the clinical relationships and referral mechanisms that exist between medical and mental health care are defined by the funding organizations. Most managed care systems have an arrangement with a panel of mental health providers offering a range of services, accessible via referral by a primary care gatekeeper, or in some systems accessed directly by the patient. Organized referral mechanisms offer patients potential improvements over the informal systems of the past, where the patient or family was left to find a mental health provider through their primary care provider or social network, a non-system which made optimal assignment of patients to clinicians with appropriate skills very difficult. These new arrangements can streamline referral from primary care to mental health services, and allow for matching of patient problems and provider skills. However, even in managed systems with organized referral systems, financial and geographical relationships between primary care and mental health care often create a disincentive for integration of medical and mental health care.

In a minority of systems, medical and mental health clinicians are located near one another or are part of a single large organization where they may have clinical relationships with each other, e.g., staff model health maintenance organization ("HMO") or multi-department medical center, creating some potential for biopsychosocial integration. However, in most managed care systems (in many preferred provider organizations, or "PPOs"), mental health services are available through a group of providers whose funding and work-site is separate from the funding and work-site of providers delivering medical services. When mental health services are delivered in a system that is geographically remote from medical services, or is part of a completely separate organization (known as a *"carve-out"* arrangement), clinical and administrative relationships are often too weak to support meaningful biopsychosocial integration.

A common scheme is for the funding for the contracting mental health provider group to be derived as a sub-contract of the capitated budget for general medical care. *"Subcapitation"*, as this is known, provides few if any incentives for collaboration and coordination of care between medical and mental health providers. Subcapitation and carve-out arrangements make a symbolic statement to providers and patients that medical and psychological problems are unrelated. Subcapitation can result in competition for funds between medical and mental health provider groups within institutions, an occurrence that only serves to weaken the climate for collaboration. Subcapitation and carve-out arrangements create a likelihood that primary care providers will try to shift mental health care to mental health specialists, avoiding expenditures from their own budget, even when the problem might be effectively treated in the primary care setting. As patients referred from primary care are asked to negotiate a second administrative system, subcapitation and carve-out arrangements also increase the risk that patients will not follow-through when referred for mental health care.

These structural impediments to biopsychosocial integration may be minimized by incentives to enhance collaboration. Even modest allocations of time or financial remuneration for communication between providers in primary care and mental health groups might enhance the quality of care. Deliberate efforts to encourage telephone conferencing or E-mail contacts may also be helpful.

Another potential problem area is that in many managed systems access to specialty mental health services includes a process of *"prior authorization"*, whereby employees of the insurance company (often known as case managers or care managers) assess the patient's mental health status over the telephone, using standardized instruments. The results of the interview are used to determine whether the patient will be referred for mental health care, what type of care they will receive, and how much care will be initially allocated. These care managers may have little or no clinical training, but they are increasingly involved in determining eligibility for mental health services. In the majority of cases these care managers may be quite helpful, but in some cases the care manager's lack of clinical training or the patient's concerns about confidentiality may result in a failure to communicate crucial medical or social information that is relevant to determining whether and how much treatment is needed.

Another administrative structure that is changing is the trend toward *combined medical and mental health clinical records.* In situations where patients have comorbid medical and mental health problems, particularly for patients receiving psychiatric medications, this can be advantageous. However, the need for exchange of clinical information must be titrated against the need to maintain confidentiality about mental health issues. Medical records may be more widely accessible, and relatively less guarded, than mental health records, creating the risk of release of potentially stigmatizing or damaging clinical information to an audience not intended to receive it. Computerized medical records offer opportunities to share clinical information more efficiently, but must include rigorous safeguards to insure that mental health information reaches only those clinicians who need it and can use it respectfully.

2. Impact of Common Managed Mental Health Benefit Restrictions on Biopsychosocial Integration

Although mental health benefits in most insurance plans have historically been more limited than medical benefits, the *lack of parity in benefit structures* has become more marked in the era of managed mental health care (29). Typical managed mental health plans offer a maximum of 20 to 30 outpatient mental health/substance treatment visits per year, and 30 to 60 days of inpatient treatment per year. Many plans limit care to "crisis" situations, and most plans only parcel out continued access to these services after detailed *"utilization review"* (hereafter referred to as "UR") of the patient's condition by a representative or committee of the insurer or financially at-risk provider group. Caps on access may result in adverse outcomes, given that many psychiatric disorders are chronic in nature.

The impact of these benefit limitations is significant, and demonstrates a bias by managed care systems against the treatment of mental health problems. These benefit limitations are not paralleled by similar limitations in the treatment of most medical disorders. Mental health benefit structures do not make allowances for more serious psychiatric diagnoses. For example, a patient who suffers recurrent episodes of mania and depression as part of bipolar disorder is subject to the same benefit limitations as a patient with moderate depressive symptoms. While UR practices result in allocation of different quantities of services to each of these patients within the overall benefit maximum, the bipolar patient might easily require more than the maximum allocable services in the course of a year. If we compare this practice to the manner in which medical benefits are managed, we note that patients with diabetes or congestive heart failure, though depression may cause as much or more functional impairment than these disorders (20), are given essentially unlimited access to medical services. While most managed medical systems would never consider limiting care for diabetes or congestive heart failure, they may turn away patients with psychiatric conditions who have used up the "maximum" number of visits, or may limit the frequency of visits to mental health providers, irrespective of patient symptomatology. Thus, managed mental health benefit packages may discriminate against patients with more severe psychiatric disorders.

Clearly, mental health and medical providers should support efforts to create parity. The current lack of parity ties the hands of both groups as they try to address potentially treatable psychopathology in patients who have exhausted their benefits.

This lack of parity between mental health and medical service benefits is also reflected in the requirement of greater degree of *cost-sharing* for mental health services, relative to cost-sharing for medical services. For example, co-payments for outpatient visits for mental health care are usually in the range from 20 to 40 dollars per visit, while medical care co-payments, including medical specialties, average 5 to 10 dollars. This discourages care-seeking for psychological problems, and is a source of special discrimination against poorer patients within any insured population. If mental health co-payments are necessary, it would seem more reasonable for cost-sharing to be progressive over time. Co-payments should be low for initial mental health contacts, so as not to create a barrier to necessary care.

Of special interest to managed care's question of whether expenditures for mental health treatment should be limited are studies in health services research of the *"medical offset effect"* (30-33). The medical offset effect hypothesizes that mental health treatment may result in reductions in use of medical services, whereby the savings in medical treatment costs may help to compensate for, or "offset", the outlay of funds for mental health treatment. This postulate stems from the observation that psychiatric distress is associated with increased medical service use. Despite a large number of studies, there remains significant contention over whether, and in what clinical situations, the offset effect holds true. Advocates for mental health treatment point to evidence that mental health treatment reduces medical costs, while managed care critics of mental health treatment point to a lack of evidence of medical cost savings as justification for curtailing mental health treatment. It is important to realize, however, that these critics are using a double standard in assessing the financial impact of mental health treatment. They do not require that the treatment of any particular medical condition reduce the cost of medical service use for unrelated medical conditions (treatment of the medical condition in question is considered an end in itself), but they suggest that mental health treatment be justified by consequent savings in medical care costs. In other words, they suggest that improvement in mental health status is not a sufficient end in itself.

Utilization review practices in many managed mental health systems emphasize biological and behavioral symptoms over psychological and social manifestations of illness. Many UR procedures involve assessment of a patient's status and rate of improvement using standardized symptom check-lists (also known as "concurrent review") that focus on easily assessed signs of illness (sleep, appetite, mood, energy level, suicidal ideation, personal hygiene, work productivity, completion of housework, etc) over more subtle but important psychological and social factors (disturbances in interactions with family and friends, despair/optimism about the future, motivation and ability to create change in current situation, etc). These measures may be helpful in tracking patient progress and in improving accountability, but the emphasis taken runs the risk of focusing on epiphenomena of the psychiatric disturbance over more fundamental, propagating psychological factors. Additionally, the UR measures themselves usually give minimal attention to the potential impact of mental health problems on medical outcomes, despite evidence that mental health and medical problems often coexist and have interactive effects on outcomes.

Patients who require continuing mental health care may, with each additional request for additional visits, find it progressively more difficult to obtain needed care. In many systems of care UR committees tend to allocate smaller numbers of visits with each subsequent application for ongoing care, even when psychopathology remains significant. The UR committees may justify this clinically by claiming that they are saving visits for the remainder of the benefit year when they may be needed, but this may be a thin facade for efforts to avoid additional expenditures on mental health care. Given that psychiatric treatments are often interpersonal, whereas medical treatments are generally pharmacologic, a medical equivalent of this scenario would be rationing analgesic medication for a patient with arthritis, so the patient would not exhaust an artificially limited supply of medication. Seen in this light, restriction of access to already limited mental health benefits seems unethical.

When patients seeking mental health care are denied initial or additional visits, the implicit message sent to the patient is that the mental health care they seek is not important or worthwhile. Since most patients have conscious and unconscious resistances to addressing emotional problems, systems that turn patients away at times when they are willing to address their problems may support resistance and increase suffering. As prior authorization and concurrent review procedures block many patients from accessing mental health services, a large number of patients are seeking mental health care outside of their insurance plans, which they pay for themselves. The resultant provision of separate medical and mental health care in these cases reinforces an already strong impact of managed mental health systems in separating the biological and the psychosocial. Encouragement of out-of-plan service use also complicates and discourages collaboration between medical and mental health providers in cases where it may be beneficial to the patient.

One way to begin to rein in overly restrictive UR procedures might be to require UR committees to include in their membership impartial mental health professionals from outside the managing entity that is at financial risk. Commentary from neutral professionals might help to restore balance between clinical and financial priorities. In addition, efforts should be taken to allow patients who are denied care the option of purchasing additional services out-of pocket, at reasonable prices, to allow continuity with their provider.

3. Impact of Managed Mental Health Clinical Treatment Methods on Biopsychosocial Integration

There have been many efforts, including some by providers working within managed care programs, to develop and evaluate innovative clinical programs that help to integrate treatment of biological, psychological, and social problems. Of particular relevance are programs focused on addressing psychological distress in medically ill populations, such as the Harvard Community Health Plan's "Ways to Wellness Program" (34) and the Stress Reduction Program at the University of Massachusetts (35). Still others have developed psychotherapy groups for patients identified in primary care as having depression or other common psychiatric problems (36). Many group-based programs provide large numbers of patients with valuable services at low cost. These programs may for some patients and for some clinical problems be as effective as individual-focused therapies, and in other situations may serve as useful and efficient supplements to more costly individual-focused care.

Other efforts with valuable potential to improve the quality of care in managed care settings include the development of new instruments and programs to screen for common psychiatric disorders (37), to educate primary care providers in the detection and treatment of specific psychiatric disorders (38), and to have primary care providers collaborate with mental health specialists in the treatment of depression (39). Clearly, biopsychosocial integration will be promoted by programs that enhance the skills of primary care providers and promote collaboration between generalists and specialists.

Managed care systems generally emphasize the use of *psychiatric medication* as part of efforts to contain costs in the treatment of depression and anxiety disorders. Developments in psychopharmacology over the past 25 years have certainly increased our ability to relieve psychiatric symptoms. However, an increasingly heavy emphasis on psychiatric medications over psychotherapy (7) is of concern, and has been justifiably questioned (40). It is significant that managed care policies often allow continued prescription of psychotropic medications, which can be fairly expensive, but do not allow ongoing psychotherapy. While medications may ameliorate symptoms over the short term, they do little to address the psychological basis for those symptoms, leaving the patient reliant on medication or otherwise at risk for recurrences of symptoms. Overemphasis on medication treatments may be based on, and may promote, a false belief that psychiatric symptoms are due more to neurochemical abnormalities than to psychodynamic and social forces. This pushes aside the multi-factorial emphasis of the biopsychosocial model, and suggests, dangerously, that physicians and patients may relegate social and psychological factors as secondary to biological factors. It is critical that managed care systems provide patients with complete information about the types of treatments available to them, including psychotherapy (40). Regardless of the degree to which a disorder may be neurochemical in nature (we rarely have definitive information about this), patients can benefit from support and exploration about the emotional significance of their suffering. In this regard, recent mergers between managed care corporations and pharmaceutical manufacturers may be particularly worrisome influences on treatment protocols within managed care organizations.

Managed mental health organizations also tend to emphasize *brief treatment* for all diagnoses, even though studies demonstrating the efficacy of brief treatments have been limited mainly to depressive and anxiety disorders. If we take the treatment of depression as an example, it is worth noting that many managed care plans allocate only 2 to 6 visits at a time, despite the fact that most brief treatment protocols require 12 to 20 visits (41,42). In recognizing that the emphasis on brief treatment is motivated by fiscal concerns, it is worth considering the likelihood that more comprehensive treatments would provide more durable improvement and lower recurrence rates, and would therefore be a worthwhile expense over the long term. In this regard, UR committees should support, as clinically appropriate, thoughtfully planned brief treatments of at least 8 to 12 visits, rather than repeated allocations of 2 to 6 visits aimed at symptom suppression in the absence of comprehensive treatment of the problem at hand.

Recent emphasis on the development of standardized *treatment guidelines* may be very useful in identifying effective and cost-efficient treatments for particular disorders, but may also obscure a clear view of the particular situations and needs of individual patients suffering from similar problems in very different settings. While the application of empirically proven treatment guidelines for medical problems may be helpful, the application of reductionistic treatment guidelines in the treatment of emotional problems of multi-factorial etiology may be less fruitful. Leon Eisenberg stated clearly, " The same disease never presents in quite the same way in successive patients. Complaints vary; severity varies; response to treatment varies" (43).

For similar reasons, a growing emphasis in managed care on *"outcome measures"* is also of concern. Although many sophisticated outcome measurement instruments have been used in research projects, few managed care systems actually use outcome measures that contribute substantively to clinical care. Rather, outcome measurements are used by managed care organizations as global performance indicators as they market their services to employer groups or public agencies.

The managed care industry's long term hope, however, is that efforts to systematically measure outcome, originating in procedure-based medicine (for example, assessment of use of a particular antibiotic to treat a specific type of infection, or assessment of efficacy of a particular type of prosthetic device in replacement of arthritic hip joints), will be generalizable to the subjective realm of human experience. This might, for example, allow monitoring of patients' progress, quantification and comparison of the status of patients with similar problems, and comparison of the efficacy of different treatments and providers. As a management strategy, this is intended to eliminate the subjective quality inherent in assessing patient progress and provider performance.

However desirable such outcome measurements may be from a management perspective, application of such an approach to any individual's mental health care may require measurement instruments of far greater sophistication than are in current use. The emphasis on outcomes is based on a scientific, rational worldview, which suggests that clinical problems may be categorized and compared in a controlled fashion. While this perspective is integral to management practices of our era, the biopsychosocial model reminds us that although we need to be rational in our approach to clinical problems, we have, with each patient, an obligation to look at the very personal and individualized interaction of biological, psychological and social realms. This interaction, in short, is what comprises individual experience. In treating mental health problems, individual experience is of paramount importance.

When primary care or mental health providers want to address mental health concerns with their patients, they find that managed care has introduced significant time pressures that interfere with attention to mental health issues. In primary care, providers are burdened by pressure to see a large number of patients, with very little time per patient. Since evaluation and treatment of psychological or social problems is relatively time intensive, compared to evaluation and treatment of most common medical problems, primary care providers have a disincentive to discuss mental health problems. Policies that give primary care providers "credit" for extra time spent dealing with psychiatric disorders might alleviate this problem. In mental health care, providers are burdened with cumbersome UR forms and the need for discussion about utilization review issues, leaving less time for actual evaluation and treatment of the presenting problem. Moreover, utilization review procedures, and the possibility of denial of additional visits, create uncertainty for both patient and provider about the future continuity of the therapeutic relationship. This strikes a particularly vulnerable chord for patients, many of whom have presented for treatment of issues that have their origin in problems of attachment, loss, or other relationship dysfunction.

Integration of Mental Health and Primary Care Services

Efforts to coordinate mental health and primary care services are of great interest at this time (39,44-46), because they present special opportunities to bring about biopsychosocial integration where it has not existed in the past. There are several factors supporting such integrative efforts. Managed care systems are requiring primary care providers to see patients more quickly, and to treat a wider variety of problems without referral to costly specialists, but primary care providers have generally not received sufficient additional education in the detection or treatment of mental health problems to take on this responsibility. In addition, undiagnosed psychiatric problems in the primary care setting may be associated with increased general health care costs, and unsuccessfully treated psychiatric problems are associated with wasted health care dollars. Taken together, these factors suggest that an efficient cooperative effort between primary care and mental health providers would benefit primary care patients with mental health problems, could enhance biopsychosocial integration in the primary care setting, and might save health care dollars.

Mental health services that are of use in the primary care realm include formal and informal on-site consultation about diagnostic and treatment matters, collaborative management of mental health problems following consultation, assistance in referring patients for specialty mental health services, and on-site specialist treatment of mental health problems for patients refusing referral to off-site mental health providers. In addition, mental health providers can help educate primary care providers about psychiatric diagnosis and treatment, and can work with primary care providers to educate patients about mental health treatments. On-site mental health providers can facilitate communication and continuity of care between primary care providers and provide bridges between medical and mental health care around inpatient (medical or mental health) treatment episodes. At the medical/psychiatric interface, special treatments can be developed for patients with psychiatric disorders common to primary care, somatization disorders (47), hypochondriasis, and particular chronic illnesses or pain syndromes. Mental health providers can become involved in developing medical treatment plans for patients with medical problems related to substance use or eating disorders. They can also advise primary care providers about the management of patients who are difficult to work with, many of whom may have personality disorders (48), and patients who are very distressed and make very frequent visits for medical care (49,50). Shared medical/mental health support of social work and psycho-education services can facilitate biopsychosocial integration, and may allow both groups to maintain social support services otherwise unaffordable to them.

In cases where medical and mental health care are separated by carve-out or sub-capitation arrangements, the support of the managed care entity and medical center or medical group administration are likely to be essential in creating incentives for cooperation between medical and mental health providers. The presence of effective and helpful mental health providers in the primary care setting can increase primary care provider's interest and enthusiasm in treating mental health problems. Ultimately, working clinical collaborations between providers will be strongest in situations where trusting personal relationships between members of both disciplines have been given opportunities to flourish. Simple factors such as joint membership on clinical treatment teams and occupancy of neighboring offices can do wonders in encouraging these personal and clinical relationships. The sharing of clinical responsibility and personal perspectives will allow individuals, and eventually institutions, to blend previously separate paradigms.

CONCLUSION

Managed care creates the theoretical possibility of an efficient, intentionally integrated, biopsychosocially oriented system of medical and mental health care, in place of the unmanaged, poorly integrated, expensive system that preceded it. In their first ten years, managed mental health systems have emphasized cost control, through a program of limited benefits and aggressive utilization management, over substantive improvements in quality of care. Though there have been some efforts at systematizing care and improving referral linkages, the focus on brief and standardized treatments aimed at symptom reduction rather than insight threatens to severely limit the depth of meaning and potential for lasting change achievable through mental health treatment. Biopsychosocially valued aspects of care, including parity of importance of medical and mental health care, individualized treatment, and the sanctity of the doctor-patient relationship have not been honored. Pathways and incentives for interdisciplinary collaboration need to be implemented to support the efforts of overburdened primary care providers, and to encourage linkage of primary care and specialty mental health services. Health care professionals and administrators must remember that accountability on economic matters should always be secondary to our ultimate responsibility: helping patients and the systems and communities we work within move toward greater health.

REFERENCES

1. Engel GL: Science 1977; 196: 129-136.

2. Robins L, Locke B, Regier D: An overview of psychiatric disorders in America, in: Robins L, Regier D, editors. *Psychiatric Disorders in America*. New York, The Free Press, 1991: 328-366.

3. Kessler L, Burns B, Shapiro S, et al. Psychiatric diagnoses of medical service users: evidence from the Epidemiologic Catchment Area Program. Am J Public Health 1987; 77: 18-24.

4. Kessler L, Cleary P, Burke J: Psychiatric disorders in primary care. Arch Gen Psychiatry 1985; 42: 583-587.

5. Hoeper E, Nycz G, Cleary P, et al: Estimated prevalence of RDC mental disorder in primary medical care. Int. J. Ment. Health 1979; 8: 6-15.

6. Wells K, Golding J, Burnam M: Psychiatric disorder in a sample of the general population with and without chronic medical conditions. Am J Psychiatry 1988; 145: 976-981.

7. Public Health Service, Agency for Health Care Policy and Research: *Depression in Primary Care: Treatment of Major Depression*. Rockville, Maryland, US Dept of Health and Human Services, 1993. AHCPR Publ 93-051.

8. Narrow W, Regier D, Rae S, et al. Use of services by persons with mental and addictive disorders. Arch Gen Psychiatry 1993; 50: 95-107

9. Miranda J, Hohmann AA, Attkisson CC, Larson DB: *Mental Disorders in Primary Care*. San Fransicso, Jossey-Bass, 1994.

10. Eisenberg L; Treating depression and anxiety in primary care. New Engl J Med 1992; 326: 1080-1084

11. Tiemens BG, Ormel J, Simon GE: Occurrence, recognition, and outcome of psychological disorders in primary care. Am J Psychiatry 1996; 153: 636-644.

12. Katon W, von Korff M, Lin E, et al.: Adequacy and duration of antidepressant treatment in primary care. Med Care 1992; 30: 67-76.

13. Perez-Stable EJ, Miranda J, Munoz RF, et al.: Depression in medical outpatients: underrecognition and misdiagnosis. Arch Int Med 1990; 150: 1083-1088.

14. Regier D, Narrow W, Rae D, et al.: The de facto US mental and addictive disorders service system. Arch Gen Psychiatry 1993; 50: 85-94.

15. Wells KB, Astrachan BM, Tischler GL, Unutzer J: Issues and approaches in evaluating managed mental health care. Milbank Quarterly 1995; 73: 57-75.

16. Jellinek MS, Nurcombe B: Two wrongs don't make a right: managed care, mental health, and the marketplace. JAMA 1993; 270: 1737-7139.

17. Wines M, Pear R: President finds he has gained even if he lost on health care. The New York Times, July 30, 1996.

18. Afield WE: Managed mental health care: curbing costs in the 1990s. Medical Interface 1990; 14: 26-34.

19. Trabin T, Freeman MA: *Managed Behavioral Healthcare*. Tiburon, California, Centralink Publishers, 1995.

20. Wells K, Stewart A, Hays R, et al. The functioning and well-being of depressed patients: results from the Medical Outcomes Study. JAMA 1989; 2627: 914-919.

21. Engel GL: The clinical application of the biopsychosocial model. Am J Psychiatry 1980; 137: 535-544.

22. Hartmann L: Reflections on humane values and biopsychosocial integration. Am J Psychiatry 1992; 149: 1135-1141.

23. Hart JT: Two paths for medical practice. Lancet 1992; 340: 772-775.

24. Lefkowitz PM: The continuum of care in a general hospital setting. Gen Hosp Psychiatry 1995; 17: 260-267.

25. Schreter RK: Ten trends in managed care and their impact on the biopsychosocial model. Hosp Comm Psychiatry 1993; 44: 325-327.

26. Lazarus A: A proposal for psychiatric collaboration in managed care. Am J Psychotherapy 1994; 48: 600-609.

27. Dolinar LJ; A historical review of outpatient consultation-liaison psychiatry. Gen Hosp Psychiatry 1993; 15: 363-368.

28. Sullivan MD, Psychosomatic clinic or pain clinic: which is more viable? Gen Hosp Psychiatry 1993; 15: 375-380.

29. Iglehart JK: NEJM 1996; 334: 131-135.

30. Borus J, Olendzki M, Kessler L, et al.: The "offset effect" of mental health treatment on ambulatory medical care utilization and charges. Arch Gen Psychiatry 1985; 42: 573-580.

31. Mumford E, Schlesinger H, Glass G, et al.: A new look at evidence about reduced cost of medical utilization following mental health treatment. Am J Psychiatry 1984; 141: 1145-1158.

32. Kessler L, Steinwachs D, Hankin J: Episodes of psychiatric care and medical utilization. Med Care 1982; 20: 1209-1221.

33. Cummings NA: The successful application of medical offset in program planning and in clinical delivery. Managed Care Quarterly 1994; 2: 1-6.

34. Budd M, presentation at Academy of Psychosomatic Medicine Conference, Palm Springs, California, November 1995

35. Kabat-Zinn J: *Full Catastrophe Living*. New York, Dell Publishing, 1991.

36. Rosenberg SA, Zimet CN: Brief group treatment and managed mental health care. Int J Group Ther 1995; 45: 367-379.

37. Spitzer RL, Williams JBW, Kroenke K, et al.: Utility of a new procedure for diagnosing mental disorders in primary care: the PRIME-MD 1000 Study. JAMA 1994; 272: 1749-1756.

38. Lin E: Primary care physician role in adherence to anti-depressant therapy; Med Care 1995; 33: 67-74

39. Katon W, Von Korff M, Lin E, et al.; Collaborative management to achieve treatment guidelines: impact on depression in primary care. JAMA 1995; 273: 1026-1031

40. Munoz RM, Holon SD, McGrath E, et al. On the AHCPR Depression in Primary Care guidelines: further considerations for practitioners. Am Psychologist 1994; 49: 42-61.

41. Crits-Christoph P: The efficacy of brief dynamic psychotherapy: a meta-analysis. Am J Psychiatry 1992; 149: 151-158.

42. Jarrett RB, Rush AJ: Short-term psychotherapy of depressive disorders: current status and future directions. Psychiatry 1994; 57: 115-132.

43. Eisenberg L: Medicine - molecular, monetary, or more than both? JAMA 1995; 274: 331-334

44. Smith GR: Determining what works in mental health care in primary care settings. Gen Hosp Psychiatry 1990; 12: 8-10.

45. Wirecki MT: How to link behavioral group practices with primary care physicians. Beh Healthcare Tomorrow 1995; Nov/Dec: 71-72.

46. Lazurus A: The role of primary care physicians in managed mental health care. Psychiatric Services 1995; 46: 343-345.

47. Smith GR: The epidemiology and treatment of depression when it coexists with somatoform disorders, somatization, or pain. Gen Hosp Psychiatry 1992; 14: 265-272.

48. Feder A, Robbins SW: Personality disorders in primary care, in: Feldman M, Christiansen J, editors, *Behavioral Medicine: A Primary Care Handbook.* Norwalk, CT: Appleton and Lange, In press.

49. Katon W, Von Korff M, Lin E, et al.: A randomized trial of psychiatric consultation with distressed high utilizers. Gen Hosp Psychiatry 1992; 14: 86-98.

50. Von Korff M, Ormel J, Katon W, Lin E: Disability and depression among high utilizers of health care: a longitudinal analysis. Arch Gen Psychiatry 1992; 49: 91-100.

CONTRIBUTORS

Stuart Beck, M.D. : Clinical Instructor in Psychiatry
University of California, San Francisco
Psychiatry Service, San Francisco Veterans Affairs Medical Center
4150 Clement Street
San Francisco, CA 94121

Stuart Eisendrath, M.D. : Professor of Clinical Psychiatry
Director, Psychiatric Consultation-Liaison Service
Department of Psychiatry, School of Medicine
University of California, San Francisco
401 Parnassus Road, San Francisco, CA 94143-0984

David Fox, M.D. : Associate Clinical Professor of Psychiatry
Department of Psychiatry,
University of California, San Francisco
2625 E. Clinton Ave, Fresno, CA 93703

M.S. Franklin : Fresno Community Alzheimer's Living Center
Community Hospitals of Central California
Fresno, CA

Avak A. Howsepian, M.D. : Department of Psychiatry
University of California, San Francisco, Fresno Division
2615 East Clinton Ave, Fresno, CA 93703

Hoyle Leigh, M.D. : Professor and Vice Chairman
Department of Psychiatry
University of California, San Francisco
Director, Fresno Division, and
Chief of Psychiatry
Fresno VA Medical Center
2615 E. Clinton Ave, Fresno, CA 93703, and
Lecturer in Psychiatry, Yale University
New Haven, CT

Vincenta Leigh, M.S.N. : Assistant Clinical Professor of Psychiatry
University of California, San Francisco
Program coordinator, Intensive Outpatient Program
Mental Health Department
Kaiser Permanente Medical Center
4785 North First Street, Fresno, CA 93726-0513

A. Knudsen, R.D. : Fresno Community Alzheimer's Living Center
Community Hospitals of Central California
Fresno, CA

S. Leiby : Fresno Community Alzheimer's Living Center
Community Hospitals of Central California
Fresno, CA

Don Lipsitt, M.D. : Clinical Professor of Psychiatry, Harvard Medical School,
Chairman, Department of Psychiatry, Mount Auburn Hospital
330 Mt. Auburn Street, Cambridge, MA 02238

Benjamin Maoz, M.D., Ph.D. : Professor of Psychiatry, Ben-Gurion University of the Negev
Beer Sheva, and Tel-Aviv University
Israel

A. Rauch : Fresno Community Alzheimer's Living Center
Community Hospitals of Central California
Fresno, CA

Seth Wigdor Robbins, M.D., M.P.H.: Clinical Instructor, Department of Psychiatry
University of California, San Francisco
2475 Washington Street
San Francisco, California 94115

Wolfram Schueffel, M.D. : Professor of Psychosomatic Medicine,
Dept. of Psychosomatic Medicine
Phillips University, Balding Strasse
35033 Marburg, Germany

Jon Streltzer, M.D. : Professor of Psychiatry
Univeristy of Hawaii at Manoa
John A. Burns School of Medicine
1356 Lusitana Street, Honolulu, HI 96813

Lowell Tong, M.D. : Assistant Clinical Professor of Psychiatry
Department of Psychiatry, School of Medicine
University of California, San Francisco
401 Parnassus Road, San Francisco, CA 94143-0984

Shimun Waldfogel, M.D.: Assistant Professor
Department of Psychiatry and Human Behavior
Behavioral Medicine Consultant
Department of Family Medicine
Jefferson Medical College
1651 Thompson Building, 1020 Sansom St,
Philadelphia, PA. 19107

Thomas Wise, M.D. : Chairman, Department of Psychiatry
The Fairfax Hospital
Professor and Vice Chair
Department of Psychiatry
Georgetown University School of Medicine
Fairfax Hospital, 3300 Gallows Rd, Falls Church, VA 22046

INDEX